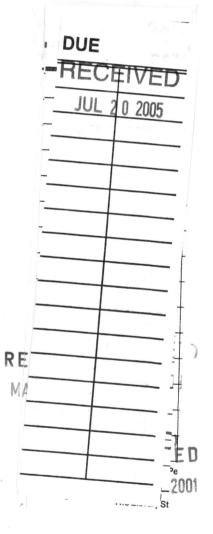

Handbook of
STRESS, MEDICINE,
and HEALTH

Edited by
CARY L. COOPER

CRC Press
Boca Raton   New York   London   Tokyo

Library of Congress Cataloging-in-Publication Data

Handbook of stress, medicine, and health / edited by Cary L. Cooper.
   p. cm.
   Includes bibliographical references and index.
   ISBN 0-8493-2908-6 (alk. paper)
   1. Medicine, Psychosomatic.   2. Stress (Physiology)   3. Stress
(Psychology)   4. Health.   I. Cooper, Cary L.
   [DNLM: 1. Stress, Psychological—complications.   2. Disease—
etiology.   3. Health.   4. Life Change Events.   WM 172 H23694 1995]
RC49.H329   1995
616.9'8—dc20
DNLM/DLC
for Library of Congress   95-7307
                                                                          CIP

Preface

Hippocrates once proclaimed that "the nature of the body can only be understood as a *whole*, for this is the great error of our day in the treatment of the human body, that physicians separate the soul from the body". Even today, centuries later, we still have some physicians who have trouble appreciating that there are direct links between the psychosocial and physical worlds of the individual, and how these linking relationships reflect themselves in health and in the disease process. Changes did begin to take place, however, at the turn of the 20th century, with physicians like Sir William Osler, who explored the relationship between angina pectoris and "a hectic pace of life". The idea that environmental forces could actually cause disease rather than just short-term ill effects was also seen in the work of Walter Cannon in the 1930s, when he studied the effects of "fight-or-flight" reactions of animals and people under stress. Cannon observed that when his subjects experienced situations of cold, lack of oxygen, and excitement, he could detect physiological changes such as adrenalin secretions.

From these beginnings, Hans Selye developed, in the 1940s, his three-stage process of stress-related illnesses: the alarm reaction, resistance, and exhaustion. Since Selye's seminal work showing the direct connection between the personality and environment and ill-health, research on the impact on the psychosocial factors has grown from strength to strength. This has taken place not only in the medical sciences but also in the physical and social sciences, in diverse disciplines like cardiology, oncology, psychology, psychiatry, medical sociology, psychosomatic medicine, social work, and so on. Much of this research is coming together in inter-disciplinary research involving medics, psychologists, occupational health physicians, and the like, helping to create a field of study which this volume hopes to christen as "stress medicine". Indeed, there is already a journal of Stress Medicine, which has over the last few years published articles from all the diverse disciplines mentioned above. It is the intention of this volume, therefore, to develop the field further by bringing together some of the most distinguished scholars in the various disciplines and to explore a range of psychosocial factors that contribute to many of today's major illnesses.

The book is divided into six sections. First, we start with chapters exploring the links between stress and health, highlighting in a generic way the role that stress plays in health generally, in cancer, in the endocrine system, in mental health, and in burnout. Next we explore the links between life events, control, coping, and ill health, with an additional chapter that explores stress and occupational exposure to HIV/AIDS. Section three examines the role of personality in illness, particularly in respect to cancer, heart disease, and immune system failures (e.g., chronic fatigue syndrome). The next section briefly provides an overview of social support, stress and illness, focusing specifically on social support and heart disease, and secure attachments and health. The final two sections examine what can be done to deal with the ill-health effects of stress, by exploring the role of social support in moderating ill health, the impact of the family in this process, and how we might treat or prevent stress-related illnesses.

All these chapters are written by active researchers and scholars in the field, from a wide range of countries, the United States, Canada, the United Kingdom, Sweden, Finland, Israel, Switzerland, Norway, and Australia. We hope that this seminal volume will help to encourage further interdisciplinary and cross-cultural research in the newly emerging field of stress medicine, so that we may better understand what William Shakespeare was alluding to in *Love's Labour's Lost* (V.ii.14-18)

> *He made her melancholy, sad, and heavy;*
> *and so she died; had she being light like you,*
> *of such a merry, nimble, stirring spirit,*
> *she might ha' been a grandma ere she died;*
> *and so may you, for a light heart lives long.*

Cary L. Cooper
University of Manchester
Institute of Science and Technology

The Editor

Professor Cary L. Cooper, Ph.D., is Professor of Organizational Psychology at the University of Manchester Institute of Science and Technology, Manchester, England. He obtained his B.S. and M.B.A. degrees from The University of California, Los Angeles, and his Ph.D. from the University of Leeds in England.

Professor Cooper is a Fellow of the British Psychological Society and was honored by the Society with the distinguished Myers Lecture in 1986. In addition, he was elected as an Honorary Member of the Psychosomatic Research Society of Great Britain, a Fellow of the Royal Society of Arts, and, in 1995, a Fellow of the Royal Society of Medicine.

He has been an adviser to two United Nations agencies: the World Health Organization on "Psychosocial Factors in Occupational Health" and the International Labor Office on "Occupational Stress and Health".

He is currently Editor-in-Chief of the international quarterly journal, *The Journal of Organizational Behavior*, and co-Editor of the medical journal, *Stress Medicine*.

He is on the Editorial Boards of many health and organizational health psychology journals and is the author of over 70 books in the occupational psychology, health psychology, and stress medicine fields. In addition, he has written over 300 scholarly articles, many of which are in occupational psychology and stress medicine journals.

He has lectured all over the world and presented major television documentaries on the fields of occupational stress and stress medicine.

Contributors

Lea Baider

Sharett Institute of Oncology
Hadassah University Hospital
Jerusalem, Israel

Christina G. Blanchard

Division of Medical Oncology
Albany Medical College
Albany, New York

John G. Bruhn

Provost and Dean
Penn State Harrisburg
Middletown, Pennsylvania

Ronald J. Burke

Faculty of Administrative Studies
York University, Ontario, Canada

Graham D. Burrows

The University of Melbourne
Department of Psychiatry
Austin & Repatriation Medical Centre
Heidelberg, Victoria, Australia

George P. Chrousos

Developmental Endocrinology Branch
National Institutes of Child Health and
    Human Development
Bethesda, Maryland

Dave DeJoy

Department of Health Promotion
    and Behavior
University of Georgia
Athens, Georgia

Pnina Ever-Hadani

Department of Medical Ecology
Hadassah Medical Center
Jerusalem, Israel

Hans J. Eysenck

Institute of Psychiatry
University of London
London, England

E. Brian Faragher

Medical Statistics Department
Withington Hospital
University of Manchester
Manchester, England

Shirley Fisher

Centre for Occupational and Health
  Psychology
Department of Psychology
University of Strathclyde
Glasgow, Scotland

Robyn M. Gershon

Department of Environmental
  Health Sciences
Johns Hopkins University School of Hygiene
  and Public Health
Baltimore, Maryland

Benjamin H. Gottlieb

Department of Psychology
University of Guelph
Guelph, Ontario, Canada

John Green

Clinical Health Psychology
St. Mary's Hospital and
National AIDS Counselling
  Training Unit
St. Charles Hospital
London, England

Gregory R. Harper

Division of Medical Oncology
Albany Medical College
Albany, New York

Stanislav V. Kasl

Department of Epidemiology
  and Public Health
School of Medicine
Yale University
New Haven, Connecticut

Atara Kaplan De-Nour

Department of Psychiatry
Hadassah University Hospital
Jerusalem, Israel

Bella Kaufman

Institute of Oncology
Hadassah University Hospital
Jerusalem, Israel

Agnes Kocsis

Department of Health Psychology
St. Mary's Hospital,
London, England

Lennart Levi

Department of Stress Research
Karolinska Institutet
University of Stockholm
Stockholm, Sweden

Suzan Lewis

Department of Psychology
  and Speech Pathology
Manchester Metropolitan University
Manchester, England

Patricia A.C. Matuszek

Department of Management
University of Texas at Arlington
Arlington, Texas

Kathleen A. Moore

School of Psychology
Deakin University
Burwood, Victoria, Australia

Lawrence R. Murphy

Applied Psychology and Ergonomics Branch
National Institute for Occupational Safety
  and Health
Cincinnati, Ohio

Debra L. Nelson

Department of Management
Oklahoma State University
Stillwater, Oklahoma

James Campbell Quick

Department of Management
University of Texas at Arlington
Arlington, Texas

Jonathan D. Quick

World Health Organization
Geneva, Switzerland

Astrid M. Richardsen

University of Tromsø
Tromsø, Norway

Paul J. Rosch

The American Institute of Stress
Yonkers, New York

Ray H. Rosenman

Mount Zion Medical Center
  of University of California
San Francisco and
SRI International
Menlo Park, California

Coleen Shannon

School of Social Work
University of Texas at Arlington
Arlington, Texas

Töres Theorell

National Institute of Psychosocial
  Factors and Health
Department of Occupational Health
Karolinska Hospital
Stockholm, Sweden

Constantine Tsigos

Developmental Endocrinology Branch
National Institutes of Child Health
    and Human Development
Bethesda, Maryland

James L. Whittington

Department of Management
University of Texas at Arlington
Arlington, Texas

Table of Contents

Introduction

Spice of life or kiss of death?

Lennart Levi

Why "stress"?

According to the *American Heritage Dictionary of the English Language* (1969), the word stress is derived from middle English *stresse* (hardship, distress), from Old French *estresse* (narrowness), from Vulgar Latin *strictia*, from Latin *strictus* (tight, narrow), from the past principle of *stringere* (to draw tight, to tighten).

In *biological and health sciences*, however, the concept derives from everyday clinical practice. Some 70 years ago, a young student sat in the lecture theater at the University of Prague and listened to his very first lecture in internal medicine (Levi, 1985). It so happened that, on that day, by way of an introduction, the students were shown several instances of the earliest stages of various infectious diseases. As each patient was brought into the lecture room, the professor carefully questioned and examined him. It turned out that each of these patients felt and looked ill, had a coated tongue, complained of more or less diffuse aches and pains in the joints, and of intestinal disturbances with loss of appetite. Most of them also had fever (sometimes with mental confusion), an enlarged spleen or liver, inflamed tonsils, and so forth. All this was quite evident, but the professor attached very little significance to any of it, focusing instead on "typical features" of each disease.

The young student, *Hans Selye*, subsequently originator of the biological concept of stress, listened to his professor and thought that every disorder certainly had such typical features—so far very inconspicuous to his untrained eye—which, of course, must be considered. But the different diseases also had features *in common* which would be just as interesting. For want of a better name, he called the latter *"The Syndrome of Just Being Sick"* (Selye, 1964).

Ten years passed. Selye had moved from Prague to Montreal, where, at the McGill University, he tried to identify a new ovarian hormone in extracts of cattle ovaries. When injected into experimental animals, all the extracts, no matter how prepared, produced the same syndrome character-

0-8493-2908-6/96/$0.00+$.50

ized by a triad of enlargement of the adrenal cortex, gastrointestinal ulcers, and involution of the thymus and lymph nodes. Although at first he ascribed all these changes to some new ovarian hormone in his extract, it soon turned out that extracts of other organs produced the same changes. Could this be due to a "tissue hormone"?

As a further control, he now injected not any organ extract but toxic substances of all kinds, like formalin, and was surprised to find the same triad once again. The experimental animals reacted in a typical way to each injection but there were also features that were common to all injections. Selye turned to one of his tutors and asked him what this peculiar *stereotypy*, this *generality* in the organism's way of reacting to such different stimuli could be due to. The senior scientist gave his young colleague a sad look and interpreted his findings as a result of *impurities* in all the extracts.

At that point, Selye suddenly remembered his classroom impression of the "syndrome of just being sick". In a flash he realized that what he had produced with his extracts and toxic drugs was an experimental replica of this condition. This model was then employed in the analysis of the stress syndrome using the adrenal enlargement, gastrointestinal ulcers, and thymico-lymphatic involution as objective indices of stress.

Based on his observations, he published his first brief article in *Nature* (Selye, 1936) on a syndrome that was produced by widely differing substances. The article is about 35 column-centimeters long and does not mention the word "stress". But it describes for the first time this generality, this stereotypy, in the organism's tendency to react to widely differing chemical and other stimuli. It was later found that if the experimental animals were exposed to cold, heat, X-rays, noise, pain, bleeding, or muscular work, the same stereotypy occurred (Selye, 1967).

What is stress?

Selye now sought a suitable name for the newly discovered phenomenon and chose an analogy from physics. Here, stress is defined as an applied force or system of forces that tends to strain or deform a body. What *happens* in the "body" in question, for example, the tensions in the girders of a bridge when a train, a column of trucks, or a number of cars cross the bridge, is called *strain*. The tensions vary from case to case but "strain" is common to all these cases. It was the corresponding biological stereotypy that Selye wanted to describe, and when he sought an analogy from engineering, he believed "the tensions in the girders of the bridge" were called "stress". This is not so. They are called "strain". But Selye, who was born in the Austro-Hungarian double monarchy, educated in Prague, and emigrated to Montreal, misunderstood the English terminology and called the phenomenon stress, thereby spoiling the analogy with everyday and technological language and—much to his own regret—causing a great deal of subsequent confusion.

What, then, is stress? According to Selye, it is the *lowest common denominator* in the organism's reactions to every conceivable kind of strain, challenge, and demand or, in other words, the stereotypy, the general features in the organism's reaction to all kinds of stresses and strains. Stress *is* thus an abstraction. It is very difficult to *observe* stress, in this sense, since Selye does not base the definition on the entire reaction but only on its *nonspecific* features, those that are common to all types of loads and demands. Another way to define and describe the phenomenon "stress" is by referring to what Selye used to call *"the rate of wear and tear in the organism"* (Selye, 1971).

Many attempts have been made since 1936 to abandon the concept of stress. Yet it is alive and flourishing all over the world, as shown by an in-depth report issued by the American National Academy of Sciences, "Stress and Human Health" (Elliot and Eisdorfer, 1982), a summary of teamwork by about 100 leading scientists. More recent reports include Kalimo et al. (1987), Karasek and Theorell (1990), Kompier and Levi (1994), and a report from the International Labor Organization (1992).

What causes stress?

Stress is caused by a multitude of demands *(stressors)*, such as an inadequate fit between what we need and what we are capable of, and what our environment offers and what it demands of us. We need a certain amount of responsibility, but our job offers less or demands more. We need a certain amount of work, but either get none at all—unemployment—or too much.

Another cause of stress lies in role conflicts. We all play several roles. We are husbands or wives, we are parents to our children, we are children to our parents, we are brothers and sisters, friends, and we are bosses, peers, and subordinates—all at the same time. And the ingredients of conflict are easy to find in trying to fill these multiple roles.

Is stress harmful? The answer is: yes and no. It all depends on the context. To use a metaphor, a car stops at a traffic light and its driver "steps on the gas". In response, the engine races, leading to increased wear and deposition of soot on the valves, without the car moving from the spot. On the other hand, stepping on the gas while driving on a motorway may be sensible and productive.

Stress in the biological sense cannot be eliminated. Without it, the process of life would cease, for the absence of stress means death. What needs to be avoided is unnecessary and noxious stress in the engineering sense. The relevant questions are: How great is it and is it appropriate to the needs of the situation?

Our *sense of control* over what is happening to us is critical. When we feel in control, stress becomes the spice of life, a challenge instead of a threat. When we lack this crucial sense of control, stress can spell crisis—bad news for us, our health, and our community. Our decision latitude, our influence over various aspects of our own lives, is a strong determinant of whether stress becomes a spice of life—or a kiss of death (Levi, 1992).

When we are exposed to stressors—such as a lack of control over our lives combined with excessive demands, unsatisfied needs, unfulfilled expectations, overstimulation, understimulation, or role conflicts—most of us experience "dysphoric" *emotional* reactions, such as anxiety, depression, uneasiness, apathy, alienation, and hypochondriasis.

Stress also causes *behavioral* reactions. Some of us start smoking or overeating. We seek comfort in alcohol or take unnecessary risks at work or in traffic. Aggressive, violent, or other types of antisocial behavior may be the outlet chosen. Many commit suicide, or try to. Many of these reactions lead to disease and premature death.

We also react *physiologically*. Take, for example, the employee who has been unjustly criticized by his or her supervisor. The employee's typical reactions are increased blood pressure, increased or irregular heart rate, muscular tension with subsequent pain in the neck, head, and shoulders, dryness of throat and mouth, and overproduction of acid gastric juice. When long-lasting, intensive and/or frequently recurring, some of these reactions can lead, for example, to hypertension, myocardial infarction, or stroke.

Although everyone can experience these reactions, those with "type A" neuroendocrinologically mediated behavior are particularly at risk. These are people leading a highly competive, hard-driving way of life, combining hostility, speed, impatience, and obsessive concern with doing more and more in less and less time, with no opportunity for unwinding and recuperation.

But these reactions can be buffered. Much depends not only on what we are exposed to but also on how we cope with the situation. We can change our environment, we can flee from our problems, we can ask for help, we can accept things as they are, or we can bury our heads in the sand by changing our appraisal of our environment (denial). Whatever our choice, it influences our stress reactions. Coping may thus mean either altering the situation or (without doing this) altering one's perception of, or adaptation to, the situation. Both approaches affect health and well-being.

Health effects

The relationships between stressors, on the one hand, and the outcome in terms of morbidity and mortality, on the other hand, have been studied by integrating the concepts and methods of psychophysiology and epidemiology. In this way, dissatisfaction, health-related behaviors and physiological stress reactions can be associated with various characteristics of our social environment, as well as with general and specific mental and physical ill health.

Disturbances in bodily functions commonly found in people exposed to stressful situations include muscular symptoms such as tension and pain; gastrointestinal symptoms such as dyspepsia, indigestion, vomiting, heartburn, constipation, and irritable colon; cardiovascular symptoms such as palpitation, arrhythmias, and inframammary pain; respiratory symptoms such as dyspnea and hyperventilation; central nervous system symptoms such as neurotic reactions, insomnia, weakness, faintness, and headaches; and sexual dysfunctions such as dysmenorrhea, frigidity, and impotence. Not only do these symptoms cause the patient much distress and suffering, they entail high cost to the community and very considerable losses in work time and productivity for the employer.

How much "say" an employee has in his/her job is a critical factor. In a study on 1600 Swedish men, heart disease symptoms were most common (with 20% of the workers affected) among those who described their work as both psychologically demanding and with a low degree of decision-making latitude (Karasek and Theorell, 1990). By contrast, workers who have reported low psychological demands and a high level of skill discretion had no symptoms of heart disease. Their jobs were associated with a much better state of health than that of the average worker.

A number of studies in different countries have shown a relationship between exposure to environmental stressors (such as high psychological demands combined with low decision-making latitude and low level of social support) and morbidity and mortality (Karasek and Theorell, 1990). Although "correlation is not causation", the evidence is strong enough to justify measures to prevent or reduce stress, at least if applied in an experimental manner and if properly evaluated (Kompier and Levi, 1994).

Stress management

There are three basic paths in order of preference:

1. Eliminate or modify the stress-producing situation or remove the individual from it; find "the right shoe for the right foot", or allow the person concerned to adjust the shoe to fit his or her foot
2. Adjust the shoe—that is, change the social situation—to fit the individual's foot
3. Strengthen the person's resilience to stress, for example, through physical exercise, meditation and relaxation techniques, and social support

Stress management has traditionally focused on individual approaches, usually by counseling individuals or small groups on ways to adapt to, or cope with, various stressors and/or their consequences. More recently, approaches have started to encourage the individual to adjust his/her environment to his or her abilities and needs, improving the person-environment fit, and advising decision makers and administrators to allow or even promote such adjustments.

Four general categories of approaches and strategies can be applied in any community:

- Improve content and organization of life conditions in order to control psychosocial risk factors
- Monitor changes in social situation, people's health, and their interrelationship, with proper feedback to all concerned
- Increase awareness, inform, train, educate
- Broaden goals and strategies of health services

Most important, we must create, for ourselves and others, those occupational and other situations that give our lives meaning, content, and structure, as well as identity, self-esteem, companions, friends, and material means. If we succeed, we will be productive without being destructive. Or, as James Thurber put it: "Old men should know, before they die, what they are running to, and from, and why".

A holistic approach

In all industrialized and most developing countries, rapid, fundamental changes are taking place in such basic social structures as the way children are reared, the types of environments in which people work, the way work is organized and conducted, and the mechanisms for taking care of the old and sick. These changes are influenced by, and influence, phenomena such as urbanization, mechanization and automation, environmental pollution, uneven distribution of resources, and shortages of work and housing. At the same time, increases in communication, education, and advertising have resulted in greater public awareness and expectations.

Singly and interacting with one another, various aspects of these phenomena are of great significance in promoting health and in causing disease. These structural problems have not been dealt with adequately in the context and scope of physical and psychosocial environmental planning, health care, and stress research.

An exception to this rule is provided in the Swedish Public Health Service Bill (1985, p. 11) in which the government declared that "our health is determined in large measure by our living conditions and lifestyle". The bill goes on to state that

> the health risks in contemporary society take the
> form of, for instance, work, traffic, and living envi-
> ronments that are physically and socially deficient,
> unemployment, abuse of alcohol and drugs, con-

sumption of tobacco, unsuitable dietary habits, as
well as psychological and social strains associated
with our relationship—and lack of relationship—
with our fellow beings. . . . These health risks . . . are
now a major determinant of our possibilities of living a healthy life. This is true of practically all the
health risks which give rise to today's most common
diseases, e.g., cardiovascular disorders, mental ill
health, tumors and allergies, as well as accidents.

As seen by the Swedish Government, therefore, "care must start from a
holistic approach. . . . By a holistic approach we mean that people's symptoms and illnesses, their causes and consequences, are appraised in both
a medical and a psychological and social perspective".

An estimate made in a World Health Organization teleconference on
October 12, 1990 indicates that such "diseases of lifestyle" are the cause of
70 to 80% of premature deaths in industrialized countries. This insight was
expressed about one decade earlier by the Secretary of Health, Education
and Welfare of the United States (Califano, 1979) in three summarizing sen-
tences about these "modern killers":

- We are killing ourselves by our own careless habits
- We are killing ourselves by carelessly polluting the environment
- We are killing ourselves by permitting harmful social conditions to
  persist

Environments and lifestyles are now changing more rapidly than ever.
Many of these changes are well-intended but still carry negative side effects.
Others are unintentional and can also lead to unforeseeable noxious effects.
Some of the changes are planned and intentional, and their noxious effects
are easily foreseeable, as in the case of exploitation of other people. Or, eventually, problems are created, not by the change, but by the lack of change,
for example, by permitting harmful conditions to persist (Levi, 1993).

Rather than describing a smooth curve, these interactions tend to be
discontinuous, besides being intertwined and uncontrolled. Their effects
in terms of health and well-being are often dramatic and destructive. The
Club of Rome correctly conceives such problems as an untidy tangle of interrelated issues (the "problematique world"). The interactions between
the different "threads" are many and varied but only dimly understood.

Against this background, a fundamental issue is whether governments, with the support of scientists and planners in all sectors and disciplines and of an informed community, will be able (and willing) to use the
new opportunities offered by advanced technologies to analyze deliberately and consciously this untidy tangle, in order to try to shape a better

society and working life. Or will they passively attempt mere adjustment, post factum, as a matter of current expediency (King, 1986)?

From research to legislation

The Swedish Government chose the former approach as related to one of the key components of the "living conditions" mentioned in its Public Health Service Bill (see above), namely the work environment. It appointed and issued its terms of reference for a Swedish Commission on the Work Environment, against a background of the Government's concern about recent trends in work-related morbidity, long-term absence due to sickness, and premature retirement. The Commission, in close collaboration with the scientific community, reviewed available evidence and presented its final report in June 1990. The report proposed amendments to the Swedish Work Environment Act.

Based on these formulations, the resulting amended Swedish Work Environment Act (1991) now states the following concerning the characteristics of the work environment:

- Working conditions shall be adapted to people's differing physical and psychological circumstances
- The employee shall be enabled to participate in the arrangement of his own job situation as well as in work on changes and developments that affect his own job
- Technology, work organization and job content shall be arranged so that the employee is not exposed to physical or mental loads that may cause ill health or accidents
- The matters to be considered in this context shall include forms of remuneration and the scheduling of working hours
- Rigorously controlled or tied work shall be avoided or restricted
- It shall be the aim for work to afford opportunities for variety, social contacts and cooperation as well as continuity between individual tasks
- It shall be the aim for working conditions to afford opportunities for personal and occupational development as well as for self-determination and occupational responsibility

These objectives can be promoted using a stick (liability to penalty) but also a carrot (financial incentives to management). Sweden has chosen to give priority to the latter approach.

Health promotion and stress-related disease prevention

Theoretically, environment and lifestyle-related disease may be prevented at any of the links in the pathogenic chain. Thus, environmental stressors might be removed, modified, or avoided by adjusting, e.g., the work environment, organization, and content. Preventive variables that interact might be increased (e.g., by improving social networks or expanding coping abilities). Emotional, behavioral, and physiological, pathogenic mechanisms might be interrupted (e.g., by blocking adrenergic beta-receptors, antismoking campaigns, psychotherapeutic counseling, tranquilizers). Precursors of disease might be treated so that they do not progress to overt disease.

Briefly, an overall program for research and environmental and health action should aim at being

- Systems oriented, addressing health-related interactions in the person-environment ecosystem (e.g., family, school, work, hospital, and old people's home)
- Interdisciplinary, covering and integrating medical, physiological, emotional, behavioral, social, and economic aspects
- Oriented to problem solving, including epidemiological identification of health problems and their environmental and lifestyle correlates, followed by longitudinal interdisciplinary field studies of exposures, reactions, and health outcomes, and then by subsequent experimental evaluation under real-life conditions of presumably health-promoting and disease-preventing interventions
- Health oriented (not merely disease oriented), trying to identify what constitutes and promotes good health and counteracts ill health)
- Intersectoral, promoting and evaluating environmental and health actions administered in other sectors (e.g., employment, housing, nutrition, traffic, and education)
- Participatory, interacting closely with potential caregivers, receivers, planners, and policymakers
- International, facilitating transcultural, collaborative, and complementary projects with centers in other countries

In order to safeguard individual rights, prevent the perpetuation of harmful or useless measures, limit losses to the community's purse, and advance knowledge of the future, any of these, or other, actions must be evaluated when implemented. Such evaluation is the modern, humane substitute for nature's slow and cruel "survival of the fittest", and is a means of enabling man to adapt with minimal trauma to a rapidly changing environment and to control some of its changes (Kagan and Levi, 1975; Levi, 1979, 1992).

References

American Heritage Dictionary of the English Language (p. 1275). Boston: American Heritage & Houghton Mifflin, 1969.

Califano, J. A., Jr.: The Secretary's Forewood. In: Healthy People. The Surgeon General's Report on Health Promotion and Disease Prevention (p. vii). Washington, D.C.: U.S. Department of Health, Education, and Welfare, 1979.

Elliott, G. R. and Eisdorfer, C. (eds.): *Research on Stress and Human Health*. National Academy of Sciences, Institute of Medicine, report. New York: Springer, 1982.

International Labor Organization (ILO): *Preventing Stress at Work*. Conditions of Work Digest No. 2, Geneva: International Labour Organization, 1992.

Kagan, A. and Levi, L.: Health and environment—psychosocial stimuli: a review. In: Levi, L. (ed.): *Society, Stress and Disease. Vol. 2: Childhood and Adolescence* (pp. 241–260). London: Oxford University Press, 1975.

Kalimo, R., El-Batawi, M. A., and Cooper, C. L. (eds.): *Psychosocial Factors at Work and Their Relation to Health*. Geneva: World Health Organization, 1987.

Karasek, R. and Theorell, T.: *Healthy Work—Stress, Productivity, and the Reconstruction of Working Life*. New York: Basic Books, 1990.

King, A.: The great transition. *World Academy of Art and Science Newsletter*. (pp. 1–6). July, 1986.

Kompier, M. and Levi, L.: *Stress at Work, Causes, Effects, and Prevention*. Dublin: European Foundation, 1994.

Levi, L. (ed.): Psychosocial factors in preventive medicine. In: Healthy People. The Surgeon General's Report on Health Promotion and Disease Prevention. Background papers (pp. 207–252). Washington, D.C.: U.S. Department of Health, Education, and Welfare, 1979.

Levi, L.: Stress: definitions, concepts and significance. *Cardiovascular Information*, 1, 10, 1985.

Levi, L.: Work Stress. *Eur. Bull. Environ. Health*, 1, 9, 1992.

Levi, L.: Conditions of life, life-styles, and health in a highly developed country. *Psychiatr. Neurol. Jpn.*, 95, 259, 1993.

Selye, H.: A syndrome produced by diverse noxious agents. *Nature*, 138, 32, 1936.

Selye, H.: *From Dream to Discovery* (p. 51). New York: McGraw-Hill, 1964.

Selye, H.: *In Vivo. The Case for Supramolecular Biology*. New York: Liveright, 1967.

Selye, H.: The evolution of the stress concept—stress and cardiovascular disease. In: Levi, L. (ed.): *Society, Stress and Disease. Vol. 1: The Psychosocial Environment and Psychosomatic Diseases* (pp. 299–311). London: Oxford University Press, 1971.

Section 1

Stress and health

chapter one

Theory of stress and health

Stanislav V. Kasl

Introduction

If one looks back over the last two decades of research on stress and health, one cannot help but be impressed by the large volume of work and the substantial accumulation of findings. The intersection of medicine and the social/behavioral sciences includes many subdisciplines—behavioral medicine, health psychology, medical sociology, psychosocial and psychiatric epidemiology, psychosomatic medicine—and for each of these, stress and health continues to be a major research topic. The ascendance of other important research themes, such as social support/networks and health, has not diminished the importance of the stress theme, since these newer concepts frequently represent, in part, an enrichment and elaboration of the stress and health topic rather than a major refocusing of investigators' interests.

That same look back at the last two decades of research on stress and health, which reveals its continued popularity, also shows that nearly all the significant issues surrounding the concept of stress remain unsettled and/or controversial. How useful is it as a scientific construct? What is the optimal conceptualization? What is the best way of measuring stress? How does it overlap with other concepts? How does it influence our research strategies? The persistence of these questions reflects the fact that no investigator (or group of investigators) has gained theoretical and/or methodological ascendance so as to persuade other stress researchers to adopt a particular set of answers to the above questions. Since the stress and health topic cuts across disciplinary boundaries, it is likely that the lack of convergence on the answers to the major methodological and conceptual issues is in part due to the inevitably different perspectives and traditions that these disciplines offer. But this is only a partial answer, since even within each discipline, many divergent formulations regarding conceptualization and measurement continue to survive and thrive. It is also likely that different investigators are comfortable with a particular stress formulation or approach because it is most useful for the type of problem they study or the type of outcomes in which they are interested. Thus, if differences in stress formulations are tied to the special characteristics of a particular discipline, as well as to the types of problems and outcomes studied, then the fact that the topic of stress and health cuts across several disciplines, and includes many different outcomes, is likely to perpetuate the diversity of formulations and approaches.

It is a fair inference from the above comments that any chapter (especially if authored by a single individual) that attempts to guide the research domain of stress and health toward greater conceptual and operational clarity, precision, and consensus will be met with widespread rejection or neglect, if not also some derision. So the goals of this chapter have to be rather modest. Specifically, I first wish to note the diversity of formulations and approaches that are currently utilized, and to comment on some of their advantages and limitations. Then I wish to adopt the strategy of trying to reformulate theoretical and conceptual concerns as methodological and research design issues. The reasons for this strategy are several. (1) Methodological ideas or principles seem to cross disciplinary boundaries more easily than concepts and theories. (2) A strong theory is less likely to rescue data based on a poor design, but a strong design is more likely to produce trustworthy or useful findings even in the absence of a strong theory. (3) The stress and health research domain is difficult enough methodologically and thus even relatively atheoretical studies generate important new questions, thereby reducing our dependence on a well-articulated theory to guide future studies.

The diversity of stress formulations

As noted already, the intent of this chapter is not to recommend or insist on changes in the conceptual status quo, but only to analyze and comment on issues that perpetuate and reinforce the current situation. Stress is obviously a broad, high-level construct which performs different functions for investigators from different disciplines, and this does not make it easy to find a single path toward clarification and explication. Three major areas of diversity or discord can be recognized: What type of a construct is it? What are its defining properties? How useful is it, or in what ways is it useful?

One important area of disagreement is that the term stress continues to be used in several fundamentally different ways:

1. Stress is an environmental condition, susceptible to an objective definition and measurement. (The term "stressor" may often be used in this context.) The emphasis is on stress as a stimulus, an independent variable, a risk factor, an exposure variable, and on its objectively measured properties.
2. Stress is a subjective perception or appraisal of an objective environmental condition. This definition, which embraces the notion that

"stress is subjective", reflects a psychological tradition which assumes that the meaning of the objectively characterized stressor will vary across individuals and that such variation determines the impact of the stressor.

3. Stress is a particular response or reaction. Included here would be a variety of proximal and distal outcomes, including dysphoric mood, psychophysiological symptoms of tension, biological parameters (e.g., neuroendocrine levels), as well as incidence of specific disease states.

4. Stress is a particular relational term linking environmental characteristics and personal characteristics, in particular, the excess of environmental demand beyond the individual's capacity to meet them. The theoretical formulation known as the Person-Environment Fit (e.g., French et al., 1982) is an example of this relational approach to concepts.

5. Stress is a process, which includes other important components such as appraisal, coping, reappraisal, and cannot be reduced to any simple stimulus-response or cause-effect formulation.

It has been argued (Cohen and Kessler, 1995) that there are at least three distinct models or approaches to stress and that these can be linked to three different disciplines: epidemiology, biology, and psychology. The *epidemiological* model utilizes the stimulus-based definition of stress and has as its broad objective the identification of environmental exposure variables that increase the risk of adverse health outcomes. The *biological* approach is viewed as focusing on a response-based definition of stress and as zeroing in on particular pathophysiological reactions (primarily those resulting from the activation of the sympathetic-adrenal medullary system and the hypothalamic-pituitary-adrenocortical axis) as possible antecedents or risk factors for adverse health outcomes. Finally, the *psychological* tradition is thought to utilize the transactional-based definition of stress in which psychological processes of appraisal of the environmental exposure and of response capabilities are crucial in understanding the mediating processes through which the exposure impacts on health.

The Cohen and Kessler (1995) analysis is quite useful in helping us understand the origins of the considerable diversity of approaches to the concept of stress. However, since most stress models or theories that focus on health and disease as outcomes (e.g., Caplan et al., 1975; Elliott and Eisdorfer, 1982) have, for some time now, been considerably broader and more integrative than any one or another of the three individual models discussed by Cohen and Kessler, then the persistence of the confusing diversity of meanings of stress is not fully explained by their analysis. It is possible, instead, that once an investigator has identified the full set of possible etiological steps from exposure to disease (via appraisal and biobehavioral and affective reactions), how the term stress gets used (if at all) is of no great relevance. This conclusion is also compatible with the observation that during the last two decades of research on stress and health, impressive evidence has been accumulated (e.g., Brown and Harris, 1989) without being hampered seriously by the continued terminological or conceptual confusion surrounding the term stress.

The above listing of the five ways of conceptualizing stress is useful beyond just serving as a reminder of the different theoretical-conceptual formulations that exist. It can also serve as a linkage to several methodological issues; these will be discussed later, in the next section.

With respect to the second question raised earlier, (what are the defining properties of stress?), we again encounter a divergence of answers or formulations. There appear to be three ways in which this question has been approached and they roughly correspond to the epidemiological, biological, and psychological models of stress noted by Cohen and Kessler (1995).

In the *epidemiological* approach, where the emphasis is on exposure conditions, the identification of defining properties of stressors is often finessed by enumerating specific environmental conditions thought to be stressful. Such a listing is probably based on some combination of intuition, empirical evidence regarding negative impact on health, and, possibly, some unarticulated notion of what that particular author means by stress. For the work setting, for example, Landy and Trumbo (1976) list: job insecurity, excessive competition, hazardous working conditions, task demands, and long or unusual working hours. In other instances, a particular concept, such as threat or uncertainty/unpredictability/uncontrollability, is invoked to justify the listing of a particular set of exemplar situations and exposures. The central concept, seldom defined with any precision, is presumably intended to represent the "essential nature" of the stress concept. In the original list of stressful life events (Holmes and Rahe, 1967), these events were all thought to indicate varying degrees of "readjustment demand."

How one evaluates this enumeration approach to defining properties of stressors depends on how seriously one takes the concept of stress and its status as a scientific construct. If stress means nothing more than the expectation that stressful exposures are likely to have adverse health consequences (and that anything labeled a stressor thus becomes more compelling as a subject of research), then we only are invoking stress as an easy shortcut to justifying the research topic and enhancing others' interest in it. This is not uncommon; such a perfunctory use of the concept appears acceptable if one acknowledges it as that. However, such an enumeration of examples of stressors cannot help us with boundary issues (e.g., are purely physical or chemical exposures also stressors?), cannot clarify linkages to other constructs, and cannot help us redefine this high-order construct in terms of more tractable, lower-level concepts.

The *biological* model of stress in the Cohen and Kessler analysis emphasizes a response-based definition of stress. In this model, finding defining properties of stress appears to be equivalent to postulating the existence of an integrated biological response pattern in the context of stress, and then selecting some specific aspects of this pattern to be criterial characteristics for denoting the presence or absence of stress. Baum (1990) and Baum and Grunberg (1995), in particular, have been cogent advocates of the view that there is sufficient specificity in the responces to a variety of stressors to make it useful to consider catecholamines and glucocorticoids as the most appropriate markers in stress research. However, they go on to note: "Some changes appear to be alerting or alarm-oriented and serve to facilitate the initiation of stress responding. Other neuroendocrine changes are supportive of general systemic response, by increasing availability of energy, potentiating response, and/or by facilitating mobilization or recovery" (Baum and Grunberg, 1995).

This suggests that, although it may be possible to identify the relevant (smallish set of) parameters that need monitoring in order to describe the stress process, it may be exceedingly difficult to coordinate the intensity and duration of the stressor exposure to individual and joint patterns of reactivity of these selected parameters. This would further suggest that it may be even more difficult to know how to take the data on complex patterns of reactions of these parameters and translate them into elevated risk for a variety of disease outcomes. This is in line with Rose's (1980) review of evidence on endocrine responses to stress, where he notes many instances in which the endocrine responses (especially cortisol), though sensitive to acute stressors, undergo extinction when the individuals are reexposed to those stressors, or are exposed to chronic stressors.

It is not clear if this should be interpreted, conceptually, that the stressor ceased to be stressful and, empirically, that the risk of disease was reduced. Instead, it could be that such endocrine variables have their own patterns of reactivity and simply are not suitable for monitoring the consequences of chronic exposures. So it would seem that, although biological parameters such as catecholamines and glucocorticoids are appropriate dependent variables in the study of aspects of the stress process, at the same time they have a much more tenuous status as risk factors for disease outcomes. Unlike other biological parameters, such as those reflecting cardiovascular functioning, which have established linkages to specific disease outcomes, neuroendocrine variables do not seem to have such direct and well-documented linkages. In addition, the linkages, such as between blood pressure and coronary heart disease, are with stable (resting, chronic) levels of the risk factors, and the results on cardiovascular reactivity, in contrast, are more difficult to translate into elevated risk of future cardiovascular disease (e.g., Krantz and Falconer, 1995).

The *psychological* model of stress is described as utilizing a transactional or psychological process definition. Thus, finding defining properties of stress is equivalent to identifying the unique properties of this transaction. One widely influential definition is that of McGrath (1970): stress is "a (perceived) substantial imbalance between demand and response capability, under conditions where failure to meet demand has important (perceived) consequences". A "generic" approach to defining stress is exemplified by Baum's (1990) definition of stress as "a negative experience that is associated with threat, harm, or demand"; the emphasis is on stress as an aversive state and on the requirement for some form of adjustment to the situation. These definitions, admittedly, have a fair amount of vagueness in them (e.g., threat, substantial imbalance), as well as the use of terms, such as demand, that may be as general and as in need of definition as stress itself. Also, the issue of boundaries is not made more precise by these definitions, nor are specific operational definitions easily suggested.

Since stress is defined from the perspective of the experience of the individual and is in some sense a phenomenological reconstruction of it, this permits a rich and complex definition of stress. In the context of the stress and health topic, this may not always be an advantage. One issue is that the psychological model of stress incorporates the negative subjective experience (distress, threat, felt need to meet demands, etc.) in the definitions. This seems to commit us to the notion that the subjective experience is essential to the etiological process linking stress and disease. A preferable strategy might be to make the negative experience part of the testable theory about stress, but not to build it into the concept itself. Another question is whether stress as a relational term (e.g., demand in relation to response capability) represents an unwise departure from the scientific strategy that even complex processes are best studied as interplays of "simple" (unidimensional) variables; creating complex study variables is likely to represent premature closure on a problem and will make it difficult to isolate crucial processes, such as those that might be needed for designing effective interventions. Thus, for example, while the Brown and Harris (1989) approach to measuring stressful life events is faithful to a rich psychological definition of stress, its use of contextual threat ratings to refine the measurement of severity of the exposure variable makes it difficult to separate event severity from other factors that may influence the probability of adverse health outcomes, such as individual characteristics of the person and of his/her social environment (Dohrenwend et al., 1993).

With respect to the third question raised earlier, (how useful is the stress concept?), we again encounter a diversity of opinions, ranging from "it is useless and an obstacle to research and scientific communication", to "it is a central concept illuminating the relationship of psychosocial variables to physical health". The issue of usefulness of a concept is not easy to analyze and discuss. How do we know we have a useful concept? How do we go about altering a concept, or the measurement of a concept, to make it more useful? At a general level one could argue that a useful concept has some such characteristics as:

1. It directs us to research topics that are important but would otherwise be neglected
2. The theory surrounding the concept helps us to see similarities and combine other concepts when appropriate, and helps us to see distinctions and break down concepts, again as appropriate
3. The concept generates operationalizations that are logistically feasible and convenient, and only trivially different from each other (when different operationalizations of the same concept exist); and they are substantially different from operationalizations for substantially different constructs

It would seem that the concept of stress has served us well in the past in directing us to additional situations and experiences and psychosocial characteristics of individuals that may be associated with adverse health outcomes and are therefore worth investigating. The field has also profited from the identification of a broad list of variables and processes, which are deemed generically relevant for the understanding of the etiology of adverse health outcomes, no matter what the specific stressor under study (e.g., Caplan et al., 1975; Dohrenwend et al., 1993; Elliott and Eisdorfer, 1982; Lazarus and Folkman, 1984; Pearlin et al., 1981). However, these aspects of usefulness of the concept may be seen as reflecting the earlier stages of research with a broad concept, when the integrative functions of a concept and the hypotheses it generates are particularly important. But as a particular research domain matures, we expect the concept to help us fine-tune the theory and to guide us toward sharper differentiation from other concepts and toward more precise measurements. However, it does not appear that in this sense the concept of stress has continued to be useful with the greater maturity of the stress and health research domain. For example, the field may be quite ready to examine the possible health effects of exposures in which the psychological reaction of distress (or threat, or felt need to meet demands) is absent. However, reliance on the broad formulation which argues that stress includes some such aversive psychological reaction may steer us away from studying that exposure and/or from utilizing stress-related concepts and formulations.

There is a stubborn persistence of two difficulties surrounding the concept of stress. One is our inability to fully remove circularity involved in defining the concept. When stress is used as a stimulus (exposure) condition, it is difficult to avoid references to adverse processes or outcomes when trying to define the characteristics of that stimulus. When stress is used as a specific reaction, it is difficult to avoid calling stimuli which cause that reaction as stressors. This persistent circularity suggests that we are unable to rise above the vernacular use of the term which, in effect, gives "surplus" meaning to selected exposures and selected outcomes. How the circularity might influence the quality of our research design methodology is discussed briefly in the next section.

Given that stress is both a very broad construct and that the term has a diversity of meanings, it is inevitable that operational definitions of stress will be problematic as well. The recent volume on measurement (Cohen et al., 1994) provides an excellent, up-to-date guide to specific measurement domains: stressful life events, daily stressors, chronic stressors, stress appraisals, affective reactions, and several biological domains (cardiovascular, neuroendocrine, and immune function). But the very diversity of these topics and the absence of any conceptual framework linking them strongly, suggest the approach "If you are interested in measuring . . . X domain . . . here are some useful guidelines", and the concept of stress recedes considerably in prominence and importance. It is not possible to raise the traditional types of questions about tests and measurements of traits and stable characteristics, such as, "what is the evidence for construct validity?", since the construct keeps eluding us and is not trait-like in any case. What we have, at best, are indirect and partial indicators of the stress process, and these indicators tend to measure both too much and not enough. Thus, a summative index of recently experienced stressful life events measures too much, since it may: (1) include events that reduce adaptive demands rather than increase them, (2) reflect stage of life cycle and social-structural characteristics, such as social class, and (3) be a function of self-selection or prior characteristics of the individuals and their lifestyles. But such a summation index does not measure enough, since it omits other sources of stress, such as chronic stressors and daily hassles. Similarly, a response-based measure, such as the perceived stress scale (Cohen et al., 1983), measures too much since it correlates so strongly with depression and is also likely to overlap heavily with trait neuroticism and/or negative affectivity. But it also does not measure enough, in that it obviously does not reflect biological processes or other components of psychological reactivity, such as appraisals of threat or anxiety reactions.

The difficulty of trying to measure stress with any one or another operational definition can be brought home to us by asking an apparently simple empirical question: Is stress among the elderly greater than among younger adults? If we use a summative life events scale, like that of Holmes and Rahe (1967), we would answer "no, it is lower", since the elderly report considerably fewer life events (e.g., Goldberg and Comstock, 1980). But since it has been argued that such a list is biased by not including enough events that are experienced in later life (e.g., Chiriboga, 1989), the implication is that we underestimate the level of stress among the elderly. But just how do we go about adding later life events to "correct" the problem without biasing the revised instrument in the other direction? Neither the concept nor the theory around it can help us out with a reasonable answer. A similar problem arises if we consider measures of chronic stressors. For retired persons, work-related stressors cannot be used. Does that mean that the elderly have less stress because of this, or does it mean we need a new instrument to measure the stresses of retirement? If the latter, then how can we create fully comparable instruments if they are going to have such widely different content? Perhaps the only way to try to answer the question is to use response-based indicators of stress. But here, too, we encounter difficulties. For example, measures based on the functioning of the immune system are likely to be biased because of the well-established age differences, which would give the appearance of higher stress among the elderly. Age differences in neuroendocrine responding, on the other hand, might suggest lower stress (reactivity) among the elderly. Measures based on psychological symptoms might be biased by the presence of a greater number of physical health problems among the elderly. In short, the simple empirical question is not so simple and becomes another way of revealing some of the difficulties with the stress concept and its measurement.

A final way of probing the usefulness of the concept of stress is to ask: What would we do if we could not use the concept and the term? Research on health effects of individual life events, such as bereavement, job loss, and retirement would not be affected very much. We already have a language for describing the exposure variable (a specific event, however complex) and we need additional knowledge about these events, not stress in general, to know what dimensions of the exposure (e.g., changed financial circumstances) are important. And even now we almost never ask, as an empirical question, do these events affect stress? Rather, we ask: does the experience affect . . . mortality, blood pressure, depression, and so on. Research with summative indices of life events (no longer called stressful) would be altered little as well. We would still debate such issues as: subjective versus "objective" weights, positive versus negative events, adequacy of the lists of events, self-selection biases, contamination between health events and health outcomes, and so on. Whether or not the concept of stress is available seems to have little influence on settling such issues. Research on the psychosocial etiology of specific diseases could no longer ask (for example): does stress contribute to the risk of heart disease? However, given the present state of accumulated evidence, this is no longer a very meaningful question, since we want to be concerned with fairly specific risk factors. That is, we need to pose such questions as: what component of type A behavior may be most pathogenic for heart disease? The question "is type A behavior a stress variable?" seems much less useful. With respect to the domain of chronic stressors, such as those applicable to the work setting, it would seem that already our measurement strategy is based on assessing specific dimensions that affect health (Kasl, 1991), not on developing a global measure that somehow transcends individual dimensions and aggregates their individual impacts. In addition, different dimensions of the work setting may be related to different outcomes, e.g., quantitative overload more to cardiovascular outcomes versus qualitative overload more to mental health outcomes. The use of a general term, stress, invites neglect of such specificity of risk-outcome associations, when in fact the accumulation of evidence should increase our concern with precision of summarizing specific risk-outcome associations.

It would seem that the one area in which the stress concept and stress theory continue to play a significant role is in encouraging us to formulate a rich model of intervening dynamics and moderating influences linking an exposure condition to a health outcome. Such a stress-linked model appears generically useful for investigating the health impact of a wide variety of exposures, even those previously poorly explored and only tentatively classified as potential stressors. Postulating the intervening role of appraisals and affective reactions, and the moderating role of social support and coping strategies, seems easier to formulate when linking the whole research effort to the stress domain of research; working only at the more specific level of individual exposures, particularly those not yet adequately conceptualized at the biobehavioral level, might leave us with a more impoverished model and design.

Methodological reformulations of theoretical issues in stress and health

In this section I wish to discuss a few *illustrative* issues that arise out of the "theory" of stress, but can usefully be formulated as issues of research design and measurement. The starting point in this discussion is the assumption that the emphasis on stress and health in this volume represents an etiological orientation, which justifies the selection of the *epidemiological* perspective as the most appropriate one. In this perspective, as noted already, stressors are classified as a class of risk factors or exposure variables that play a role in the etiology of a particular disease outcome.

It is useful to formulate, as a start, an idealized observational (nonexperimental) research design, which can then help us discuss issues that arise as design compromises are inevitably forced upon us. A skeleton of such a design can be suggested with the following characteristics:

1. The cohort assembled is free of the disease of interest
2. The cohort is in a "steady state", prior to exposure or anticipation of exposure, and baseline variables (including potential confounders and vulnerability factors) are assessed
3. The exposure variable (environmental condition) is objectively defined and measured
4. Self-selection into exposure conditions is minimized, if possible, by choice of research opportunities ("natural experiments") and examined with reference to baseline data
5. Initial reactions to exposure and later stages of adaptation are monitored with biological, behavioral, and affective parameters in order to understand the process whereby some individuals develop the disease the others do not

6. The period of follow-up is sufficiently long so that the exposed cohort has reached a stable adaptation and so that new clinical events, attributable to the exposure, will have developed
7. Data analysis describes the main effect of the exposure variable, net of the contribution of baseline confounders, and the interactive effects of exposure with any predisposing and (postexposure) precipitating variables.

When the above idealized design is not feasible, but options exist regarding allocation of resources to strengthen different aspects of design, then we need explicit priorities to guide us further. From the epidemiological perspective the highest priority would seem to be the establishment of secure etiological (risk factor or cause-effect) relationships. This is generally based on prospective designs and monitoring for incidence of clinical disease. However, such a priority might mean that we give up on also trying to understand the steps in the mediating processes or even that we do not understand the exact nature of the exposure variable. From a psychological perspective, we might give up on a strong design (e.g., opt for a case/control study) in order to collect more comprehensive data on the exposure variable and how it is appraised. From a biological perspective, we might put our emphasis on biological reactivity which might involve only short-term monitoring around the transition into exposure status. However, such reactivity might have very little to do with long-term risk of disease development.

These issues are not easy to resolve, and methodological, not theoretical, considerations play the important role. For example, establishing securely that the exposure is truly a risk factor would seem such an obvious first priority. However, if (1) we intend to proceed directly to intervention studies and thus need as complete an understanding of the exposure variable as possible, and (2) the plausible confounders can be handled to some extent in the case/control design, then the strong but expensive prospective study design may not need to be our highest priority. Similarly, if our incomplete understanding of the nature of the exposure variable in the prospective study can be remedied in a later step involving small cross-sectional studies fine-tuning the concept and its measurement, then such a two-step strategy seems reasonable. However, if the reconceptualized and newly operationalized exposure variable would need a second-generation prospective study to reestablish its status as a risk factor, then our initial prospective study needs to put more resources into assessing the exposure.

Another theoretical issue that can profit from a methodological perspective is the issue of relative emphasis on objective versus subjective measurement of exposure (e.g., Frese and Zapf, 1988). There are a number of (somewhat overlapping) considerations that would lead us to prefer the *objective* approach. For example:

1. It provides for a more direct identification of the environmental condition that would need to be modified if we are considering techniques for reducing the risk
2. It provides a clearer picture of etiology, since subjective appraisals can be under the influence of many variables, including preexisting stable traits
3. It is associated with less measurement confounding if our outcomes are based on self-reports and involve similar psychological processes to the subjective appraisals
4. It allows for a clearer and more appropriate separation of stimuli and responses, of independent and dependent variables, since the subjective appraisal may be just the first step in a number of tightly linked reactions. Then the proper goal of study is to predict differential appraisals from the exposure, not the link from appraisal to the next step, such as affective reaction. For example, if the loss of a job is appraised as "I don't have enough skills to hold on to a job" (versus "No one wants to buy their product"), then it is rather trivial to use appraisal as the independent variable for predicting loss of self-esteem, depression, and job-seeking behavior.

On the other hand, there are circumstances in which more *subjective* approaches to measuring exposure are to be preferred. Some examples:

1. The objective measurement may completely remove the exposure variable from the causal chain; thus, actual crime rates in different urban neighborhoods may have little impact on fears and behaviors of elderly residents if they are not known to the residents and are not communicated in any formal or informal way
2. The objective measurement of exposure, alone, is completely insensitive to the differential "meanings" it may have; for example, objective measurement of characteristics of retirement communities or settings (e.g., the complete absence of children and young adults) is not likely to predict satisfaction and leisure behaviors of the retirees if we do not also consider the type of retirement setting characteristics the individual retirees preferred and sought
3. If modification of a particular environmental condition is not possible and the planned intervention strategy is based on reactions of individuals, then subjective assessments seem to be the more important strategy
4. If important moderator variables, such as social support processes, are linked to subjective appraisals but not to the objective environmental conditions, then a proper exploration of the role of social support cannot be carried out with objective measurements alone

The basic import of the above discussion of objective versus subjective measurements is that theoretical formulations have many immediate re-search design, methodological consequences, and that in the stress and health research domain methodological considerations frequently need to dominate over theoretical ones. The above discussion also suggests that what is an optimal strategy for one problem may not be optimal for the next one. Thus, high-level stress theory is not as good a guide to optimal research strategies as low-level theoretical and empirical analysis applied to the specific problem and the specific goals of a study.

Research in the stress and health domain is inevitably committed to the importance of studying intervening processes and moderating influences, not just the overall risk factor-disease outcome linkages. However, classi-cal epidemiologic methods do not serve us adequately in the stress and health domain, because they traditionally address only the overall expo-sure-disease association. The appropriate research model to emulate in stress and disease is the way biomarkers, including molecular biomarkers, are beginning to influence epidemiologic research strategies (Hulka et al., 1990; McMichael, 1994). These biomarkers, in effect, become powerful tools for studying intervening processes and moderating influences: (1) they can help with the measurement of the internal dose, which links it to the ex-ternal exposure; (2) they can help assess the "biologically effective" dose; (3) they can identify an early state of biologic response to the exposure; and (4) they can identify individual susceptibilities and effect-modifying host characteristics. Of course, molecular epidemiology is a model for stress and health research by analogy only, since we do not normally work with DNA as the target tissue or with mutations of the p53 gene, and since in stress and disease we move back and forth between the biological and the psy-chological levels of measurement and analysis as if these were fully inter-changeable steps in the causal chain. In the future, it will be important to take concepts such as "internal dose" and "early state of responding" more seriously so that we can more clearly distinguish changes that are part of the stress process but are mere epiphenomena for disease causation, from changes that represent the steps in progression toward disease outcomes.

References

Baum, A. (1990). Stress, intrusive imagery, and chronic distress. *Health Psychol.*, 9, 653–675.

Baum, A. and Grunberg, N. E. (1995). Neuroendocrine measures of stress response. In S. Cohen, R. C. Kessler, and L. G. Gordon (eds.), *Measuring Stress: A Guide for Health and Social Scientists.* pp. 175–192. New York, Oxford University Press.

Brown, G. W. and Harris, T. O. (eds.) (1989). *Life Events and Illness.* New York, The Guilford Press.

Caplan, R. D., Cobb, S., French, J. R. P., Jr., Van Harrison, R., and Pinneau, S. R., Jr. (1975). *Job Demands and Worker Health.* Publication No. (NIOSH) 75–160. Washington, D.C., U.S. Department of Health, Education and Welfare.

Chiriboga, D. A. (1989). The measurement of stress exposure in later life. In K. S. Markides and C. L. Cooper (eds.), *Aging, Stress, and Health*. pp. 13–41. New York, Wiley.

Cohen, S., Kamarck, T., and Mermelstein, R. (1983). A global measure of perceived stress. *J. Health Social Behav.*, 24, 385–396.

Cohen, S. and Kessler, R. C. (1995). Strategies for measuring stress in studies of psychiatric and physical disorders. In S. Cohen, R. C. Kessler, and L. G. Gordon (eds.), *Measuring Stress: A Guide for Health and Social Scientists*. pp. 3–26. New York, Oxford University Press.

Cohen, S., Kessler, R. C., and Gordon, L. G. (eds.) (1994). *Measuring Stress: A Guide for Health and Social Scientists*. New York, Oxford University Press.

Dohrenwend, B. P., Raphael, K. G., Schwartz, S., Stueve, A., and Skodol, A. (1993). The structured event probe and narrative rating method for measuring stressful life events. In L. G. Goldberger and S. Breznitz (eds.), *Handbook of Stress*. pp. 174–199. New York, Free Press.

Elliott, G. R. and Eisdorfer, C. (eds.) (1982). *Stress and Human Health*. New York, Springer.

French, J. R. P., Jr., Caplan, R. D., and Van Harrison, R. (1982). *The Mechanism of Job Stress and Strain*. Chichester, Wiley.

Frese, M. and Zapf, D. (1988). Methodological issues in the study of work stress: objective vs. subjective measurement of work stress and the question of longitudinal studies. In C. L. Cooper and R. Payne (eds.), *Causes, Coping, and Consequences of Stress at Work*. pp. 375–411. New York, Wiley.

Goldberg, E. L. and Comstock, G. W. (1980). Epidemiology of life events: frequency in general populations. *Am. J. Epidemiol.*, 111, 736–752.

Holmes, T. H. and Rahe, R. H. (1967). The social readjustment scale. *J. Psychosom. Res.*, 11, 213–218.

Hulka, B. S., Wilcosky, T. C., and Griffith, J. D. (1990). *Biological Markers in Epidemiology*. New York, Oxford University Press.

Kasl, S. V. (1991). Assessing health risks in the work setting. In H. E. Schroeder (ed.), *New Directions in Health Psychology Assessment*. pp. 95–125. New York, Hemisphere Publishing.

Krantz, D. S. and Falconer, J. J. (1995). Using cardiovascular measures in stress research: an introduction. In S. Cohen, R. C. Kessler, and L. G. Gordon (eds.), *Measuring Stress: A Guide for Health and Social Scientists*. pp. 193–212. New York, Oxford University Press.

Landy, F. J. and Trumbo, D. A. (1976). *Psychology of Work Behavior*. Homewood, IL, Dorsey Press.

Lazarus, R. S. and Folkman, S. (1984). *Stress, Appraisal, and Coping*. New York, Springer.

McGrath, J. E. (1970). A conceptual formulation for research on stress. In J. E. McGrath (ed.), *Social and Psychological Factors in Stress*. pp. 10–21. New York, Holt, Rinehart, Winston.

McMichael, A. J. (1994). Invited commentary—"molecular epidemiology": new pathway or new travelling companion? *Am. J. Epidemiol.*, 140, 1–11.

Pearlin, L. I., Lieberman, M. L., Menaghan, E., and Mullan, J. T. (1981). The stress process. *J. Health Social Behav.*, 22, 337–356.

Rose, R. M. (1980). Endocrine responses to stressful psychological events. *Psychiatr. Clin. North Am.*, 3, 251–276.

chapter two

Stress and cancer: disorders of communication, control, and civilization

Paul J. Rosch

> *Whatever happens in the mind of man, is always*
> *reflected in the diseases of his body.*
> René Dubos

> *The mind is its own place, and in itself,*
> *Can make a heaven of hell, a hell of heaven.*
> John Milton

> *Mind moves matter.*
> Virgil

In 1977, Hans Selye's International Institute of Stress cosponsored, with the Sloan Kettering Institute in New York, a symposium entitled "Cancer, Stress, and Death". Selye and I had developed a close friendship since my Fellowship at his Institute in 1951, when we coauthored articles dealing with his novel concepts.[1,2] Over the intervening years, he had invited me to prepare updated reviews, we corresponded frequently, and tried to meet when mutually convenient.[3,4] He had come to New York in connection with the symposium, and during dinner, indicated that he had a very personal interest in this subject. Five years previously, a tumor in his thigh was diagnosed as histiocytic reticulosarcoma, a normally fatal malignancy, from which he apparently completely recovered. He had refused chemotherapy, and attributed his good fortune not to any other treatment received, but rather his very firm determination to continue living so that he could complete his important research activities. Based on anecdotal reports of similar experiences and spontaneous remissions, he was convinced that a firm faith and fierce determination could retard or reverse cancer growth. Conversely, he wondered whether stress might contribute

0-8493-2908-6/96/$0.00+$.50
© 1996 by CRC Press, Inc.

to the development of certain malignancies, or accelerate their growth and metastases. He recalled that I had previously suggested that cancer might represent another of his "Diseases of Adaptation" and asked if I could contribute a paper that would support this. It was difficult for me to refuse anything that Selye requested, but I politely pointed out a variety of potential pitfalls in attempting to prove such a link. In addition, I had been completely involved in clinical practice for the past 20 years, and no longer had the time, training, or resources to adequately address this subject. We reminisced about other things, and I assumed the matter was closed.

Several weeks later, however, I received a large parcel, filled with an assortment of articles dealing with various pertinent experimental and clinical reports. It fortuitously arrived just before I was going on vacation, so I took it with me and had an opportunity to leisurely review its contents. Selye had written comments on many of the reprints to support his position, or questions designed to pique my curiosity. He also suggested that I contact various authorities concerning their opinion or experiences with respect to possible relationships between stress and cancer, but this did not prove very helpful. The President and Director of Sloan Kettering, which cosponsored the symposium, replied, "I have no information about stress and cancer," although he conceded that the topic was "most important".[5] I found it fascinating, became increasingly inveigled by its possibilities and challenges, and eventually acquiesced.[6]

Since then, there has been an explosion of interest and articles on every aspect of this subject. Advances in our understanding of psychoneuroimmunologic relationships have also provided important insights that suggest possible mechanisms that could explain some anecdotal observations.[7,8] Unfortunately, some pop psychologists and self-help zealots have gone overboard, by implying that certain types of cancer are usually stress related. Nothing could be crueler than adding to the stress and guilt of cancer patients, by insinuating that their illness, or failure to improve with treatment, is due to some deficiency in their character.[9] Many of these claims confirm the questions and concerns I originally conveyed to Selye, and should be kept in mind when evaluating extravagant allegations. A "baker's dozen" of these caveats include:

1. How can we satisfactorily define "stress"?
2. How can we scientifically measure "stress"?
3. How can we define or distinguish between acute and chronic stress, since Selye had demonstrated they were so different in his General Adaptation Syndrome?
4. How can we ascertain when or where a malignancy first begins?
5. How can we determine the duration between initial onset and clinical detection?
6. Do all cancers share some common etiologic component?

7. How can we reconcile conflicting animal studies and clinical reports demonstrating that stress can both accelerate and retard malignant growth?
8. What are the mechanisms that might mediate relationships between stress and cancer?
9. What does "the immune system" consist of and where are its constituents located?
10. What are the best ways to measure immune system function, with respect to responses to stress and susceptibility to cancer?
11. While certain types of stress appeared to lower immune system measurements thought to reflect resistance to cancer (natural killer cell and T cell mitogenic activity), other stressors have an opposite effect.
12. Stress stimulates some endocrine responses that accelerate the growth of certain tumors, but also others that have inhibitory effects.
13. How can we explain the observation that all the interventions we use to treat cancer (radiation, hormones, and chemotherapy), also facilitate the development of malignancy?

The most obvious question is "What Is Stress?" There is still no satisfactory scientific definition, despite decades of attempts to decipher this dilemma.[10] Stress is a useless term for pragmatic researchers, because it represents different things to different people, really is different for each of us, and most importantly, often cannot be measured with any significant degree of accuracy. Stress is used interchangeably to denote physical stressors, such as pain, noise, and opposite extremes of temperature, but also emotional states varying from depression and loneliness, to anxiety, anger, and hostility. Do all of these have common characteristics that are relevant to cancer?

Similarly, "What Is Cancer?" Although the term refers to undisciplined and uncontrollable cellular growth, a basal cell carcinoma of the skin is quite different from adenocarcinoma of the lung, prostate, or breast, brain tumors, lymphomas, leukemias, and other malignancies. These all differ markedly with respect to growth rates, metastatic tendencies, and sensitivity to neuroendocrine or immune system influences, particularly those that might be modulated by stress. There are critical concerns when it comes to determining exactly how long a cancer has been present. If a lump in the breast is found to be malignant, when did the cancer start? A month, six months, or years before clinical detection? Such information would be crucial to establish any temporal relationship with antecedent stress.

Even if we could confirm stress-induced neuroendocrine, immune system, or other pathways that induce malignant changes, this is not proof that stress can cause cancer. It is essential to emphasize that association never proves causation.[11] Although there are well-defined risk factors for certain malignancies, this simply signifies some statistical association, rather than proving a causative, or even contributory, role.[12] However, although it may never be possible to prove that stress can initiate or modify malignant growth, supportive evidence from different disciplines is impressive and compelling.[13] Since space limitations preclude documenting all of these, ample supplemental references have been provided to supply additional information on specific topics.

Neurohumoral, immune, and subtle energy influences

Any attempt to explain how stress could affect malignant growth would have to demonstrate germane effects on systemic activities possessing this potential. There is abundant support with respect to immune, humoral, and central nervous system influences. These three integrative networks are intimately involved in regulating adaptive reactions to stress by surveillance of the status of specific parameters, and responding in an expedient and coordinated fashion.[14-18] The numerous interactions between the central nervous and immune systems and their links to stress can be found in several reviews.[19-24] The hypothalamus plays a crucial role in mediating these as well as endocrine responses.[25-28] Many brain neurotransmitters that can influence malignant growth also participate in the humoral response to stress, including melatonin, serotonin, dopamine, and the endorphins.[29-40]

Some types of cancer are very sensitive to hormonal influences. Estrogens, androgens, progestins, glucocorticoids, insulin-like growth factor, prolactin, and iodothyronines can directly modulate neoplastic growth, and influence other hormones that affect cancer cells.[41-43] Some of these actions may be direct, such as estrogen suppression of follicle stimulating hormone, whereas others influence hormonal binding or immune responses.[44-50] Breast and prostate cancer are notoriously hormone dependent, and manipulating the hormonal environment is a cornerstone of treatment. Steroidal sex hormones can affect tumor growth factors and other immune system activities, and are sometimes used in the treatment of autoimmune disorders.[51-53] Stress profoundly effects key hypothalamic and pituitary peptides that regulate the activity of target endocrine glands that can modify tumor growth.[54]

Glucocorticoids and their congeners dramatically influence the progression of leukemias and lymphomas, and levels produced in response to stress can provide similar clinical benefits. The composer Bela Bartok is often cited as an illustration. While dying in the terminal stages of advanced leukemia, he was approached by Serge Koussevitsky, the Conductor of the Boston Symphony Orchestra, who offered him a commission for a new work. He promptly went into an inexplicable remission, which persisted only until the composition had been completed, after which he promptly succumbed to the disease.[55] There are numerous other anecdotes similar to this which support Selye's contention about the benefits of a firm faith and powerful purpose. It is doubtful that these are all mediated by increased glucocorticoid activity, but there are other possible explanations.

Lowered immune defenses clearly predispose to the development of malignancy, and conversely, heightened immune resistance is presumed to provide protection. Consequently, reports attempting to show some relationship between stress and cancer try to support this conclusion by demonstrating suppression or stimulation of "the immune system".[56,57] As noted, stress is a semantic snakepit for scientists, who also have concerns about categorizing different cancers as a collective entity with common characteristics. Similar confusion surrounds the immune system. There is an unfortunate tendency to assume that by giving something a name, we have now somehow defined it, and therefore agree on, or understand, what it means. Although the term is used freely and authoritatively, we have only a sketchy grasp of what the immune system comprises, or where each of its varied components are located. There is no distinct global measurement of immune system function. We can assess levels and ratios of T cells, B cells, helper cells, suppressor cells, natural killer cells, and responses to various blastogenic stimuli. We can measure specific immunoglobulins and antibodies in blood, saliva, urine, and cerebrospinal fluid, thymosin, interferons, interleukins, properdin, and other elements or markers. Humoral immune responses occur in minutes or seconds, whereas those that are cell mediated may not be evident for days and weeks. The same stressor might cause some immune measures to increase while others are simultaneously suppressed or unaffected. The nature of the stressor, its severity, duration, prior exposure, age, sex, race, nutritional considerations, health status, and hereditary factors may all influence immune responses that have been associated with cancer activity.[58-61] It is essential to consider such variables when evaluating claims about the effects of stress on "immune system function". Very divergent conclusions could be reached depending upon such modifiers, and which particular parameters of immune system function were selected.

In addition to central nervous system, humoral, and immune mechanisms, weak electromagnetic forces may also accelerate or depress malignant growth. Nordenström has postulated that there is an electrical circulatory system in the body.[62] Based on this, he has developed an effective treatment program for lung and breast malignancies using very feeble electrical forces, and these impressive results have now been replicated in other centers.[63,64] Other investigators have now also confirmed that such energies, in conjunction with conventional therapy, can markedly retard or reverse head and neck cancers and brain tumors previously resistant to treatment.[65-67] It is not inconceivable that similar subtle forces generated within the body may have comparable consequences that could explain spontaneous regression, as well as a variety of other reported relationships between stress and cancer. The concept that there may be psychoelectroneuroimmunologic responses has been proposed, and may be useful in exploring this possibility.[68]

Historical support

The belief that stress could cause various diseases or influence their course has always been a popular notion. It can be found in all ancient religions and philosophies, and was emphasized in Ayurvedic principles and practices that have persisted for more than 3500 years.[69] The notion that cancer might in some way be related to emotional stress is as old as the history of recorded medicine. Cancer, is derived from *karkinos*, the Greek word for crab, which in Latin became "cancer". This apparently stemmed from the observation that the large veins surrounding a tumor resembled the claws of a crab, as evidenced by Galen's description:

> As a crab is furnished with claws on both sides of the body, so in this disease the veins which extend from the tumor represent with it a figure much like a crab.

Four centuries later, Paul of Aegina suggested:

> Cancer is so called because it adheres with such obstinacy to the part it seizes, that like the crab, it cannot be separated from it without great difficulty.[70]

Middle English astronomers unfortunately used the term to describe the constellation between Leo the Lion and Gemini the Twins. Thus, the Tropic of Cancer marks the most northern latitude at which the sun can be seen directly overhead, usually at noon around June 22. Although the use of cancer in astrology has no connection with its medical meaning, some superstitious people still believe that anyone born under this Zodiac sign is more predisposed to die of cancer.

In his treatise on tumors, *De Tumoribus*, Galen observed that melancholy women were particularly prone to cancer of the reproductive organs because they had an excess of black bile (Gr. *mélas chole*). This may clarify why the earliest (1601) English definition explained that:

> Cancer is a swelling or sore coming of melancholy bloud, about which the veins appeare of a blacke or swert colour spread in the manner of a creifish (crayfish) claws.

Galen believed that such humors, vital spirits, imagination, blood, muscle, and nerves were all closely linked with one another, in some hierarchical fashion. Thus, thoughts and feelings were constantly circulating through the body, exerting their effects by direct physical contact with particular parts of our anatomy. This was 2000 years before the development of psychoneuroimmunology as a discipline.

In 1701, the English physician Gendron emphasized the effect of "disasters of life as occasion much trouble and grief" in the causation of cancer.[71] Eighty years later, Burrows attributed the disease to "the uneasy passions of the mind, with which the patient is strongly affected for a long time."[72] Nunn was impressed with the influence of emotional factors on breast tumors,[73] and Stern similarly noted that cancer of the cervix in women was more common in sensitive and frustrated individuals.[74] In the mid-1800s, Walshe's *The Nature and Treatment of Cancer* called attention to

> the influence of mental misery, sudden reverses of fortune and habitual gloomings of the temper on the disposition of carcinomatous matter. If systematic writers can be credited, these constitute the most powerful cause of disease.[75]

Towards the end of the century, in a study of more than 250 patients at the London Cancer Hospital, Snow concluded that "the loss of a near relative" was an important factor in the development of cancer of the breast and uterus.[76] Numerous additional citations attest to the firm belief of 18th- and 19th-century physicians that stressful states and emotions predisposed to cancer.[77-79]

I attach particular importance to these commentaries, because the practice of medicine in the last two centuries was quite different from today. This is particularly important with respect to patient encounters, which were much more personalized. Those physicians had to rely more upon eliciting and appraising the significance of the patient's history, environment, emotional makeup, and lifestyle, in contrast to contemporary diagnostic workups, which emphasize sophisticated laboratory tests and imaging procedures. Their education was much more apt to include a strong background in literature, philosophy, history, and other branches of learning concerned with human thought and relations, rather than the prevailing preoccupation with a basic science curriculum. They undoubtedly spent much more time observing patients, and talking to them about intimate family, social, and work relationships, and other potentially pertinent psychosocial influences. Thus, by virtue of educational enlightenment, cultural orientation, and a more personalized approach, they might well be expected to have had a greater sensitivity to any subtle relationships between stress and cancer, than is possible in the frenetic pace of today's high-tech, and often apathetic, practice environment.

Interest was rekindled in this subject in the 20th century with the advent of psychiatry as a specialty, and its emphasis on individual psychodynamics. Evans, a Jungian psychoanalyst, again called attention to the link between loss of a close emotional relationship and cancer.[80] Kissen first noted that there appeared to be similar personality traits in patients with lung cancer that differentiated them from those with other pulmonary diseases, simply by taking a detailed personal history, and later extended these observations to other malignancies.[81-85] Schmale and Iker were intrigued with the relationship between antecedent stress and cancer of the cervix.[86] Merely by reviewing a personality questionnaire completed by asymptomatic women with suspicious pap smears, they were able to predict, with almost 75% accuracy, those who would subsequently develop cancer. Malignancy was most likely to surface in women with a "helplessness-prone personality" or overwhelming sense of frustration due to some emotional loss or conflict during the preceding six months, and this has recently been reconfirmed.[87-90] Greene carefully studied the life histories of three sets of identical twins, one of whom had died of leukemia. He noted that each one with the disease had experienced an antecedent emotional upheaval not shared by the survivor.[91] In another 15-year study of patients with lymphoma or leukemia, he found that the disease was more apt to occur following emotional loss or separation, which had engendered sustained feelings of anxiety, anger, sadness, or hopelessness.[92]

Thomas's 40-year prospective health study of medical students was designed to determine whether there were any emotional patterns or stressful antecedents that might predict the development of hypertension in later life. It included a variety of psychological assessment techniques, including figure drawing and extensive personal and family interviews. Follow up revealed that there were personality profiles not only for hypertension, but also suicide, mental illness, coronary heart disease, and cancer.[93] Physicians who subsequently developed tumors often tended to be lonely individuals, who had figuratively "lost their parent", or had difficulties in adequately expressing their emotions.[94] Le Shan was impressed with similar characteristics seen in cancer patients, and particularly their possible contributory role.[95-97] Based on a thorough review of the literature and more than two decades of detailed interviews, he concluded that there were four key types of personality characteristics that tended to precede the onset of malignancy:

1. The loss of an important emotional relationship
2. An inability to express anger or resentment
3. An unusual amount of self-dislike and distress
4. Feelings of hopelessness and helplessness.[98]

The first item appears to be of particular importance. Various writers and poets have also emphasized this theme, including Tolstoy,[99] Auden,[100] and Sontag.[101] Even the emotional loss of political defeat has been suggested as contributing to the cancers of Napoleon, Ulysses S. Grant, Robert Taft, Hubert Humphrey, and The Shah of Iran.[102]

Animal research support

Animal studies have also demonstrated links between stress and cancer. Investigators in Pavlov's laboratory reported that dogs subjected to severe and chronic stress had a marked tendency to develop malignancies of the internal organs.[103] Riley studied a strain of mice carrying the Bittner mammary tumor virus. Under normal circumstances, 70 to 80% can be expected to develop breast cancer within one year. However, routine conditions in animal laboratories can be quite stressful, even in the absence of painful procedures. There is often unexpected and excessive noise, a confined environment, and frequent, jarring movement of the racks holding the cages. Such animals have been shown to have much higher levels of stress-related hormones than others maintained under peaceful and quiet conditions. Exposure to pheromones that signal stressful states might also contribute to this. Riley found that when he protected these mice by placing then in protective housing that completely insulated them from all laboratory commotion and potentially stressful stimuli, only 7% had evidence of tumors at the end of a year. Conversely, the stress of simply periodically rotating litter mates on a turntable resulted in a 92% incidence of breast cancer.[104] The growth of transplanted mammary tumors can also be markedly increased by stressing experimental animals with electric shocks.[105–107]

Stress is an unavoidable consequence of life, but is most damaging when it is perceived to be completely beyond control. This is an important issue with respect to relationships with cancer, best illustrated by "yoked testing" experiments. In one such study, two matched groups of rats were housed in separated soundproof chambers and subjected to identical electrical shocks delivered in an erratic fashion with respect to time intervals and duration. When a rat in the first group depressed a small lever, it terminated the shock received by it. In the second group, pressing a similar lever did nothing. A third matched group, living under normal laboratory conditions, received no shocks, serving as controls to reflect normal tumor growth in the absence of this stressful stimulus. All of the animals were injected with a dosage of Walker[256]sarcoma virus calculated to induce malignancies in 50% of recipients, to determine whether the physical stress of the shock could influence tumor growth. Three out of four rats in the second group, who received shocks over which they had no control, developed malignant tumors. As expected, the incidence of tumors was 50% in the non-shocked group of rats. However, in the first group of rats, who had received identical shocks as the second but were able to exert some control over them, tumors could be found in only one third. The rats in this group had less than half as many tumors as litter mates subjected to the same stress over which they had no control, and one third less than those who had received no shocks at all![108]

A "fighting attitude" can retard the development of experimental leukemia in mice, and transplanted mammary tumors in female mice who spontaneously developed an antagonistic or fighting behavior, were also smaller and slower growing, than those in more submissive litter mates.[109] A similar phenomenon has been observed in "feisty" females with breast cancer.[110-112] This may have therapeutic implications, and again suggests that the feeling of being in control can inhibit malignant growth.[113,114] Other significant effects of stress on the development and growth of cancer in experimental animals have been summarized elsewhere.[115] However, not all researchers agree. Some supportive animal and clinical studies have been criticized because of their design, failure to control for pertinent variables, and contrary findings with respect to results, or presumed mechanisms of action.[116-123]

Personality and psychosocial stress as precursors to cancer

In addition to the historical citations noted, more recent reports are also replete with references linking stress and cancer. Depression is most frequently cited, and is supported by evidence of concomitant reduction of natural killer cell and other immune system activities.[124-128] Feelings of helplessness, hopelessness, and suppression of emotions, particularly anger, may predispose to cancer.[129-132] Suppression of anger is associated with higher serum immune globulin-A levels, which have been shown to correlate with metastases and mortality rates in breast cancer.[133,134] Stress can also affect the metastatic spread of other tumors.[135-138]

Increased antecedent stress as assessed by the magnitude of life change events has been reported to be associated with a greater subsequent incidence of certain cancers.[139-141] The most stressful life change event is the death (loss) of a spouse, and significantly higher mortality rates for cancer and other leading causes of death have been reported in bereaved survivors over the following 6 to 12 months.[142-144] Several studies have demonstrated concurrent impaired immune function, especially depression of T cell mitogenic and natural killer cell activity during this time period.[145-148] The next three most stressful life change events, divorce, marital separation, and death of a close family member, also reflect emotional losses, and are similarly associated with higher cancer mortality rates.[149-151] Decreased immune defenses may accompany such losses, and can even be seen in workers who lose their job and remain unemployed.[152-156] Psychosocial stresses such as poverty, social isolation, and low societal status, appear to be risk markers for malignancy.[157-166] Conversely, the incidence of cancer appears to be unusually low in schizophrenic and certain other psychiatric patients, possibly because they do not consider such situations as stressful, or may be unable to experience the normal feelings and emotions associated with loss and separation.[167-170]

Various constellations of personality traits seem to be connected with increased cancer tendencies, and possibly predispose to behaviors and lifestyles that are risk factors, or render individuals more susceptible to the effects of stressful life change events.[171-182] So called "Type C" cancer-prone patients have been characterized as cooperative, conforming, compliant, and unassertive, with a tendency to suppress negative emotions, particularly anger.[183-185] This characteristic of "pathological niceness" is commonly encountered in malignant melanoma, which is also often associated with increased antecedent stress.[186-188]

African antelopes and the teleology of evolution

The loss of important emotional relationships clearly constitutes the most stressful life change events. As emphasized above, they also represent the most common emotional and psychological precursors of cancer. Could there be some causal relationship between psychological loss and cancer? Implicit in Cannon's "fight or flight" theory is the teleological premise that our automatic and uncontrollable responses to stress have been steadily sharpened over the lengthy course of evolution. It is posited that they represent adaptive changes that were essential for the survival of our antedeluvian ancestors, when faced with life-threatening, physical challenges. The outpouring of adrenalin and stimulation of the sympathetic nervous system resulted in pupillary dilatation to promote better vision, quickened clotting to reduce blood loss from lacerations or internal hemorrhage, a rise in blood pressure and heart rate to increase blood flow to the brain and facilitate decision making, increased blood sugar and lipid levels from the breakdown of carbohydate and fat stores furnished more fuel for energy, and numerous other responses that were purposeful for primitive man. The shunting of blood flow away from the gut, where it was not immediately needed for digestive purposes, to the large muscles of the arms and legs, provided greater strength for fight in combat, or flight from a scene of potential peril.

However, the nature of stress for modern man is not some physical encounter with a saber toothed tiger or warring tribe every few months, but rather an array of psychological and emotional threats and challenges which may occur several times daily. The tragedy is that these trigger automatic, archaic, "fight or flight" responses, which are no longer purposeful or appropriate. Repeatedly invoked, it is not difficult to understand how they could contribute to such "Diseases of Civilization" as hypertension, diabetes, heart attack, stroke, peptic ulcer, muscle spasm, etc. Many of our responses to stress seem senseless, and it may be difficult to appreciate how they could ever have been beneficial. When severely frightened, some people feel their "flesh crawl", develop "goose bumps", or the hairs on the back of the neck "stand up". Although all of these are useless for us, the "flying fur" on the arched back of an aroused cat makes it appear more ferocious to an assailant. Similarly, the stimulation of those same arrector pili muscles is responsible for the "bristling quills" of the porcupine, which is a very effective defense mechanism. Thus, all of our instantaneous, instinctive, reflexive responses to stress undoubtedly served some useful purpose during the lengthy course of human evolution. It is equally apparent that we may often overreact to a stressful stimulus with healing consequences that prove harmful. We see this in the occasional development of disfiguring keloids due to excessive scar formation, and when lip cancer develops in clay pipe smokers, in an attempt to repair heat-damaged tissue.

There are other instances where adaptational evolutionary responses may ultimately prove pernicious. In a review article on Selye's concepts of "Stress" and "Diseases of Adaptation" over 35 years ago, I referred to the theory of "opportunism" in the evolutionary process.[3] This refers to the organism's response to fill a need with whatever means are available, even if the long-term consequences proved undesirable. The illustration cited at that time was the tremendous variation in the development of distinctive horns by some 23 species of African antelopes. The horns of the kudu are prohibitively unwieldy, while those of the duiker are obviously too small to be effective. As one examines the different deviations that have evolved in others, their divergent anatomical configurations and functional capabilities do not appear to serve any rational adaptive purpose. If I were to rewrite that article today, I would choose the development of malignancy in man as perhaps a more dramatic example of "opportunism" in the evolutionary process, for the following reasons.

As one descends the phylogenetic scale, the incidence of malignancy decreases progressively. Cancer does not occur in primitive forms of life. Conversely, the ability of the organism to regenerate injured or lost tissues increases proportionately. Simple organisms, including some invertebrates, have the ability to sever parts of their anatomy when they are injured. This capability would have survival value only if the animal possessed an equally remarkable ability to regenerate the cast off portion from available cell remnants. A starfish can restore a lost appendage, and the newt will grow a new tail or leg if it is severed, or can even cause its mechanical release to escape a predator. This restorative capability is not retained in humans, although the spleen does possess unusual regenerative potential.

I believe that some malignant responses in man may represent an atavistic, vestigial remnant of this primordial, purposeful, regenerative trait. When we suffer a loss or injury, attempts at replacement could well be activated, as they are in lower life forms. Unfortunately, this new growth (neoplasia) may prove to be harmful rather than helpful. Experiments with chemicals that cause cancer when applied to the human skin or injected into rodents support this hypothesis. When these same carcinogens are injected into the leg of a newt, a new accessory limb starts to grow at that site, rather than a tumor. If injected into the epithelial iris tissue of the eye, the newt will regenerate a new lens. Thus, the identical carcinogenic stimulus can produce either purposeful regeneration or a malignant growth, depending upon the evolutionary development of the organism.[189–192]

It is interesting that the sole exception to this in humans is the spleen. Years after its surgical removal, remnants of functioning splenic tissue are often found, a phenomenon that has been referred to as the "born again spleen".[193] The spleen is also the only organ in humans that does not give rise to spontaneous cancer, suggesting that its response to loss has been preserved as purposeful regeneration. Small accessory spleens, or spleniculi, are not uncommon, and in rare cases, several hundred may be present in or around the gastrointestinal tract. This represents a reversion to a more primitive condition, in which splenic tissue is not located in a single organ, but instead is scattered throughout the gut. Thus, from the standpoint of embryology and comparative anatomy, the spleen retains certain ancient attributes that may explain its unique freedom from cancer, as well as its remarkable regenerative capacity.

The leap from physical to emotional loss should not be too troublesome. The ability to regenerate lost or injured tissue in lower forms of life obviously involves something more than a simple local response. The message that tissue has been lost, irritated, or damaged must be relayed to higher centers in the central nervous system. These could initiate coordinated restorative activities, most likely involving the integration of central nervous system, humoral, and immune system mechanisms. With man's highly developed cerebral cortex, emotional loss may well be perceived as being an equally significant or even greater stress than physical privation. The same reparative signals may be activated, but our responses are anomalous and aberrant. Our strivings to stimulate purposeful replacement are futile and fruitless, and any resultant new growth is apt to be in the form of malignant neoplasia.

Selye was unusually enthusiastic about this theory, and emphasized it and associated concepts in his Foreword to *Cancer, Stress and Death*:

> Perhaps, as Paul Rosch of New York has suggested, cancer might even be an attempt by the human organism to regenerate tissues and organs and even limbs, as lower animals are able to do spontaneously. Going further, one might say that "the ultimate health of the organism, like that of society, appears to depend on how well or appropriately its constituent units communicate with one another.[194]

Cancer and civilization

In keeping with Selye's assignment, the title of my paper was "Stress and Cancer: A Disease of Adaptation?". In retrospect, "A Disease of Civilization" might have been a more appropriate subtitle. This may suggest some allusion to smoking, air pollution, the proliferation of putative cancer-causing substances such as asbestos, depletion of the ozone layer, radiation hazards, or other current carcinogenic concerns. However, what I wish to refer to are psychosocial stresses that were evident long before these 20th-century problems. This concept is not new, and was proposed over 150 years ago in Tanchou's 1843 *"Memoir on the Frequency of Cancer"* delivered to the French Academy of Sciences:

> M. Tanchou is of the opinion that cancer, like insanity, increases in a direct ratio to the civilization of the country and of the people. And it is certainly a remarkable circumstance, doubtless in no small degree flattering to the vanity of the French *savant*, that the average mortality rate from cancer in Paris during 11 years is about 0.80 per 1000 living annually, while it is only 0.20 in London! Estimating the intensity of civilization by these data, it clearly follows that Paris is four times more civilized than London![195]

Bainbridge's *The Cancer Problem*, noted:

> Man in his primeval condition has been thought to be very little subject to new growth, particularly to those of a malignant character. With changed environment, it is claimed by some, there came an increase in susceptibility to cancerous disease, this susceptibility becoming more marked as civilization develops.[196]

Hoffmann's treatise *The Mortality of Cancer Throughout the World*, a global survey conducted under the auspices of the Prudential Life Insurance Company, emphasized:

> The rarity of cancer among native races (primitive races) suggests that the disease is primarily induced by the conditions and methods of living which typify our modern civilization. . . . A large number of medical missionaries and other trained medical observers, living for years among native races throughout the world, would long ago have provided a more substantial basis of fact regarding the frequency of occurrence of malignant disease among the so-called uncivilized races, if cancer were met with among them to anything like the degree common to practi-

cally all civilized countries. Quite the contrary, the
negative evidence is convincing that, in the opinion
of qualified medical observers, cancer is exception-
ally rare among the primitive peoples including the
North American Indians and the Eskimo population
of Labrador and Alaska.[197]

This was substantiated by the African medical missionary, Dr. Albert
Schweizer:

> On my arrival in Gabon in 1913, I was astonished to
> encounter no cases of cancer. I cannot, of course, say
> positively that there was no cancer at all; but like
> other frontier doctors, I can only say that if any cases
> existed, they must have been quite rare. In the
> course of the years, we have seen cases of cancer in
> growing numbers in our region. My observations
> incline me to attribute this to the fact that the na-
> tives are living more and more after the manner of
> the whites.[198]

Similarly, the celebrated anthropologist and Arctic explorer, Vilhjalmur
Stefansson, in his book which actually was titled, *Cancer: Disease of
Civilization?*, noted the absence of cancer in the Eskimos upon his arrival
in the Arctic, but a subsequent increase in the incidence of the disease as
closer contact with white civilization was established.[199] He quoted Sir
Robert McCarrison, a physician who had studied 11,000 Hunza natives in
Kashmir from 1904 to 1911. They not only enjoyed unusual longevity, but
preserved their youthful physique and appearance well into their sixties
and seventies. McCarrison attributed the absence of cancer to the fact that
they were "endowed with a nervous system of notable stability" (resistant
to stress), and "far removed from the refinement of civilization".

Hay's *Cancer: A Disease of Either Election or Ignorance*, commented:

> A study of the distribution of cancer, among the races
> of the entire earth, shows a cancer ratio in about pro-
> portion to which civilization living predominates; so
> evidently something inherent in the habits of civi-
> lization is responsible for the difference of cancer in-
> cidence compared with the uncivilized races and
> tribes. Climate has nothing to do with this difference,
> as witness the fact that tribes living naturally will
> show a complete absence until mixture with more
> civilization, even so does cancer begin to show its
> head.[200]

In *Malignancy and Evolution*, Roberts wrote, "I take the view commonly held that, whatever its origin, cancer is very largely a disease of civilization".[201] He was referring to opinions such as those expressed in Moore's *The Antecedents of Cancer*, that "connect the progress of civilization with the increase of cancer which has remained an incontestable theory to the present day"; Banks' contention that "cancer is on the increase in this country. Is it possible that this is coincident with our full habit of living as a people?"; Powell's *The Pathology of Cancer*: "There can be little doubt that the various influences grouped under the title of civilization play a part in producing a tendency to Cancer"; and Hooker's *Eclecticism in Cancer Therapy*, which urged less emphasis upon research in artificially induced cancer in laboratory animals, and more emphasis upon the observation of people:

> There is, as a matter of fact, a growing group of independent thinkers both lay and professional, who are anything but impressed with the story of the discovery and isolation of the "cancer germ". Mr. Ellis Barker has also written reiterating his views, in common with those of Sir William Arbuthnot Lane, my own and many others, that cancer is a disease of civilization.[202,203]

One of the most persuasive arguments is to be found in Berglas' *Cancer; Its Nature, Cause and Cure*. Throughout this book runs the theme that cancer is a disease from which primitive peoples are relatively or wholly free, and that we are

> threatened with death from cancer because of our inability to adapt to present day living conditions . . . Over the years, cancer research has become the domain of specialists in various fields. Despite the outstanding contributions of scientists, we have been getting farther away from our goal, the curing of cancer. This specialized work, and the knowledge gained through the study of individual processes, has had the peculiar result of becoming an obstacle to the whole. More than thirty years in the field of cancer research have convinced me that it is not to our advantage to continue along this road of detailed analysis. I have come to the conclusion that cancer may perhaps be just another intelligible natural process whose cause is to be found in our environment and mode of life.[204]

In addition to cancer, simple and stable societies are relatively resistant to diabetes, hypertension, peptic ulcer, and other "Diseases of Civilization". However, as Donnison reported in *Civilization and Disease*, this resistance is rapidly lost when established norms and traditions are swept aside by the pressures of civilization.[205] Since the advent of Cro-Magnon, societal groups have progressively increased in size, and changed dramatically with respect to interpersonal relationships and values. Appropriate adaptive alterations have not kept pace with these evolutionary advances with respect to the acquisition of psychological and emotional assets that could facilitate acclimatization to swiftly shifting sociocultural environments.[206] "Social disruption" may also increase susceptibility to tuberculosis and other infectious diseases.[207] It is the rapidity of change which particularly predisposes to inappropriate and damaging coping responses that eventually result in reduced resistance to both physical and emotional disorders.[208,209]

Recent government statistics show a puzzling increase in the incidence of breast cancer in middle-aged females, which may also be related to certain new stresses of "civilization". It has been well established that the younger a woman is when she has her first child or even becomes pregnant, the less likely she is to develop breast cancer. Pregnancy lowers prolactin, which stimulates breast tissue growth and promotes breast cancer in experimental animals. As more and more women enter the workforce, they tend to remain single, marry later in life, and decide not to have children, or do so only when they are much older. Similarly, the incidence of deadly ovarian cancer is 14 times higher in career-oriented, single working women, compared to a matched group of homemakers. Job stress itself may be a factor, as many women workers have to juggle job responsibilities with being a wife, supermom, single parent, or providing custodial duties for an aged relative. Superimposed on this, there may be sexual harassment, lower compensation than male counterparts despite superior ability and experience, and a dead end when they try to reach the upper rungs of the corporate ladder.

Other demographic groups, including children, adolescents and the elderly, are subjected to unique stresses not experienced generations ago, as a consequence of changes imposed by the pressures of contemporary civilization. Key among these are the rapid sociocultural changes that have eroded close family and religious ties, and the sense of belonging, so deftly described by Wolf in his studies of Roseto.[210,211] These also represent loss of meaningful emotional relationships that may not be fully appreciated, because they are not sudden and dramatic detachments. For today's younger generations, social ties are more often apt to lie in rooting for the same sports team, or being a fan of some rock group, or celebrity, rather than religion, family, or humane and redeeming relationships which are oriented towards, and have the capacity to relieve loss and suffering.

Biopsychosocioecological communication, control, and subtle energies

Similarly, civilization also seems to have been responsible for a progressive loss of communication with the cosmos, or nature. Life on earth consists of a hierarchy of living systems that range upward from atoms, molecules, cells, and organs, to people, families, corporations, and societies.[212] Poorly understood communication channels continually connect all these components, as meaningful messages are sent up and down the line. Homeostasis and health are entirely dependent on good communication— good communication not only within the constituency of the internal environment of each system, but also with the external environment at higher and lower levels (Figure 1). These dynamic interrelationships are essential for the preservation of balance, harmony, and homeostasis in the universe. Such a biopsychosocioecologic perspective must be appreciated to comprehend the complex connections between psychosocial stress and cancer.

As Yamasaki has elegantly demonstrated, the basic problem with the cancer cell is that it no longer communicates properly:

> Cancer can be regarded as a rebellion in an orderly society of cells when they neglect their neighbors and grow autonomously over surrounding normal cells. Since intercellular communication plays an important role in maintaining an orderly society, it must be disturbed in the process of carcinogenesis. Evidence suggests that blockage of intercellular communication is important in the promotion process of carcinogenesis.[213]

Selye had previously described this need for cooperative communication in more humanistic terms:

> The indispensability of this disciplined, orderly mutual cooperation is best illustrated by its opposite— the development of a cancer, whose most characteristic feature is that it cares only for itself.[194]

But how does communication take place in the body? The nervous system communicates by direct contact, as adrenergic or cholinergic molecules are released at nerve endings and synapses. Endocrine secretions and neurotransmitter secretions are carried via the bloodstream to selected receptor sites on cell walls at distant locations. Much less is known about the immune system, although it is clear that its conversations include both humoral and hard wired connections. However, in the final analysis, all of these messages are transmitted by means of weak energy transfers across

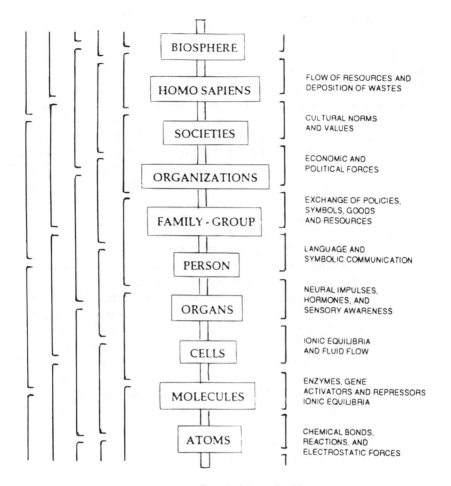

Figure 1   Information flow in hierarchial living systems.

cell membranes. These occur at an atomic rather than a molecular level. It has also become increasingly apparent that the cell membrane is more than a protective shield studded with receptor sites for antibodies, small neuropeptides, and other molecules. It appears to be a powerful signal amplifier that provides an interactive window through which the cell senses and responds to its environment. Some substances can pass freely back and forth through certain channels, but for others, the cell membrane is an impenetrable barrier. When designated molecules fit into special receptor sites, a subtle signal produces a sudden change in electrical tension between the interior and exterior of the cell, allowing a new channel to open for a few thousandths of a second. During this period, although millions of ions pass back and forth, the total current generated is only a few billionths of an ampere!

As previously proposed, I believe that cell membranes may have receptor sites for subtle energy signals which react exactly as they would to chemical/molecular stimuli. Electrical stimulation of highly specific areas in the pain pathway produces analgesia, and microinjections of morphine at these precise sites have the identical effect. Injection or stimulation a few millimeters away is worthless. However, combining suboptimal doses of morphine or electrical stimulation, which alone are too weak to reduce pain, results in a synergistic effect that does provide analgesia. This suggests that for some receptors, the effects of weak electrical stimulation are completely congruent with those of morphine. Furthermore, the specific locations at which either molecular or electrical signals relieve pain are precisely the sites of action of the endorphins.[214]

If feeble electrical forces can produce such profound physiologic effects, this might account for the association of malignancy with proximity to high power lines, increased birth defects when electric blankets are used during pregnancy, and a variety of psychophysiologic effects due to geomagnetic influences, including cancer.[215] Such observations cannot be explained in terms of Newtonian physics, or any form of chemical/molecular communication. It is quite likely that energies of similar magnitude can be generated in the body, that could also affect cell growth and malignant change. Electroencephalogram (EEG) waves may reflect more than the noise of the machinery of the brain, and possibly represent signals being sent to other parts of the body. Since it is possible to move a cursor on a computer screen solely by deep concentration, it does not seem unreasonable to postulate that mental activities could also affect activities in the body that are sensitive to weak energy stimuli, such as cellular growth. We need to move from the current chemical/molecular concept of communication, to a physical/atomic model. Such a paradigm might explain not only regression or spontaneous remission of cancer in patients with a strong determination, but also the placebo effect, faith healing, "therapeutic touch", psychokineseis, telepathic and other widely acknowledged, but poorly understood, phenomena.

Pribram[216] and Bohm[217] propose that the universe consists of swirls of energy fields that operate in dimensions far beyond our conventional senses. They view the brain as a holographic instrument which mathematically constructs concrete realities, by interpreting these energies from another dimension that transcends our current comprehension of time and space. A similar concept was expressed by William Wordsworth in his *Ode On The Intimations Of Immortality From Recollections Of Early Childhood*, and in recent years, Sheldrake has provided some scientific support for such beliefs.[218] The Chinese conceptualization of *"chi"* energy, and its role in health and disease has persisted for thousands of years, and is increasingly attracting scientific interest and support. However, *chi* is not only an energy system that flows through acupuncture meridians in the body, but is found in trees, rocks, and all of nature. Hence, the need to add an ecological component to our current biopsychosocial model of health.

Although we cannot define stress, all of our research confirms that the sense of being out of control is always distressful. That also happens to be an accurate definition of the cancer cell. It is a cell that is out of control, because it does not communicate properly with its neighbors, or the rest of the organism. A domineering and dogmatic determination, firm and forceful faith, and aggressive attitude, all reflect the development of a strong sense of control. These are common themes in reports of patients who triumphed over seemingly fatal malignancies.[219-221] Can this message of control be communicated to cancer cells through unsuspected energy pathways to alter their undisciplined activities? Is it possible to listen in on this conversation? If we understood its vocabulary, could we learn how to emulate, simulate, or stimulate such subtle signals, and to utilize our innate and awesome potential for self-healing?

How can one explain the numerous well-documented cases of spontaneous remission of cancer? Careful studies of such patients suggest that a firm faith and a strong positive belief system is the most common denominator.[222,223] Anecdotal, but irrefutable, reports of cancer cures from shrines, faith healers, laetrile®, coffee enemas, acupuncture, macrobiotic diets, and other alternative treatments are difficult to explain. There are numerous reports of cancer regression through the use of various stress reduction or mind altering techniques, including intense meditation, visual imagery, and hypnosis.[224-235] Yet, like spontaneous remission, all these cures are extremely rare, and benefits are entirely unpredictable in any given patient. Here again, having a strong faith in anything the individual believes in, and which provides a sense of control, might offer the best explanation. But how are the salutary rewards of faith healing, "therapeutic touch", and the placebo effect mediated? Is there such a thing as psychic healing? How can one explain the well-documented benefits associated with the development of strong social support in patients with cancer and other problems?[236-241] Conversely, what are the mechanisms involved in the numerous reports of reactivation of dormant cancer following an extremely stressful event, particularly sudden loss?[242-245] No consistent immune, neuroendocrine, or central nervous system changes have been demonstrated in connection with such effects.[246,247] Could the answer lie in some latent energy force? Is it possible to learn how to harness this?

The endemiology of cancer

We are exposed daily to a host of potential physical carcinogens in the air we breathe or the foods we eat. However, not all smokers develop lung cancer, which also occurs in nonsmokers without any family history of malignancy or other conceivable contributory factor. I would suggest that there may be equally powerful psychosocial carcinogens that exist both in our external and internal milieus. Our current focus is on the epidemiology of cancer, the roots of which connote some external stressor that the individual has been subjected to. What we must now also acknowledge is what might be referred to as the endemiology of cancer, and those factors that influence health which are generated in our internal environment.[248]

Good health is entirely dependent on maintaining the constancy or stability of the internal environment during stress. Walter Cannon coined the term "homeostasis", from the Greek *homios* (similar), and *stasis* (position), to refer to this "steady state".[249] However, the concept of the importance of the internal environment, and the term itself (*milieu intérieur*) originated a half century earlier with the celebrated French physiologist, Claude Bernard,[250] often called "The Father of Physiology". Louis Pasteur was a powerful proponent of external causes of disease, because of his discovery of pathogenic bacteria. He engaged in many debates about this with Claude Bernard at the prestigious *Académie Française*, where they sat next to one another. However, on his deathbed, Pasteur allegedly stated "*Bernard avait raison. Le germe n'est rien, c'est le terrain qui est tout.*" [Bernard was right. The microbe is nothing, the soil is everything.][251]

Sir William Osler reported the spontaneous shrinkage of metastases from breast cancer in two women in 1901.[252] It is interesting that the term "spontaneous" is so often used to describe this phenomenon, rather than "unexplained". Spontaneous refers to occurrences that happen without apparent external cause, and are therefore self-generated, as in "spontaneous combustion". Osler often commented that it was more important to know what went on in a patient's head than in his chest, to determine the clinical course of tuberculosis. He also paraphrased Parry's perception that "It is much more important to know what sort of a patient has a disease, than what sort of a disease the patient has."[253,254] This observation, as well as the important role of stress, is being increasingly confirmed in patients with hypertension, coronary heart disease, peptic ulcer, allergic conditions, psoriasis, low back pain, and a variety of mental and emotional disorders. As suggested in this presentation, it may be appropriate to insert cancer near the top of this list of "Diseases of Civilization".

References

1. Selye H. and Rosch, P. J., Integration of endocrinology, in *Glandular Physiology and Therapy*, J. B. Lippincott, Philadelphia, 1946, 1–100.
2. Selye H. and Rosch, P. J., The renaissance in endocrinology, in *Medicine and Science*, International University Press, New York, 1954, 30–49.
3. Rosch, P. J., Growth and development of the stress concept and its significance in clinical medicine, in *Modern Trends in Endocrinology*, Hoeber, P. B., Ed., Butterworths, London, 1958, 278–297.
4. Rosch, P. J., Stress: its relationship with illness, in *Traumatic Medicine and Surgery For the Attorney*, III, part 6, Cantor, P.D., Ed., Butterworths, Washington, D.C., 1960, 261–364.

5. Good, R., A., personal communication.
6. Rosch, P. J., Stress and cancer: a disease of adaptation?, in *Cancer, Stress, and Death*, Tache, J., Selye, H., and Day, S. B., Eds., Plenum Publishing, New York, 1979, 187–212.
7. Ader, R., Felten, D. L., and Cohen, N., Eds., *Psychoneuroimmunology*, Academic Press, San Diego, 1991.
8. Herbert, T. B. and Cohen, S., Stress and immunity in humans: a meta-analytic review, *Ann. Behav. Med.*, 55, 364–379, 1993.
9. Rosch, P. J., Mind over cancer: some caveats, *Stress Med.*, 10, 71, 1994.
10. Selye, H., Forty years of stress research: principal remaining problems and misconceptions, *Can. Med. Assoc. I.*, 115, 53–56, 1976.
11. Rosch, P. J., Stress, cholesterol, and coronary heart disease, *Lancet*, ii, 851–852, 1983.
12. Rosch, P. J., Ridiculous risk factors and heart attacks: diet-cholesterol dogma versus stress, *Stress Med.*, 9, 203–205, 1993.
13. Pettingale, K. W., Towards a psychobiologic model of cancer: biological considerations, *Soc. Sci. Med.*, 20, 779–787, 1985.
14. Bulloch, K., Neuroendocrine-immune circuitry: pathways involved with the induction and persistence of humoral immunity, *Diss. Abstr. Int.*, 41, 4447-B, 1981.
15. Stein, M., Stress, brain and immune function, *Gerontologist*, 22, 203, 1982.
16. Besedovsky, H. O. and Sorkin, E., Network of immune-neuroendocrine interactions, *Clin. Exp. Immunol.*, 27, 1–12, 1977.
17. Besedovsky, H. O. and Sorkin, E., Network of immune-neuroendocrine interactions, in *Hormonal Control of Immune Processes*, James, V. H. T., Ed., Oxford University Press, Amsterdam, 1977, 504–513.
18. Rosch, P. J., Illness syndromes: high disability, in *Psychiatry in the Medical Specialties*, Dunbar, F., Ed., McGraw-Hill, New York, 1959, 152–317.
19. Felton, D. L., Cohen, N., Ader, R., Felten, S. E., Carlson, S. L., and Roszman, T. L., Central neural circuits involved in neural-immune interactions, in *Psychoneuroimmunology*, Ader, R., Felten, D. L., and Cohen, N., Eds., Academic Press, San Diego, CA, 1991, 3–18.
20. Holland, J. C., Behavioral and psychosocial risk factors in cancer: human studies, in *Handbook of Psychooncology*, Holland, J. C. and Rowland, J. H., Eds., Oxford University Press, New York, 1989, 612–627.
21. Kiecolt-Glaser, J. K., Garner, W., Speicher, C. et al., Psychosocial modifiers of immune competence in medical students, *Psychosom. Med.*, 46, 7–14, 1984.
22. Kiecolt-Glaser, J. K., Glaser, R., Strain, E. C. et al., Modulation of cellular immunity in medical students, *J. Behav. Med.*, 9, 5–21, 1986.
23. Glaser, R., Rice, J., Stout, J. C., Speicher, C. E., and Kiecolt-Glaser, J. K., Stress depresses interferon production by leukocytes concomitant with a decrease in natural killer cell activity, *Behav. Neurosci.*, 100, 675–678, 1986.
24. Bardos, P., Biziere, K., De Genne, D., and Renoux, G., Regulation of natural killer activity by the cerebral neocortex, in *Natural Killers: Fundamental Aspects and Role in Cancer*, Serron, B. and Herberman, R. B., Eds., Elsevier, Amsterdam, 1983, 346–359.
25. Stein, M., Keller, S., and Schleifer, S., Role of the hypothalamus in mediating stress effects on the immune system, in *Mind and Cancer Prognosis*, Stoll, B. A., Ed., John Wiley & Sons, New York, 1979.

26. Keller, S. E. et al., Suppression of lymphocyte stimulation by anterior hypothalamic lesions in the guinea pig, *Cell. Immunol.*, 52, 334–340, 1980.
27. Besedovsky, H. O., Sorkin, E., Felix, D., and Haas, H., Hypothalamic changes during the immune response, *Eur. J. Immunol.*, 7, 323–325, 1977.
28. Cross, R. J., Markesbery, W. R., Brooks, W. H., and Rozman, T. L., Hypothalamic-immune interactions. The acute effect of anterior hypothalamic lesions on the immune response, *Brain Res.*, 196, 79–87, 1980.
29. Lippman, M. E., Yarbro, G. K., and Leventhal, B. G., Effects of glucocorticoids on F_c receptors of a human granulocyte cell line, *Cancer Res.*, 38, 4251–4256, 1978.
30. Heijnen, C. J., Kavelaars, A., and Ballieux, R., Corticotropin-releasing hormone and proopiomelanocortin-derived peptides in modulation of immune function, in *Psychoneuroimmunology*, 2nd ed., Ader, R., Felten, D. L., and Cohen, N., Eds., Academic Press, San Diego, CA, 1991, 429–446.
31. Irwin, M. R., Vale, W., and Britton, K. T., Central corticotropin-releasing factor suppresses natural killer cytotoxicity, *Brain Behav. Immun.*, 1, 81–87, 1987.
32. Irwin, M. R., Hauger, R. L., Brown, M. R., and Britton, K. T., CRF activates autonomic nervous system and reduces natural killer cytotoxicity, *Am. J. Physiol.*, 255, R744–R747, 1988.
33. Irwin, M., Brain corticotropin-releasing hormone- and interleukin-1 beta-induced suppression of specific antibody production, *Endocrinology*, 133, 1352–1360, 1993.
34. Irwin, M., Hauger, R., and Brown, M., Central corticotropin-releasing hormone activates the sympathetic nervous system and reduces immune function: increased responsivity of the aged rat, *Endocrinology*, 131, 1047–1053, 1992.
35. Johnson, H. M., Smith, E. M., Torres, B. A., and Blalock, J. E., Regulation of the *in vitro* antibody response by neuroendocrine hormones, *Proc. Natl. Acad. Sci. U.S.A.*, 79, 4171–4174, 1982.
36. Ben-Eliyahu, S., Yirmiya, R., Shavit, Y., and Liebeskind, J. C., Stress-induced suppression of natural killer cell cytotoxicity in the rat: a naltrexone-insensitive paradigm, *Behav. Neurosci.*, 104, 235–238, 1990.
37. Yirmiya, R., Shavit, Y., Ben-Eliyahu, S., Gale, R. P., Liebeskind, J. C., Taylor, A. N., and Weiner, H., Modulation of immunity and neoplasia by neuropeptides released by stressors, in *Stress, Neuropeptides, and Systemic Disease*, McCubbin, J. A., Kaufmann, P. G., and Nemeroff, C. B., Eds., Academic Press, San Diego, CA, 1991, 261–279.
38. Zagon, I. S. and McLaughlin, P. J., Endogenous opioid systems, stress and cancer, in *Enkephalins and Endorphins: Stress and the Immune System*, Plotnikoff, N. P., Faith, R. E., Murgo, A. J., and Good, R. A., Eds., Plenum, New York, 1986, 81–100.
39. Lapin, V., Pineal influences on tumor, *Prog. Brain Res.*, 52, 523–533, 1979.
40. Dilman, V. M., Anisimov, V. N., Ostroumova, M. N., Morozov, V. G., Khavinson, V. K., and Azarova, M. A., Study of the anti-tumor effect of polypeptide pineal extract, *Oncology*, 36, 274–280, 1979.
41. Lippman, M. E., Yarbro, G. K., and Leventhal, B. G., Effects of glucocorticoids on F_c receptors of a human granulocyte cell line, *Cancer Research*, 38, 4251–4256, 1978.

42. Lippman, M. E., Endocrine responsive cancers in man, in *Textbook of Endocrinology*, Williams, R., Ed., W. B. Saunders, Philadelphia, 1985, 286–302.
43. Lippman, M. E., Strobl, J., and Allegra, J. C., Effects of hormones in human breast cancers cells in tissue culture, in *Cell Biology of Breast Cancer*, McGrath, C., Brennan, M., and Rich, M., Eds., Academic Press, Orlando, FL, 1980, 218–234.
44. Kakidani, H. et al., Cloning and sequence analysis of cDNA for procine B-neo-endorphin/dymorphin precursor, *Nature*, 298, 245–249, 1982.
45. Berczi, I. and Nagy, E., A possible role of prolactin in adjuvant arthritis, *Arthritis Rheum.*, 25, 591–594, 1982.
46. Fauci, A. S., Mechanisms of the immunosuppressive and anti-inflammatory effects of glucocorticoids, *J. Immunopharmacol.*, 1, 1–25, 1978.
47. Gisler, R. and Schenkel-Hulliger, L., Hormonal regulation of the immune response. II. Influence of pituitary and adrenal activity on immune responsiveness in vitro, *Cell Immunol.*, 2, 646–657, 1971.
48. McCruden, A. B. and Stimson, W. H., Sex hormones and immune function, in *Psychoneuroimmunology*, 2nd ed., Ader, R., Felten, D. L., and Cohen, N., Eds., Academic Press, San Diego, CA, 1991, 475–477.
49. Munck, A. and Guyre, P. M., Glucocorticoids and immune function, in *Psychoneuroimmunology*, 2nd ed., Ader, R., Felten, D. L., and Cohen, N., Eds., Academic Press, San Diego, CA, 1991, 447–460.
50. Nagy, E., Berczi, I., and Friesen, H. G., Regulation of immunity in rats by lactogenic and growth hormones, *Acta Endocrinol.*, 102, 351–357, 1983.
51. Ikeda, T. and Sirbasku, D. A., Purification and properties of a mammary-uterine pituitary tumor cell growth factor from pregnant sheep uterus, *Biol. Chem.*, 259, 4049–4064, 1984.
52. Kappas, A., Jones, H. E. H., and Roitt, I. M., Effects of steroid sex hormones on immunological phenomena, *Nature*, 198, 902, 1963.
53. Van Vollenhorn, R. F. and McGuire, J. L., Estrogen, progesterone and testosterone: can they be used to treat autoimmune disease?, *Cleveland Clin. J. Med.*, 61, 276–284, 1994.
54. Brown, G., Seggle, J., and Ettigi, P., Stress, hormone responses, and cancer, in *Cancer, Stress, and Death*, Tache, J., Selye, H., and Day, S. B., Eds., Plenum, New York, 1979, 29–39.
55. Lippman, M. E., Yarbro, G. K., and Leventhal, B. G., Effects of glucocorticoids on F_c receptors of a human granulocyte cell line, *Cancer Research*, 38, 4251–4256, 1978.
56. Levy, S., Herberman, R., Maluish, A. et al., Prognostic risk assessment in primary breast cancer by behavioral and immunological parameters, *Health Psychol.*, 4, 99–113, 1985.
57. Levy, S., Herberman, R., Lippman, M. et al., Correlation of stress factors with sustained depression of natural killer activity and predicted prognosis in patients with breast cancer, *J. Clin. Oncol.*, 5, 348–353, 1987.
58. Bovbjerg, D. H. and Valdimarsdottir, H., Familial cancer, emotional distress, and low natural cytotoxic activity in healthy women, *Res. Nurse Health*, 16, 395–404, 1993.
59. Shamberger, R. J., Tytko, S. A., and Willis, C. E., Antioxidants in cereals and in food preservatives and declining cancer mortality, *Cleveland Clin. O.*, 39, 119–124, 1972.

60. Horrobin, D. F., Manku, M. S., Oka, M., Morgan, R. O., Cunnane, S. C., Ally, A. I., Ghayur, T., Schweitzer, M., and Karmali, R. A., The nutritional regulation of T lymphocyte function, *Med. Hypotheses*, 5, 969–985, 1979.
61. Wynder, E. L., Dietary habits and cancer epidemioloy, *Cancer*, 43, 1955–1961, 1979.
62. Nördenstrom, B. E. W., *Biologically Closed Electric Circuits: Clinical Experimental and Theoretical Evidence for an Additional Circulatory System*, Nordic Medical Publications, Stockholm, 1983, 358.
63. Azavedo, E., Svane, G., and Nördenstrom, B., Radiological evidence of response to electrochemical treatment of breast cancer, *Clin. Radiol.*, 43, 84–87, 1991.
64. Nördenstrom, B. E., Impact of biologically closed electric circuits (BCEC) on structure and function, *Integr. Physiol. Behav. Sci.*, 27, 285–303, 1992.
65. Belehradek, M., Domenge, C., Luboinski, B., Orlowski, S., Belehradek, J., and Mir, L. M., Electrotherapy, a new antitumor treatment. First clinical phase I–II trial, *Cancer*, 72, 3694–3700, 1993.
66. Belehradek, J., Orlowski, S., Poddevin, B., Paoletti, C., and Mir, L. M., Electrotherapy of spontaneous mammary tumours in mice, *Eur. J. Cancer*, 27, 73–76, 1991.
67. Salford, L. G., Persson, B. R., Brun, A., Ceberg, C. P., Kongstad, P. C., and Mir, L. M., A new brain tumor therapy combining bleomycin with in vivo electropermeabilization, *Biochem. Biophys. Res. Commun.*, 194, 938–943, 1993.
68. Rosch, P. J., Future directions in psychoneuroimmunology: psychoelectroneuroimmunology?, in *Stress, the Immune System and Psychiatry*, Leonard, B. and Miller, K., Eds., John Wiley & Sons, Chichester, 1995.
69. Sanyal, P. K., *History of Medicine and Pharmacy in India*, Amitava Sanyal, Calcutta, 1964.
70. Cramer, D. L., The semantics of cancer, *Int. Med.*, 2, 9, 1981.
71. Gendron, D., *Enquiries Into The Nature, Knowledge And Cure Of Cancer*, London, 1701.
72. Burrows, J., *A New Practical Essay on Cancer*, London, 1783.
73. Nunn, T. W., *On Cancer of the Breast*, J & A Churchill, London, 1882, 123.
74. Stern, R., as quoted in Suess, R., Kinzel, V., and Scribner, J. P., *Cancer—Experiments and Concepts*, Springer-Verlag, New York, 1973.
75. Walshe, W. H., *The Nature and Treatment of Cancer*, Taylor & Walton, London, 1846.
76. Snow, H., *Cancer and the Cancer Process*, Churchill, London, 1893.
77. Kowal, S. J., Emotions as a cause of cancer: eighteenth and nineteenth century contributions, *Psychoanal. Rev.*, 42, 217–227, 1955.
78. Guy, R., *An Essay On Schirrhous Tumours And Cancer*, W. Owen, London, 1759.
79. Gibson, W. T., *The Etiology and Nature of Cancerous and Other Growths*, John Bale Sons & Danielsson, London, 1909.
80. Evans, E., *A Psychological Study Of Cancer*, Dodd-Mead and Co., New York, 1926.
81. Kissen, D. M., Personality characteristics in males conducive to lung cancer, *Br. J. Med. Psychol.*, 36, 27–36, 1963.
82. Kissen, D. M., Psychosocial factors, personality and lung cancer, *Br. J. Med. Psychol.*, 40, 29–43, 1967.

83. Kissen, D. M., Brown, R. I. F., and Kissen, M. A., A further report on personality and psychosocial factors in lung cancer, *Ann. NY Acad. Sci.*, 164, 535–545, 1969.

84. Kissen, D., Psychosocial factors, personality and lung cancer in men aged 55–64, *Br. J. Med. Psychol.*, 40, 29–43, 1967.

85. Kissen, D., The present status of psychosomatic cancer research, *Geriatrics*, 24, 129, 1969.

86. Schmale, A. H. and Iker, H. P., The affect of hopelessness and the development of cancer. I. The prediction of uterine cervical cancer in women with atypical cytology, *Psychosom. Med.*, 28, 714–721, 1966.

87. Schmale, A. H. and Iker, H. P., The affect of hopelessness and the development of cancer, *Psychosom. Med.*, 28, 714–721, 1966.

88. Schmale, A. H. and Iker, H. P., The psychological setting of uterine cervical cancer, *Ann. NY Acad. Sci.*, 25, 807–813, 1966.

89. Schmale, A. H. and Iker, H., Hopelessness as a predictor of cervical cancer, *Soc. Sci. Med.*, 5, 95–100, 1971.

90. Lambley, P., The role of psychological processes in the aetiology and treatment of cervical cancer: a biopsychological perspective, *Br. J. Med. Psychol.*, 66, 43–60, 1993.

91. Greene, W. A. and Miller, G., Psychological factors and reticuloendothelial disease, *Psychosom. Med.*, 20, 124–144, 1958.

92. Greene, W. A., The psychosocial setting of the development of leukemia and lymphoma, *Ann. NY Acad. Sci.*, 125, 794–801, 1966.

93. Thomas, C. B. and Duszynski, K. R., Closeness to parents and the family constellation in a prospective study of five disease states: suicide, mental illness, malignant tumour, hypertension and coronary heart disease, *Johns Hopkins Med. J.*, 134, 251–270, 1974.

94. Thomas, C. B., Duszynski, K. R., and Shaffer, J. W., Family attitudes reported in youth as potential predictors of cancer, *Psychosom. Med.*, 41, 287–302, 1979.

95. Le Shan, L. and Worthington, R. E., Some recurrent life history patterns observed in patients with malignant disease, *J. Nerv. Ment. Dis.*, 124, 460–465, 1956.

96. Le Shan, L. L., An emotional life-history pattern associated with neoplastic disease, *Ann. NY Acad. Sci.*, 164, 546–557, 1969.

97. Le Shan, L., Psychological states as factors in the development of malignant disease: a critical review, *J. Natl. Cancer Inst.*, 22, 1–18, 1959.

98. Le Shan, L., *You Can Fight For Your Life*, M. Evans, New York, 1977.

99. Tolstoy, L., *The Death of Ivan Ilyitch*, Solotaroff, L., Ed., Bantam, New York, 1981.

100. Auden, W. H., *Collected Poems*, Random House, New York, 1991.

101. Sontag, S., *Illness as Metaphor*, Farrar, Straus, and Giroux, New York, 1977.

102. Rosch, P. J., Some thoughts on the epidemiology of cancer, in *Readings in Oncology*, Day, S. B., Sugarbaker, E. V., and Rosch, P. J., Eds., The International Foundation for Biosocial Development and Human Health, New York, 1980, 1–6.

103. Rosch, P. J., Stress and cancer, in *Psychosocial Stress and Cancer*, Cooper, C. L., Ed., John Wiley & Sons, London, 1984, 3–19.

104. Riley, V., Mouse mammary tumors: alteration of incidence as apparent function of stress, *Science*, 189, 465–467, 1975.

105. Riley, V., Cancer and stress: overview and critique, *Cancer Detection Prevention*, 2, 163–195, 1979.
106. Riley, V., Psychoneuroendocrine influences on immunocompetence and neoplasia, *Science*, 212, 1100–1109, 1981.
107. Kissen, D., Psychosocial factors, personality and lung cancer in men aged 55–64, *Br. J. Med. Psychol.*, 40, 29–43, 1967.
108. Visintainer, M. A., Volpicelli, J. R., and Seligman, M. E. P., Tumor rejection in rats after inescapable or escapable shock, *Science*, 216, 437–439, 1982.
109. Lemonde, P., Influence of fighting on leukemia in mice, *Proc. Soc. Exp. Biol. Med.*, 102, 292–295, 1959.
110. Greer, S. and Morris, T., Psychological attributes of women who develop breast cancer: a controlled study, *J. Psychosom. Res.*, 19, 147, 1975.
111. Greer, S., Morris, T., and Pettingale, K. W., Psychological response to breast cancer: effect on outcome, *Lancet*, 2, 785–787, 1979.
112. Greer, S., Morris, T., Pettingale, K., and Haybittle, J., Mental attitudes to cancer: an additional prognostic factor, *Lancet*, 1, 750, 1985.
113. Greer, S., Moorey, S., Baruch, J. D. R., Watson, M. et al., Adjuvant psychological therapy for patients with cancer: a prospective randomized trial, *Br. Med. J.*, 304, 675–680, 1992.
114. Holden, C., Cancer and the mind: how are they connected?, *Science*, 200, 1363–1368, 1978.
115. Peters, L. J. and Mason, K. A., Influence of stress on experimental cancer, in *Mind and Cancer Prognosis*, Stoll, B. A., Ed., John Wiley & Sons, New York, 1979, 104–124.
116. Cassileth, B. R., Lusk, E. J., Miller, D. S. et al., Psychological correlates of survival in advanced malignant disease?, *N. Engl. J. Med.*, 312, 1551–1555, 1985.
117. Jamison, R. N., Burish, T. G., and Wallston, K. A., Psychogenic factors in predicting survival of breast cancer patients, *J. Clin. Oncol.*, 5, 772–798, 1987.
118. Levenson, J. L. and Bernis, C., The role of psychological factors in cancer onset and progression, *Psychosomatics*, 32, 124–132, 1991.
119. Fox, B. H., Premorbid psychological factors as related to cancer incidence, *J. Behav. Med.*, 1, 45–133, 1978.
120. Fox, B. H. and Newberry, B. H., *Impact of Psychoendocrine Systems in Cancer and Immunology*, C.J. Hogrefe, Lewiston, NY, 1984.
121. Riley, V., Introduction: stress-cancer contradictions—a continuing puzzlement, *Cancer Detect. Prev.*, 2, 159–162, 1979.
122. Greer, S. and Morris, T., The study of psychological factors in breast cancer: problems of method, *Soc. Sci. Med.*, 12, 129–134, 1978.
123. Miller, T. and Spratt, J. S., Critical review of reported psychological correlates of cancer prognosis and growth, in *Mind and Cancer Prognosis*, Stoll, B. A., Ed., John Wiley & Sons, New York, 1979, 31–37.
124. Bieliauskas, L. A. and Garron, D. C., Psychological depression and cancer, *Gen. Hosp. Psychiatry*, 4, 187–195, 1982.
125. Shekelle, R. B., Raynor, W. J., Ostfeld, A. M., Garron, D. C., Bieliauskas, L. A., Liu, S. C., Maliza, C., and Paul, O., Psychological depression and 17-year risk of death from cancer, *Psychosom. Med.*, 43, 117–125, 1981.
126. Nerozzi, D., Santoni, A., Bersani, G. et al., Reduced natural killer cell activity in major depression: neuroendocrine implications, *Psychoneuroendocrinology*, 14, 295–301, 1989.

127. Irwin, M., Patterson, T., Smith, T. L. et al., Reduction of immune function in life stress and depression, *Biol. Psychiatry*, 27, 22–30, 1990.
128. Linn, B. S., Linn, M. W., and Jensen, J., Degree of depression and immune responsiveness, *Psychosom. Med.*, 44, 128–129, 1982.
129. Gossarth-Maticek, R., Bastiaans, J., and Kanazin, D. T., Psychosocial factors as strong predictors of mortality from cancer, ischemic heart disease and stroke: the Yugoslav prospective study. *J. Psychosom. Res.*, 29, 167–176, 1985.
130. Grossarth-Maticek, R., Psychosocial predictors of cancer and internal diseases: an overview, *Psychother. Psychosom.*, 33, 122–128, 1980.
131. Greer, S. and Watson, M., Towards a psychobiological model of cancer: psychological considerations, *Soc. Sci. Med.*, 20, 773–777, 1985.
132. Morris, T., Greer, S., Pettingale, K. W., and Watson, M., Patterns of expression of anger and their psychological correlates in women with breast cancer, *J. Psychosom. Res.*, 25, 111–117, 1981.
133. Pettingale, K. W., Greer, S., and Tee, D. E. H., Serum IGA and emotional expression in breast cancer patients, *J. Psychosom. Res.*, 21, 395–399, 1977.
134. Traue, H. C. and Pennebaker, J. W., *Emotion Inhibition and Health*, Hogrefe & Huber Publishers, Kirkland, WA, 1993.
135. Balitsky, K. P., Shmalko, Y. P., and Pinchuk, V. G., Stress, cancer: stress modulation of the metastatic process, in *Cancer, Stress, and Death*, 2nd ed., Day, S. B., Ed., Plenum Publishing, New York, 1986, 113–129.
136. Bammer, K., Stress, spread and cancer, in *Stress and Cancer*, Bammer, K. and Newberry, B. H., Eds., C. J. Hogrefe, Toronto, 1981, 137–163.
137. Spiegel, D. and Sands, S. H., Psychological influences on metastatic disease progression, in *Progressive States of Malignant Neoplastic Growth*, Kaiser, H. E., Ed., Martinus Nijhoff, Dordrecht, The Netherlands, 1985, 74–89.
138. Derogatis, L. R., Abeloff, M. D., and Melisaratos, N., Psychological coping mechanisms and survival time in metastatic breast cancer, *JAMA*, 242, 1504–1508, 1979.
139. Lehrer, S., Life change and lung cancer, *J. Hum. Stress*, 7, 7–11, 1981.
140. Lehrer, S., Life change and gastric cancer, *Psychosom. Med.*, 42, 499–502, 1980.
141. Stephenson, J. H. and Grace, W. J., Life stress and cancer of the cervix, *Psychosom. Med.*, 16, 287–294, 1954.
142. Helsing, K. J. and Szklo, M., Mortality after bereavement, *Am. J. Epidemiol.*, 114, 41–52, 1981.
143. Stroebe, W. and Stroebe, M. S., *Bereavement and Health*, Cambridge University Press, Cambridge, 1987.
144. Schneider, J., *Stress, Loss and Grief*, University Park Press, Baltimore, 1984.
145. Bartrop, R. W., Luckhurst, E., Lazarus, L, Kiloh, L. G., and Penny, R., Depressed lymphocyte function after bereavement, *Lancet*, 1, 834–836, 1977.
146. Schleifer, S. J., Keller, S. E., Camerino, M. et al., Suppression of lymphocyte stimulation following bereavement, *JAMA*, 250, 374–377, 1983.
147. Pettingale, K. W. and Hussein, M., Changes in immune status following conjugal bereavement, *Stress Med.*, 10, 145–150, 1994.
148. Pettingale, K. W., Watson, H., Tee, D. E. H., Inayat, Q., and Alhaq, A., A pathological grief, psychiatric symptoms and immune status following conjugal bereavement, *Stress Med.*, 5, 77–83, 1989.

149. Holmes, T. H. and Rahe, R. H., The social readjustment rating scale, *J. Psychosom. Med.*, 11, 213–218, 1967.
150. Kune, S., Kune, G. A., Watson, L. F., and Rahe, R. H., Recent life change and large bowel cancer: data from the Melbourne Colorectal Cancer Study, *J. Clin. Epidemiol.*, 44, 57–68, 1991.
151. Kune, S., Stressful life events and cancer, *Epidemiology*, 4, 395–397, 1993.
152. Irwin, M., Daniels, M., and Weiner, H., Immune and neuroendocrine changes during bereavement, *Psychiatr. Clin. North Am.*, 10, 449–465, 1987.
153. Irwin, M., Daniels, M., Smith, T. L., Bloom, F., and Weiner, H., Impaired natural killer cell activity during bereavement, *Brain Behav. Immun.*, 1, 98–104, 1987.
154. Stein, M., Miller, A. H., and Trestman, R. L., Depression, the immune system, and health and illness. *Arch. Gen. Psychiatry*, 48, 171–177, 1991.
155. Kronfol, Z., Silva, J., Greden, J., Dembinski, S., and Carroll, B. J., Cell-mediated immunity in melancholia, *Psychosom. Med.*, 44, 304, 1982.
156. Marriott, D., Kirkwood, B. J., and Stough, C., Immunological effects of unemployment, *Lancet*, 344, 269–270, 1994.
157. Kegeles, S. S., Relationship of sociocultural factors to cancer. In *Cancer: The Behavioral Dimensions*, Cullen, J. W., Fox, B. H., and Isom, R. N., Eds., Raven Press, New York, 1976, 108–125.
158. Adelstein, A. M., Life-style in occupational cancer, *J. Toxic. Environ. Health*, 6, 953–962, 1980.
159. Jenkins, C. D., Social environment and cancer mortality in men, *N. Engl. J. Med.*, 308, 395–398, 1983.
160. Shaffer, J. W., Graves, P. L., Swank, R. T. et al., Clustering of personality traits in youth and the subsequent development of cancer among physicians, *J. Behav. Med.*, 10, 441–447, 1987.
161. Rosch, P. J., Mind and cancer, *Lancet*, 1, 1302, 1979.
162. Rosch, P. J., Lifestyle and cancer, *NY State Med. J.*, 80, 2031–2038, 1980.
163. Trichopoulos, D., MacMahon, B., and Brown, J., Socioeconomic status, urine estrogens, and breast cancer risk, *J. Natl. Cancer Inst.*, 64, 753–755, 1980.
164. Morrison, F. R., Psychosocial factors in the etiology of cancer, *Diss. Abstr. Int.*, 42, 155B, 1981.
165. Cox, T. and Mackay, C., Psychosocial factors and psychophysiological mechanisms in the aetiology and development of cancers, *Soc. Sci. Med.*, 16, 381–396, 1982.
166. Kiecolt-Glaser, J. K. and Glaser, R., Stress and immune function in humans, in *Psychoneuroimmunology*, 2nd ed., Ader, R., Felten, D. L., and Cohen, N., Eds., Academic Press, San Diego, CA., 1991, 849–867.
167. Warren, S. and Canavan, M. M., Frequency of cancer in the insane, *N. Engl. J. Med.*, 210, 739, 1934.
168. Ananth, J. and Bernstein, M., Cancer less common in psychiatric patients, *Psychosomatics*, 18, 44–46, 1977.
169. Derogatis, L. R., Morrow, G. R., Fetting, J., Penman, D., Piasetsky, S., Schmale, A. M., Henrichs, M., and Carnicke, C. L., Jr., The prevalence of psychiatric disorders among cancer patients, *JAMA*, 249, 751–757, 1983.
170. Levitan, L. J., Levitan, H., and Levitan, M., The incidence of cancer in psychiatric patients: cancer and the emotions: a review, *Mt. Sinai J. Med.*, 47, 627–631, 1980.

171. Kune, G. A., Kune, S., Watson, L. F., and Bahnson, C. B., Personality as a risk factor in large bowel cancer: data from the Melbourne Colorectal Cancer Study, *Psychol. Med.*, 21, 29–41, 1991.

172. Bahnson, C. B., Stress and cancer: the state of the art. I, *Psychosomatics*, 21, 975–981, 1980; Stress and cancer: the state of the art. II; *Psychosomatics*, 22, 207–220, 1981.

173. Brown, F., The relationship between cancer and personality, *Ann. NY Acad. Sci.*, 125, 865–875, 1966.

174. Dattore, P. J., Shontz, F. C., and Coyne, L., Premorbid personality differentiation of cancer and non-cancer groups: a test of the hypothesis of cancer proneness, *J. Consult. Clin. Psychol.*, 48, 388–394, 1980.

175. Dunbar, F., *Emotions and Bodily Changes*, 4th ed., Columbia University Press, New York, 1954.

176. Hagnell, O., The premorbid personality of persons who develop cancer in a total population investigated in 1947 and 1957, *Ann. NY Acad. Sci.*, 125, 846–864, 1966.

177. Kissen, D. M., The significance of personality in lung cancer in men, *Ann. NY Acad. Sci.*, 125, 820–826, 1966.

178. Le Shan, L. L. and Worthington, R. E., Personality as a factor in the pathogenesis of cancer, *Br. J. Med. Psychol.*, 29, 49–56, 1956.

179. Eysenck, H. J., Personality, stress, and motivational factors in drinking as determinants of risk for cancer and coronary heart disease, *Psychol. Rep.*, 69, 1027–1043, 1991.

180. Eysenck, H. J., Grossarth-Maticek, R., and Everitt, B., Personality, stress, smoking, and genetic predisposition as synergistic risk factors for cancer and coronary heart disease, *Integr. Physiol. Behav. Sci.*, 26, 309–322, 1991.

181. Cooper, C. L. and Faragher, E. B., Psychosocial stress and breast cancer: the inter-relationship between stress events, coping strategies and personality, *Epidemiol. Rev.*, 15, 163–168, 1993.

182. Cooper, C. L., The social-psychological precursors to cancer, *J. Hum. Stress*, 10, 4–11, 1984.

183. Temoshok, L. and Dreher, H., *The Type C Connection: The Behavioral Links to Cancer and Your Health*, Penguin, New York, 1993.

184. Temoshok, L., Heller, B. W., and Sageviel, R. W. et al., The relationship of psychological factors of prognostic indicators in cutaneous malignant melanoma, *J. Psychosom. Res.*, 29, 139–153, 1985.

185. Kneier, A. W. and Temoshok, L., Repressive coping reactions in patients with malignant melanoma as compared to cardiovascular patients, *J. Psychosom. Res.*, 28, 145–155, 1984.

186. Renneker, R., Cancer and psychotherapy, in *Psychotherapeutic Treatment of Cancer Patients*, Goldberg, J., Ed., Free Press, New York, 1981, 131–166.

187. Gibertini, M., Reintgen, D. S., and Baile, W. F., Psychosocial aspects of melanoma, *Ann. Plast. Surg.*, 28, 17–21, 1992.

188. Havlik, R. J., Vukasin, A. P., and Ariyan, S., The impact of stress on the clinical presentation of melanoma, *Plast. Reconstr. Surg.*, 90, 57–61, 1992.

189. Breedis, C., Induction of accessory limbs and of sarcoma in the newt with carcinogenic substances, *Cancer Res.*, 12, 861–866, 1952.

190. Eguchi, E. and Watanabe, K., Elicitation of lens formation from the ventral iris epithelium of the newt by a carcinogen N-methyl-N-nitro-N-nitrosoguanidine, *J. Embryol. Exp. Morphol.,* 30, 63–71, 1973.

191. Seilerrn-Aspeng, F. and Kratochwil, K., Relation between regeneration and tumor growth, in *Regeneration in Animals and Related Problems,* Kioutsis, V. and Transpusch, H., Eds., North Holland, Amsterdam, 1965, 452–473.

192. Donaldson, D. J. and Mason, J. M., Cancer related aspects of regeneration research: a review, *Growth,* 39, 475–496, 1975.

193. Pearson, H. A., Johnston, D., Smith, K. A., and Touloukian, R. J., The bornagain spleen. Return of splenic function after splenectomy for trauma, *N. Engl. J. Med.,* 298, 1389–1392, 1978.

194. Selye, H., Foreword, in *Cancer, Stress, and Death,* Taché, J., Selye, H., and Day, S. B., Eds., Plenum Publishing, New York, 1979, xii.

195. LeConté, J., Statistical researches on cancer, *South. Med. Surg. J.,* 4, 273–274, 1846.

196. Bainbridge, W. S., *The Cancer Problem,* Macmillan, New York, 1914.

197. Hoffman, F. L., *Mortality From Cancer Throughout The World,* Prudential Press, Newark, 1916.

198. Schweitzer, A., *Forest Hospital of Lamborene,* Holt, Oxford, 1931.

199. Stefansson, V., *Cancer: Disease of Civilization?,* Hill and Wang, New York, 1960.

200. Hay, W. H., Cancer: A disease of either election or ignorance, *Am. J. Cancer,* 6, 410–422, 1927.

201. Roberts, M., *Malignancy and Evolution,* Grayson, New York, 1934.

202. Moore, C. H., *The Antecedents of Cancer,* London, Longmans, 1865.

203. Powell, C., *The Pathology of Cancer,* Macmillan, New York, 1908.

204. Berglas, A., *Cancer: Its Nature, Cause and Cure,* Pasteur Institute, Paris, 1957.

205. Donnison, C. P., *Civilization and Disease,* William Wood, Baltimore, 1938.

206. Halliday, J., L., *Psychosocial Medicine: A Study of the Sick Society.,* W. W. Norton, New York, 1948.

207. Dubos, R., Biological and social aspects of tuberculosis., *Bull. NY Acad. Med.,* 27, 351, 1951.

208. Cassell, J., The contribution of the social environment to host resistance, *Am. J. Epidemiol.,* 104, 7–13, 1976.

209. Antonovsky, A., *Health, Stress, and Coping: New Perspectives on Mental and Physical Well-Being,* Jossey-Bass, San Francisco, 1979.

210. Wolf, S., Herrenkohl, R. C., Lasker, J., Egloff, J., Philips, B. U., and Bruhn, J. G., Roseto, Pennsylvania, 25 years later—highlights of a medical and sociological survey, *Trans. Am. Clin. Climatol. Soc.,* 100, 57–67, 1988.

211. Bruhn, J. and Wolf, S., *The Roseto Story: An Anatomy of Health,* University of Oklahoma Press, Norman, 1978.

212. Miller, J., *Living Systems,* McGraw-Hill, New York, 1978.

213. Yamasaki, H., Aberrant expression and function of gap junctions during carcinogenesis, in *Nongenotoxic Mechanisms in Carcinogenesis,* Butterworth, B. E. and Slaga, T. J., Eds., Cold Spring Harbor Laboratory, Cold Spring Harbor, NY, 1987, 297–316.

214. Rosch, P. J., Stress and electromedicine, *Med. Electron.,* 19(4), 124–128, 1989.

215. Tromp, S. W., Meteorological stress and cancer, in *Stress and Cancer*, Bammer, K. and Newberry, B. H., Eds., C. J. Hogrefe, Toronto, 1981, 164–185.
216. Pribram, K., *Rethinking Neural Networks: Quantum Fields and Biological Data*, L. Erlbaum, New York, 1993.
217. Bohm, D., *Wholeness and the Implicate Order*, Routledge and Kegan Paul, London, 1980.
218. Sheldrake, R., *Rebirth of Nature*, Bantam, New York, 1992.
219. Kobasa, S., Maddi, S., and Kahn, S., Hardiness and health: a prospective study, *J. Personality Soc. Psychol.*, 42, 168–177, 1982.
220. Achterberg, J., Matthews, S., and Simonton, O. C., Psychology of the exceptional cancer patient—a description of patients who outlive predicted life expectancies, *Psychother. Theory Res. Practice*, 9, 1–21, 1976.
221. Kune, G. A., Kune, S., and Watson, L. F., Perceived religiousness is protective for colorectal cancer: data from the Melbourne Colorectal Cancer Study, *J. R. Soc. Med.*, 86, 645–647, 1993.
222. Ikemi, Y., Akagawa, S., Nakagawa, T., and Sugita, M., Psychosomatic considerations on cancer patients who have made a narrow escape from death, *Dynam. Psychiatry*, 31, 77–92, 1975.
223. Cole, W. H., Spontaneous regression of cancer. The metabolic triumph of the host? *Ann. NY Acad. Sci.*, 230, 111, 1974.
224. Meares, A., A form of intensive meditation associated with the regression of cancer, *Am. J. Clin. Hypn.*, 25, 114–121, 1982.
225. Meares, A., Regression of osteogenic sarcoma metastases associated with intensive meditation, *Med. J. Aust.*, 2, 433, 1978.
226. Meares, A., Remission of massive metastasis from undifferentiated carcinoma of the lung associated with intensive meditation, *J. Am. Soc. Psychosom. Dent. Med.*, 27, 40–41, 1980.
227. Meares, A., Regression of recurrence of carcinoma of the breast at mastectomy site associated with intensive meditation, *Aust. Fam. Physician*, 10, 218–219, 1981.
228. Meares, A., Regression of cancer after intensive meditation, *Med. J. Aust.*, 2, 184, 1976.
229. Meares, A., The quality of meditation effective in the regression of cancer, *J. Am. Soc. Psychosom. Dent. Med.*, 25, 129–132, 1978.
230. Meares, A., Vivid visualization and dim visual awareness in the regression of cancer in meditation, *J. Am. Soc. Psychosm. Dent. Med.*, 25, 85–88, 1978.
231. Bolen, J. S., Meditation and psychotherapy in the treatment of cancer, *Psychic*, 4, 19–22, 1973.
232. Achterberg, J. and Lawlis, G. F., *Imagery of Cancer*, Institute for Personality and Ability Testing, Champaign, IL, 1978.
233. Clawson, T. A. and Swade, R., The hypnotic control of blood flow and pain: the cure of warts and the potential for the use of hypnosis in the treatment of cancer, *Am. J. Clin. Hypn.*, 17, 160–169, 1975.
234. Hall, H. R., Hypnosis and the immune system: a review with implications for cancer and the psychology of healing, *Am. J. Clin. Hypn.*, 25, 92–103, 1982.
235. Hedge, A. R., Hypnosis in cancer, *Br. J. Med. Hypn.*, 12, 2–5, 1960.
236. Funch, D. P. and Marshall, J., The role of stress, social support and age in survival from breast cancer, *J. Psychosom. Res.*, 27, 177–183, 1983.

237. Funch, D. P. and Mettlin, C., The role of support in relation to recovery from breast surgery, *Soc. Sci. Med.*, 16, 91–98, 1982.
238. Eli, K., Nishimoto, R., Mediansky, L., Mantell, J., and Hamovitch, M., Social relations, social support and survival among patients with cancer, *J. Psychosom. Res.*, 36, 531–541, 1992.
239. Bagenal, F. S., Easton, D. F., Harris, E., Chilvers, C. E. D., and McElwain, T. J., Survival of patients with breast cancer attending Bristol cancer help centre, *Lancet*, 336, 606–610, 1990.
240. Spiegel, D., Bloom, J. R., and Yalom, I. D., Group support for patients with metastatic cancer: a randomized prospective outcome study, *Arch. Gen. Psychiatry*, 38, 527–533, 1981.
241. Spiegel, D., Bloom, J. R., Kraemer, H. C., and Gottheil, E., Effects of psychosocial treatment on survival of patients with metastatic breast cancer, *Lancet*, 2, 888–891, 1989.
242. Ogilvie, H., The human heritage, *Lancet*, ii, 42, 1957.
243. Gordon-Taylor, G., The incomputable factors in cancer prognosis, *Br. Med. J.*, 1, 455, 1959.
244. Pendergrass, E. P., Host resistance and other intangibles in the treatment of cancer, *Am. J. Roentgenol. Radium Ther.*, 85, 891, 1961.
245. Miller, T. R., Psychophysiologic aspects of cancer, *Cancer*, 39, 413, 1977.
246. Levy, S. M., Herberman, R. B., Whiteside, T. et al., Perceived social support and tumor estrogen/progesterone receptor status as predictors of natural killer cell activity in breast cancer patients, *Psychosom. Med.*, 52, 73–85, 1990.
247. Rosch, P. J., Stress: cause or cure of cancer, in *Psychotherapeutic Treatment of Cancer Patients*, Goldberg, J., Ed., Free Press, New York, 1981, 39–57.
248. Rosch, P. J., Some thoughts on the endemiology of cancer, *Cancer, Stress, and Death*, 2nd ed., Day, S. B., Ed., Plenum Publishing, New York, 1986, 293–300.
249. Cannon, W. B., *The Wisdom of the Body*, W. W. Norton, New York, 1932.
250. Bernard, C., *Introduction to the Study of Experimental Medicine*, Flammarion, Paris, 1945 (Original edition 1865).
251. Pasteur, L., quoted in Selye, H., *The Stress of Life*, p. 205, McGraw-Hill, New York, 1956.
252. Osler, W., quoted in Lewison, E. F., Spontaneous regression of breast cancer., *Natl. Cancer Inst. Monogr.*, 44, 23, 1976.
253. Osler, W., *Aequanimitas*, p. 258, McGraw-Hill, New York, 1906.
254. Parry, C. H., quoted in Margetts, E. L., Historical notes on psychosomatic medicine, in *Recent Developments in Psychosomatic Medicine*, Vol. 1, Wittkower, E. D. and Cleghorn, R. A., Eds., Pitman and Sons, London, 1954, 56.

chapter three

Stress, endocrine manifestations, and diseases

Constantine Tsigos and George P. Chrousos

Introduction

Life exists by maintaining a complex dynamic equilibrium, or *homeostasis*, that is constantly challenged by intrinsic or extrinsic adverse forces or *stressors*. Stress is, thus, defined as a state of threatened homeostasis or dysharmony and is counteracted by a complex repertoire of physiologic and behavioral responses that reestablish homeostasis. In this overview, we focus on the neuroendocrine, cellular, and molecular infrastructure of the adaptive responses to stress and discuss the altered regulation or dysregulation of these responses in various physiologic and pathophysiologic states.

Stress syndrome—phenomenology

The stress system receives and integrates a great diversity of neurosensory (visual, auditory, somatosensory, nociceptive, visceral), blood-borne, and limbic signals, which arrive through distinct pathways. Activation of the stress system leads to behavioral and physical changes that are remarkably consistent in their qualitative presentation (Table 1). These changes are normally adaptive and improve the chances of the individual for survival.[1] Behavioral adaptation includes increased arousal, alertness, vigilance, and cognition, focused attention, and enhanced analgesia, with concurrent inhibition of vegetative functions, such as feeding and reproduction. Concomitantly, physical adaptation occurs principally to promote an adaptive redirection of energy. Thus, oxygen and nutrients are shunted to the central nervous system (CNS) and the stressed body site(s), where they are needed the most. Increases in cardiovascular tone, respiratory rate, and intermediate metabolism (gluconeogenesis, lipolysis) all work in concert to promote availability of vital substrates. Moreover, the ability of the individual to quickly develop the restraining forces that prevent an overresponse is also essential for a successful general adaptive response. If the restrain-

Table 1   Behavioral and Physical Adaptation During Stress

Behavioral Adaptation

Adaptive redirection of behavior
    Increased arousal and alertness
    Increased cognition, vigilance, and focused attention
    Suppression of feeding behavior
    Suppression of reproductive behavior
    Containment of the stress response

Physical Adaptation

Adaptive redirection of energy
    Oxygen and nutrients directed to the CNS and stressed body site(s)
    Altered cardiovascular tone, increased blood pressure and heart rate
    Increased respiratory rate
    Increased gluconeogenesis and lipolysis
    Detoxification from toxic products
    Inhibition of growth and reproductive systems
    Containment of the stress response
    Containment of the inflammatory/immune response

Adapted from Chrousos G. P. and Gold P. W., *JAMA*, 267, 1244, 1992.

ing or counteracting forces of the body fail to control the elements of the stress response in a timely manner, the adaptive responses may turn maladaptive and contribute to the development of pathology.

Often stress is of a magnitude and nature that allows the perception of control by the individual. Thus, stress can commonly be rewarding and pleasant, even exciting, providing positive stimuli to the individual for emotional and intellectual growth and development.[2] It is of note that the activation of the stress system during feeding and sexual activity, both *sine qua non* functions for survival, is also primarily linked to pleasure.

Stress syndrome—physiology

Neuroendocrine effectors of the stress response

Modulation of the activity of the hypothalamic-pituitary unit and the central and peripheral components of the autonomic nervous system are central for a successful adaptive response during stress. The central components of the stress system are located in the hypothalamus and the brainstem and include the parvocellular corticotropin-releasing hormone (CRH) and arginine-vasopressin (AVP) neurons of the paraventricular nuclei (PVN) of the hypothalamus, and the CRH neurons of the paragigantocellular and parabranchial nuclei of the medulla, as well as the locus coeruleus (LC) and other catecholaminergic cell groups of the medulla and pons (central sympathetic system).[3,4] The hypothalamic-pituitary-adrenal (HPA) axis, together with the efferent sympathetic/adrenomedullary system, represent the peripheral limbs of this system.

CRH/AVP/Catecholaminergic neurons

CRH, a 41-amino-acid peptide, was first isolated as the principal hypothalamic stimulus to the pituitary-adrenal axis by Vale et al.[5] in 1981. The subsequent availability of synthetic CRH and of inhibitory analogues opened huge vistas for the investigation of stress. Thus, CRH and CRH receptors were found in many extrahypothalamic sites of the brain, including parts of the limbic system, the basal forebrain, and the central arousal-sympathetic systems (LC-sympathetic systems) in the brainstem and spinal cord.[6,7] In addition, central administration of CRH was shown to set into motion a coordinated series of physiologic and behavioral responses, which included activation of the pituitary-adrenal axis and the sympathetic nervous system, as well as characteristic stress behaviors.[8,9] CRH appears, therefore, to have a broader role in coordinating the stress response than had been suspected previously.[3,4] In fact, this neuropeptide seems to reproduce the phenomenology of the stress response as it is summarized in Table 1.

The central neurochemical circuitry responsible for activation of the stress system has been studied extensively and is summarized in Figure 1. There are apparently multiple sites of interaction among the central components of the stress system. Reciprocal reverberatory neural connections exist between the CRH and catecholaminergic neurons of the central stress system, with CRH and norepinephrine (NE) stimulating each other, the latter primarily through α1-noradrenergic receptors.[10–12] Autoregulatory ultra-short negative feedback loops also exist in both the PVN CRH and brainstem catecholaminergic neurons,[13,14] with collateral fibers inhibiting CRH and catecholamine secretion, respectively, via presynaptic CRH and α2-noradrenergic receptors.[15] Both the CRH and catecholaminergic neurons also receive stimulatory innervation from the serotonergic and cholinergic systems[16,17] and inhibitory input from the gamma-aminobutyric acid (GABA)/benzodiazepine (BZD) and the opioid neuronal systems of the brain,[18,19] as well as by the end-product of the HPA axis glucocorticoids.[20]

It is noteworthy that neuropeptide Y (NPY) stimulates the CRH neuron, whereas it inhibits the central sympathetic system.[21–23] This may be of particular relevance to changes in stress system activity in states of dysregulation of food intake and obesity. Interestingly, glucocorticoids stimulate hypothalamic NPY gene expression.[26] Substance P (SP), on the other hand, has reciprocal actions to those of NPY, since it inhibits the CRH neuron,[25] whereas it activates the central catecholaminergic system.[26] Presumably, substance P is elevated centrally when there is peripheral activation of somatic afferent fibers[27] and may, thus, have relevance to changes in the stress system activity in inflammatory states.

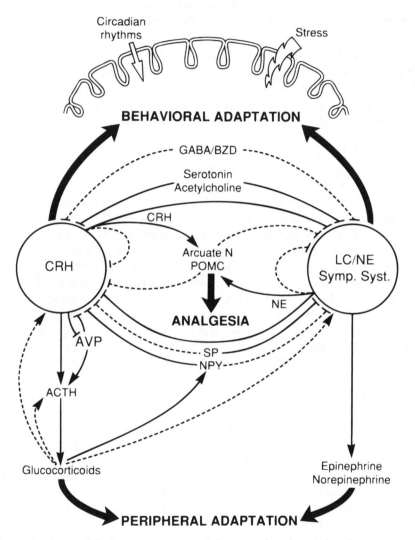

Figure 1 A simplified representation of the central and peripheral components of the stress system, their functional interrelations, and their relationships to other central nervous systems involved in the stress response. CRH, corticotropin releasing hormone; LC/NE Symp. Syst., locus ceruleus/norepinephrine-sympathetic system; POMC, proopiomelanocortin; AVP, arginine vasopressin; GABA, γ-aminobutyric acid; BZD, benzodiazepine; ACTH, corticotropin; NPY, neuropeptide Y; SP, substance P. Activation is represented by solid lines and inhibition by dashed lines. (Adapted from Chrousos, G. P. and Gold, P. W., *JAMA*, 267, 1244, 1992.)

A subset of parvocellular neurons synthesize and secrete both CRH and AVP. The relative proportion of this subset increases significantly with stress. Another group of PVN CRH neurons also sends projections to pro-opiomelanocortin (POMC)-containing neurons in the arcuate nucleus of the hypothalamus, which in turn reciprocally project to the PVN CRH neurons, and innervate the catecholaminergic neurons of the central stress system in the brainstem, as well as descending pain control neurons of the hind brain and spinal cord. Thus, activation of the stress system stimulates hypothalamic β-endorphin and other POMC-peptide secretion, which reciprocally inhibits the activity of the stress system, produces the so-called "stress-induced" analgesia and may influence the emotional tone (Figure 1).

The hypothalamic-pituitary-adrenal axis

CRH released into the hypophysial portal system is the principal regulator of anterior pituitary corticotroph ACTH secretion.[4] It is permissive for secretion of ACTH, while AVP, though a potent synergistic factor of CRH, has very little ACTH secretagogue activity by itself.[28,29] Further, it appears that there is a reciprocal positive interaction between CRH and AVP at the level of the hypothalamic-pituitary unit (Figure 1). Thus, AVP stimulates CRH secretion, while CRH causes AVP secretion *in vitro*.[30] In nonstressful situations both CRH and AVP are secreted in the portal system in a circadian and highly concordant pulsatile fashion.[31,32] The amplitude of the CRH and AVP pulses increases in the early morning hours, resulting eventually in increases of both the amplitude and frequency of ACTH and cortisol secretory bursts in the general circulation.[33,34]

The circadian release of CRH/AVP/ACTH/cortisol in their characteristic pulsatile manner appears to be controlled by one or more pacemakers,[35] whose location is not known in humans to date. These diurnal variations are perturbed by changes in lighting, feeding schedules, and activity, and are disrupted when a stressor is imposed. During acute stress, the amplitude and synchronization of the CRH and AVP pulsations increases, with additional recruitment of PVN CRH and AVP secretion. Also, with strong physical stress, recruitment of AVP of magnocellular neuron origin secreted into both the HPS via collateral neuraxons and into the systemic circulation takes place. In addition, depending on the stressor, angiotensin II, as well as various cytokines and lipid mediators of inflammation are secreted and act on hypothalamic, pituitary, and/or adrenal components of the HPA axis, mostly to potentiate its activity.

The adrenal cortex is the principal target organ of pituitary-derived circulating ACTH. The latter is the key regulator of glucocorticoid and adrenal androgen secretion by the zonae fasciculata and reticularis, respectively, while it also participates in the control of aldosterone secretion by the zona glomerulosa.[36] However, there is evidence that other hormones and/or cytokines, either originating from the adrenal medulla or coming from the systemic circulation, and/or neuronal information from the autonomic innervation of the adrenal cortex, may also participate in the regulation of cortisol secretion.

Glucocorticoids are the final effectors of the HPA axis. These hormones are pleiotropic and exert their effects through their ubiquitously distributed intracellular receptors.[37] The nonactivated glucocorticoid receptor resides in the cytosol in the form of a heterooligomer with heat shock proteins and immunophilin.[38] Upon ligand binding, the glucocorticoid receptors dissociate from the rest of the heterooligomer, they homodimerize, and translocate into the nucleus, where they interact with specific glucocorticoid responsive elements (GREs) within the DNA to transactivate appropriate hormone-responsive genes.[39] The activated receptors also inhibit the c-jun/c-fos heterodimer, a positive regulator of transcription of several genes involved in the activation of immune and other cells,[40,41] and they suppress the activity of NF-KB,[42] another positive regulator of specifically immune cell genes. They also change the stability of mRNAs and, hence, the translation rates of several glucocorticoid-responsive proteins. Further, glucocorticoids influence the secretion rates of specific proteins and alter the electrical potential of neuronal cells, through mechanisms that have not yet been defined.

Glucocorticoids play a key regulatory role in the basal control of HPA axis activity and in the termination of the stress response, by acting at extrahypothalamic regulatory centers, the hypothalamus and the pituitary gland.[43] The inhibitory glucocorticoid feedback on the ACTH secretory response acts to limit the duration of the total tissue exposure to glucocorticoids, thus minimizing the catabolic, lipogenic, antireproductive, and immunosuppressive effects of these hormones. Interestingly, a dual receptor system exists for glucocorticoids in the CNS, including the glucocorticoid receptor type I, or mineralocorticoid receptor, which responds to low levels of glucocorticoids and is primarily activational, and the classic glucocorticoid receptor (type II), which responds to higher levels of glucocorticoids and is dampening in some systems and activational in others.[43]

Sympathetic/adrenomedullary and parasympathetic systems

The autonomic nervous system provides a rapidly responding mechanism to control a wide range of functions. Cardiovascular, respiratory, gastrointestinal, renal, endocrine, and other systems are regulated by either the sympathetic nervous system or the parasympathetic system or both.[44] Generally, the parasympathetic system can both assist sympathetic functions by withdrawing and antagonize them by increasing its activity (see below).

Sympathetic innervation of peripheral organs is derived from the efferent preganglionic fibers whose cell bodies lie in the intermediolateral column of the spinal cord. These nerves synapse in the bilateral chain of sympathetic ganglia with postganglionic sympathetic neurons, which innervate widely vascular smooth muscle, kidney, gut, fat, and many other organs.[45] The preganglionic neurons are primarily cholinergic, whereas the postganglionic neurons release mostly noradrenaline. However, both types of neurons also secrete neuropeptides, such as NPY, CRH, or somatostatin (see below). The sympathetic system also has a humoral contribution from circulating epinephrine and, to a lesser extent, norepinephrine released from the adrenal medulla, which can be considered as a modified sympathetic ganglion.

In addition to the "classic" neurotransmitters acetylcholine and norepinephrine, both sympathetic and parasympathetic subdivisions of the autonomic nervous system contain several subpopulations of target-selective and neurochemically coded neurons that express a variety of neuropeptides and, in some cases, adenosine triphosphate (ATP), nitric oxide, or lipid mediators of inflammation.[46] Thus, CRH, NPY, somatostatin, and galanin are colocalized in noradrenergic vasoconstrictive neurons, whereas vasoactive intestinal polypeptide (VIP) and, to a lesser extent, substance P and calcitonin gene-related peptide (CGRP) are colocalized in cholinergic neurons. Transmission in sympathetic ganglia is also modulated by neuropeptides released from preganglionic fibers and short interneurons (e.g., enkephalin, neurotensin) and primary afferent (e.g., substance P, VIP) collaterals.[47] Thus, the particular combination of neurotransmitters in sympathetic neurons is strongly influenced by central and local factors, which may trigger or suppress specific genes.

Stress system interactions with other CNS components

In addition to setting the level of arousal and influencing the vital signs, the stress system also interacts with two other major CNS elements, the mesocorticolimbic dopaminergic system and the amygdala/hippocampus.[48-50] Both of these are activated during stress and, in turn, influence the activity of the stress system. Both the mesocortical and mesolimbic components of the dopaminergic system are innervated by the LC-NE/sympathetic noradrenergic system and are activated by it during stress. The mesocortical system, which contains neurons in the ventral tegmentum that send projections to the prefrontal cortex, is thought to be involved in anticipatory phenomena and cognitive functions.[49] The mesolimbic system, which consists of neurons also in the ventral tegmentum that innervate the nucleus accumbens, is believed to play a principal role in motivational/reinforcement/reward phenomena.

The amygdala/hippocampus complex is activated during stress primarily by ascending catecholaminergic neurons originating in the brainstem, or by inner emotional stressors, such as conditioned fear, possibly from cortical association areas.[50] Activation of the amygdala is important for retrieval and emotional analysis of relevant information for any given stressor. In response to emotional stressors, the amygdala can directly stimulate both central components of the stress system, as well as the mesocorticolimbic dopaminergic system. Interestingly, there are CRH peptidergic neurons in the amygdala which respond positively to gluco-corticoids and whose activation leads to anxiety. The hippocampus exerts an important inhibitory influence on the activity of the amygdala, as well as of the PVN/CRH and LC/sympathetic systems.

HPA axis—other endocrine axes interactions

Reproductive axis

The reproductive axis is inhibited at all levels by various components of the HPA axis (Figure 2). Thus, either directly or via arcuate POMC neuron β-endorphin, CRH suppresses the gonadotropin hormone releasing hormone (GnRH) neuron. Glucocorticoids, on the other hand, exert inhibitory effects at the level of the GnRH neuron, the pituitary gonadotroph, and the gonads themselves and render target tissues of sex steroids resistant to these hormones.[51-53] Cytokines also suppress reproductive function at several levels. Thus, steroidogenesis is directly inhibited at both ovaries and testes, with concomitant inhibition of the pulsatile secretion of the gonadotropin releasing hormone from the hypothalamus. The latter effect is exerted both directly and by activating hypothalamic neural circuits that contain CRH and POMC.

The interaction between CRH and the gonadal axis appears to be bidirectional. The presence of estrogen responsive elements in the promoter area of the CRH gene and direct stimulatory estrogen effects on CRH gene expression were shown recently.[54] This finding implicates the CRH gene and, therefore, the HPA axis, as a potentially important target of ovarian steroids and a potential mediator of gender-related differences in the stress response/HPA axis activity.[55] On the other hand, the activated estrogen receptor interacts with, and on occasion potentiates, the c-jun/c-fos heterodimer, which mediates several cytokine effects. In addition, estrogen appears to stimulate adhesion molecules and their receptors in immune and immune accessory cells. This may explain why autoimmune diseases afflict more females than males.

Growth axis

The growth axis is also inhibited at many levels during stress (Figure 3). Prolonged activation of the HPA axis leads to suppression of growth hormone secretion and inhibition of somatomedin C and other growth factor effects on their target tissues by glucocorticoids,[56-58] the latter presumably mediating by inhibition of the c-jun/c-fos heterodimer. However, acute elevations of growth hormone concentration in plasma may occur at the onset of the stress response in man and after acute administration of glucocorticoids, presumably through stimulation of the growth hor-

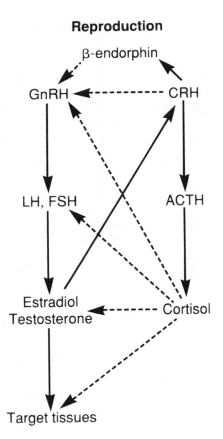

Figure 2 A schematic representation of the interactions between the HPA axis and the reproductive axis. GnRH, gonadotropin releasing hormone; LH, luteinizing hormone; FSH, follicle stimulating hormone. (Adapted from Chrousos, G. P. and Gold, P. W., *JAMA*, 267, 1244, 1992.)

mone gene by glucocorticoids through its GREs.[59] In addition to direct effects of glucocorticoids, which are pivotal in the suppression of growth observed in prolonged stress, increases in somatostatin secretion caused by CRH, with resultant inhibition of growth hormone secretion, have also been implicated as a potential mechanism of stress-related suppression of growth hormone secretion.[60] The redirection of nutrients and vital substrates to the brain and other areas where they are needed most during stress is the apparent teleology for the adverse effects of chronic stress on growth.

Thyroid axis

A corollary phenomenon to growth axis suppression is the stress-related inhibition of thyroid axis function (Figure 3). Activation of the HPA axis is

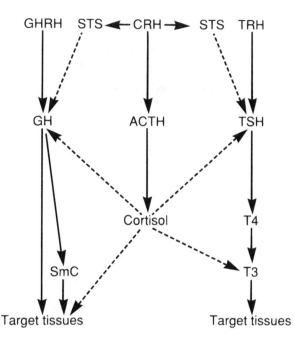

Figure 3 Effects of the HPA axis on growth and thyroid function. GHRH, growth hormone releasing hormone; STS, somatostatin; TRH, thyrotropin releasing hormone; GH, growth hormone; TSH, thyroid stimulating hormone; T_4, thyroxine; T_3, triiodothyronine; SmC, somatomedin C. (Adapted from Chrousos, G. P. and Gold, P. W., *JAMA*, 267, 1244, 1992.)

associated with decreased production of thyroid stimulating hormone (TSH) and inhibition of conversion of the relatively inactive thyroxine to the more biologically active triiodothyronine in peripheral tissues (the "euthyroid sick" syndrome).[61,62] Although the exact mechanism(s) for these phenomena is not known, both phenomena may be caused by the increased levels of glucocorticoids and may serve to conserve energy during stress. Inhibition of TSH secretion by CRH-stimulated increases in somatostatin might also participate in the central component of thyroid axis suppression during stress. In the case of inflammatory stress, inhibition of TSH secretion and enhancement of somatostatin production may be in part through the action of cytokines on the hypothalamus and/or the pituitary.

Fat, muscle, and bone metabolism

Glucocorticoids not only have profound inhibitory effects on growth hormone and sex steroid production, but also antagonize the actions of these hormones on fat tissue catabolism (lipolysis), and muscle and bone anabolism (Figure 4). Thus, chronic activation of the stress system would be

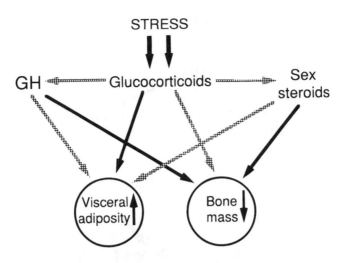

Figure 4   Detrimental effects of chronic stress on adipose tissue metabolism and bone mass; GH, growth hormone. Stimulation is represented by solid lines and inhibition by dashed lines.

expected to increase visceral adiposity, decrease lean body (bone and muscle) mass, and suppress osteoblastic activity. Interestingly, this phenotype is shared by patients with Cushing's syndrome, some patients with melancholic depression (pseudo-Cushing syndrome), and patients with metabolic syndrome X (visceral obesity, hyperlipidemia, hypertension), all of whom are characterized by increased activity of the HPA axis and a similar somatic and biochemical phenotype.[63–66]

Gastrointestinal function

An increasing body of evidence suggests that CRH is involved in the central mechanisms by which stress influences gastrointestinal function (Figure 5). Thus, PVN CRH induces both inhibition of gastric emptying and stimulation of colonic motor function, independently of the associated stimulation of the HPA axis. This is via inhibition of the vagus nerve and ensuing selective inhibition of gastric motility, and via stimulation—through the locus ceruleus/sympathetic system—of the sacral parasympathetic system, with ensuing selective stimulation of colonic motility.[67] Thus, CRH may be implicated in mediating the gastric stasis that results from the stress of surgery or from high levels of central interleukin-1.[68] CRH may also be implicated in the stress-induced colonic hypermotility of patients with the irritable bowel syndrome. Colonic contraction in these patients may activate LC/sympathetic neurons forming, thus, a vicious cycle, which may help explain the chronicity of the condition.

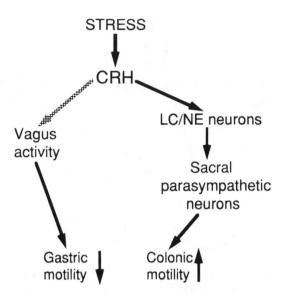

Figure 5 Effects of stress on gastrointestinal function. CRH, corticotrophin releasing hormone; LC/NE, locus ceruleus/norepinephrine. Stimulation is represented by solid lines and inhibition by dashed lines.

HPA axis—immune system interactions

Effects of the immune system on the HPA axis

The immune system exerts its surveillance-defense function constantly and mostly unconciously for the individual. It has been known for several decades that immune/inflammatory insults in the form of an infectious disease, an active autoimmune inflammatory process, or an accidental or operative trauma, are associated with concurrent activation of the HPA axis. More, recently it also became apparent that immune cytokines and other humoral mediators of inflammation are potent activators of central stress-responsive neurotransmitter systems, constituting the afferent limb of the feedback loop though which the immune/inflammatory system and the CNS communicate (Figure 6). This way, the peripheral immunologic apparatus signals the brain to participate in maintaining immunological and behavioral homeostasis.[69,70]

The three "inflammatory cytokines" tumor necrosis factor-alpha (TNF-α), interleukin-1 (IL-1), and interleukin-6 (IL-6), all produced at inflammatory sites and elsewhere in a cascade-like fashion, can cause stimulation of the HPA axis *in vivo*, alone, or in synergy with each other.[71,72] This can be blocked significantly with CRH-neutralizing antibodies, prostanoid synthesis inhibitors, and glucocorticoids. In addition, all three cytokines directly stimulate hypothalamic CRH secretion *in vitro*, an action also suppressed by glucocorticoids and prostanoid synthesis inhibitors.[73–75] There is evidence to suggest that IL-6, the main endocrine cytokine, plays the primary role in the immune stimulation of the human HPA axis, at least in the long term. Thus, in humans, IL-6 is an extremely potent activator of the axis, importantly without the vascular leak-promoting and hypotensive side-effects of the other two inflammatory cytokines.[76] The elevations of ACTH and cortisol attained by IL-6 are well above those observed with maximal stimulatory doses of CRH, suggesting that parvocellular AVP and other ACTH secretagogues are also stimulated by this cytokine. At high doses, IL-6 also stimulates peripheral elevations of AVP, presumably as a result of a stimulatory effect on magnocellular AVP-secreting neurons.[77] This suggests that IL-6 may be involved in the genesis of the syndrome of inappropriate antidiuretic hormone secretion (SIADH), which is observed during the course of infectious/inflammatory disease, or during trauma.

Some of the activating effects of inflammation on the HPA axis may be exerted indirectly, by stimulation of the central catecholaminergic pathways by the inflammatory cytokines and other humoral mediators of inflammation. Also, activation of peripheral nociceptive, somatosensory, and visceral afferent fibers would lead to stimulation of both the catecholaminergic and CRH neuronal systems via ascending spinal pathways. Interestingly, in chronic inflammatory states, where chronic central elevations of substance P may take place, an impairment of HPA axis responsiveness to stimuli or stress is observed, probably because of the suppressive effect of substance P on the CRH neuron.[24] Such an impairment has been observed in trypanosomiasis and extensive burns in humans and in chronic animal models of inflammation.[27,78]

Other inflammatory mediators may also participate in the activation of the HPA axis, in addition to the three inflammatory cytokines. Thus, several eicosanoids, platelet activating factor (PAF), serotonin, show strong CRH-releasing properties.[17,79,80] It is not clear, however, which of the above effects are endocrine and which are paracrine. Direct effects, albeit delayed, of most of the above cytokines and mediators of inflammation on pituitary ACTH secretion, on the other hand, have also been shown,[81–83] and direct effects of these substances on adrenal glucocorticoid secretion appear also to be present.[84]

Effects of the HPA axis on the immune/inflammatory reaction

Conversely, activation of the HPA axis has profound inhibitory effects on the inflammatory immune response, because virtually all the components of the immune response are inhibited by cortisol (Figure 6). At the cellular level, alterations of leukocyte traffic and function, decreases in production of cytokines and mediators of inflammation, and inhibition of the latters' effects on target tissues are among the main anti-inflammatory and

Immune Function

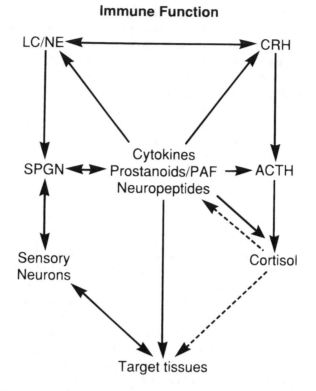

Figure 6 Interactions between the stress and immune systems. LC/NE, locus ceruleus/norepinephrine; SPGN, sympathetic postganglionic neurons; CRH, corticotropin releasing hormone; ACTH, corticotropin; PAF, platelet activating factor. Stimulation is represented by solid lines and inhibition by dashed lines.

immunosuppressive effects of glucocorticoids.[37] These effects are exerted at both the resting, basal state and during inflammatory stress, when the circulating concentrations of glucocorticoids are elevated. Thus, a circadian activity of several immune functions has been demonstrated in reverse-phase synchrony with that of plasma glucocorticoid levels.

A large infrastructure of anatomical, chemical, and molecular connections allows communication, not only within, but between the neuroendocrine and immune systems. The efferent sympathetic/adrenomedullary system apparently participates in a major fashion in the interactions of the HPA axis and the immune/inflammatory stress by being reciprocally connected with the CRH system, by receiving and transmitting humoral and nervous immune signals from the periphery, by densely innervating both primary and secondary lymphoid organs, and by reaching all sites of inflammation via the postganglionic sympathetic neuron.[85,86] Thus, leukocytes and macrophages contain receptors for and respond functionally to neurotransmitters, neuropeptides, and neurohormones and are also capable of making many of these substances.

When activated during stress, the autonomic system exerts its own direct effects on immune organs, which can be immunosuppressive, such as inhibition of natural killer cell activity, or both immunopotentiating and immunosuppressive, by inducing secretion of IL-6 in the systemic circulation.[87]

HPA axis—pathophysiology

Generally, the stress response with the resultant activation of the HPA axis is meant to be acute or at least of a limited duration. The time-limited nature of this process renders its accompanying catabolic and immunosuppressive effects temporarily beneficial and of no adverse consequences. Chronicity of stress system activation, on the other hand, would lead to the syndromal state that Selye described in 1936.[1] Since CRH coordinates behavioral, neuroendocrine, autonomic, and immunologic adaptation during stressful situations, increased and prolonged production of CRH could explain the pathogenesis and all the manifestations of the chronic stress syndrome, including the psychiatric, circulatory, metabolic, and immune components.

The syndrome of melancholic depression represents a prototypical example of dysregulation of the generalized stress response, leading to dysphoric hyperarousal, chronic activation of the HPA axis and the sympathetic nervous system, and relative immunosuppression.[88,89] Indeed, cortisol excretion is elevated and plasma ACTH response to exogenous CRH is decreased.[64] These abnormalities are state-related and resolve coincident to waning psychopathology. Hypersecretion of CRH has been shown in depression and suggests that CRH may participate in the initiation and/or perpetuation of a vicious cycle. Recently, depressed patients were found on autopsy to have increased numbers of PVN CRH neurons.[90] Whether this is genetically determined, environmentally induced, or both is unclear at the present time.

In addition to melancholic depression, a spectrum of other conditions may be associated with increased and prolonged activation of the HPA axis (Table 2). These include anorexia nervosa and malnutrition,[91–93] obsessive-compulsive disorder,[94] panic anxiety,[95] excessive exercising,[96] chronic active alcoholism,[97] alcohol and narcotic withdrawal,[98,99] diabetes mellitus, especially when complicated by diabetic neuropathy,[100,101] central (visceral) obesity,[63,66] childhood sexual abuse,[102] and, perhaps, hyperthyroidism[103] and the premenstrual tension syndrome.[104] In addition, Cushing's syndrome is characterized by autonomous excess production of glucocorticoids, which interrupts the integrity of the HPA axis by suppressing PVN CRH and by increasing the exposure of tissues to glucocorticoids. It is of interest that

Table 2 States Associated with Altered Hypothalamic-Pituitary-Adrenal Axis
Activity and Altered Regulatory or Dysregulation of Behavioral and/or
Peripheral Adaptation

Increased HPA axis	Decreased HPA axis
Chronic stress	Adrenal insufficiency
Melancholic depression	Atypical/seasonal depression
Anorexia nervosa	Chronic fatigue syndrome
Obsessive-compulsive disorder	Fibromyalgia
Panic disorder	Hypothyroidism
Excessive exercise (obligate athleticism)	Nicotine withdrawal
Chronic active alcoholism	Postglucocorticoid therapy
Alcohol and narcotic withdrawal	Post-Cushing syndrome cure
Diabetes mellitus	Postpartum period
Central obesity (metabolic syndrome X)	Postchronic stress
Childhood sexual abuse	Rheumatoid arthritis
Hyperthyroidism	
Premenstrual tension syndrome	
Cushing's syndrome	
Pregnancy	

Updated from Chrousos G. P. and Gold P. W., *JAMA*, 267, 1244, 1992.

anorexia nervosa and malnutrition are characterized by increased levels of CSF NPY, which could provide an explanation as to why the HPA axis in these subjects is activated, while the LC/sympathetic system shows clear evidence of profound hypoactivity. Glucocorticoids, by stimulating NPY, and by inhibiting the NE/sympathetic system, would produce the hyperphagia and obesity observed in Cushing's syndrome.

Pregnancy is another condition characterized by hypercortisolism of a degree similar to that observed in severe depression, anorexia nervosa, and mild Cushing syndrome, and is the only known physiologic state in humans in which CRH circulates in plasma at levels high enough to cause activation of the HPA axis.[105,106] Although circulating CRH, which is of placental origin, is bound with high affinity to CRH-binding protein,[107,108] it appears that the circulating free fraction is sufficient to explain the observed escalating hypercortisolism when the concentration of CRH-binding protein starts to gradually decrease in plasma after the 35th week of pregnancy.[109]

Hypoactivation of the stress system, rather than sustained activation, in which chronically reduced secretion of CRH may result in pathological hypoarousal, characterizes another group of states (Table 2). Patients with seasonal depression and the chronic fatigue syndrome fall in this category.[110,111] In the depressive (winter) state of the former and in the period of fatigue in the latter, there is chronically decreased activity of the HPA axis. Similarly, patients with fibromyalgia have decreased urinary free cortisol excretion and frequently complain of fatigue.[112] Hypothyroid patients also have clear evidence of CRH hyposecretion.[102] Interestingly, one of the major manifestations of hypothyroidism is depression of the "atypical" type. Withdrawal from smoking has also been associated with decreased cortisol and catecholamine secretion.[113,114] Decreased CRH secretion in the early period of nicotine abstinence could explain the hyperphagia and weight gain frequently observed in these patients. It is interesting that in Cushing syndrome, the clinical picture of hyperphagia and weight gain, as well as fatigue and anergia, is consistent with the suppression of the CRH neuron by the associated hypercortisolism.[64,115] The period after cure of hypercortisolism, the postpartum period, and periods following cessation of stress are also associated with suppressed PVN CRH secretion and decreased HPA axis activity.[116]

Theoretically, an excessive HPA axis response to inflammatory stimuli would mimic the stress or hypercortisolemic state and would lead to increased susceptibility of the individual to a host of infectious agents or tumors, but enhanced resistance to autoimmune/inflammatory disease;[117] in contrast, a defective HPA axis response to such stimuli would reproduce the glucocorticoid-deficient state and would lead to relative resistance to infections and neoplastic disease, but increased susceptibility to autoimmune/inflammatory disease.[118] Indeed, such properties were unraveled in an interesting pair of near-histocompatible, highly inbred rat strains, the Fischer and Lewis rats, both genetically selected out of Sprague-Dawley rats for their resistance or susceptibility, respectively, to inflammatory disease.[119,120] Setting off from the findings in this animal model, there is an increasing body of evidence that patients with rheumatoid arthritis have a mild form of central hypocortisolism, as they have reduced 24-h cortisol excretion, less pronounced diurnal rhythm of cortisol secretion, and blunted adrenal responses to surgical stress.[121,122] Thus, dysfunction of the HPA axis may actually play a role in the development and/or perpetuation of autoimmune disease, rather than being an epiphenomenon.

References

1. Chrousos, G. P. and Gold, P. W., The concepts of stress system disorders: overview of behavioral and physical homeostasis, *JAMA*, 267, 1244, 1992.
2. Dorn, L. D. and Chrousos, G. P., The endocrinology of stress and stress system disorders in adolescence, *Endocrinol. Metab. Clin. North. Am.*, 22, 685, 1993.
3. Chrousos, G. P., Regulation and dysregulation of the hypothalamic-pituitary-adrenal axis: the corticotropin releasing hormone perspective, *Endocrinol. Metab. Clin. North Am.*, 21, 833, 1992.
4. Tsigos, C. and Chrousos, G. P., Physiology of the hypothalamic-pituitary-adrenal axis in health and dysregulation in psychiatric and autoimmune disorders, *Endocrinol. Metab. Clin. North Am.*, 23, 451, 1994.
5. Vale, W. W., Spiess, S., Rivier, C. et al., Characterization of a 41-residue ovine hypothalamic peptide that stimulates secretion of corticotropin and beta-endorphin, *Science*, 213, 1394, 1981.

6. Aguilera, G., Millan, M. A., Hauger, R. L., and Catt, K. J., Corticotropin-releasing factor receptors: distribution and regulation in brain, pituitary, and peripheral tissues, *Ann. NY Acad. Sci.*, 512, 48, 1987.

7. DeSouza, E. B., Insel, T. R., Perrin, M. H. et al., Corticotropin-releasing factor receptors are widely distributed within the rat central nervous system, *J. Neurosci.*, 5, 3189, 1985.

8. Cole, B. and Koob, G. F., Corticotropin-releasing factor, stress, and animal behavior, in *Stress, Neuropeptides and Systemic Disease*, McCubbin, J. A., Kaufman, P. G., and Nemeroff, C. B., Eds, Academic Press, New York, 1991, 119.

9. Dunn, A. J. and Berrigde, C. W., Physiological and behavioral responses to corticotropin-releasing factor administration: is CRF a mediator of anxiety or stress response?, *Brain Res. Rev.*, 15, 71, 1990.

10. Calogero, A. E., Gallucci, W. T., Gold, P. W. et al., Multiple regulatory feedback loops on hypothalamic corticotropin releasing hormone secretion, *J. Clin. Invest.*, 82, 767, 1988.

11. Valentino, R. J., Foote, S. L., and Aston-Jones, G., Corticotropin-releasing hormone activates noradrenergic neurons of the locus ceruleus, *Brain Res.*, 270, 363, 1983.

12. Kiss, A. and Aguilera, G., Participation of α_1-adrenergic receptors in the secretion of hypothalamic corticotropin-releasing hormone during stress, *Neuroendocrinology*, 56, 153, 1992.

13. Calogero, A. E., Gallucci, W. T., Chrousos G. P. et al., Effect of the catecholamines upon rat hypothalamic corticotropin releasing hormone secretion in vitro: clinical implications, *J. Clin. Invest.*, 82, 839, 1988.

14. Silverman, A., Hou-Yu, A., and Chen, W. P., Corticotropin releasing factor synapses within the paraventricular nucleus of the hypothalamus, *Neuroendocrinology*, 49, 291, 1989.

15. Aghajanian, G. K. and Van der Maelen, C. P., α_2-Adrenoreceptor mediated hyperpolarization of locus ceruleus neurons: intracellular studies in vivo, *Science*, 215, 1394, 1982.

16. Calogero, A. E., Bagdy, G., Szemeredy, K. et al., Mechanisms of serotonin agonist-induced activation of the hypothalamic-pituitary-adrenal axis in the rat, *Endocrinology*, 126, 1888, 1990.

17. Fuller, R. W., The involvement of serotonin in regulation of pituitary-adrenocortical function, *Front. Neuroendocrinol.*, 13, 250, 1992.

18. Calogero, A. E., Gallucci, W. T., Chrousos, G. P. et al., Interaction between gabaergic neurotransmission and rat hypothalamic corticotropin releasing hormone in vitro, *Brain Res.*, 463, 28, 1988.

19. Overton, J. M. and Fisher, L. A., Modulation of central nervous system actions of corticotropin-releasing factor by dynorphin-related peptides, *Brain Res.*, 488, 233, 1989.

20. Keller-Wood, M. E. and Dallman, M. F., Corticosteroid inhibition of ACTH secretion, *Endocr. Rev.*, 5, 1, 1984.

21. Kamilaris, T. C., Calogero, A. E., and Ehrlich, Y. H., Effect of neuropeptide Y (NPY) on hypothalamic-pituitary-adrenal function in the rat, 19th Annual Meeting of the Society for Neuroscience, Phoenix, AR, 1989 (Abstr 58.9).

22. Egawa, M., Yoshimatsu, H., and Bray, G. A., Neuropeptide Y suppresses sympathetic activity to interscapular brown adipose tissue in rats, *Am. J. Physiol.*, 260, R328, 1991.

23. Oellerich, W. F., Schwartz, D. D., and Malik, K. U., Neuropeptide Y inhibits adrenergic transmitter release in cultured rat superior cervical ganglion cells by restricting the availability of calcium through a pertussis toxin-sensitive mechanism, *Neuroscience*, 60, 495, 1994.

24. White, B. D., Dean, R. G., Edwards, G. L., and Martin, R. J., Type II corticosteroid receptor stimulation increase NPY gene expression in basomedial hypothalamus of rats, *Am. J. Physiol.*, 266, R1523, 1994.

25. Larsen, P. J., Jessop, D., Patel, H., Lightman, S. L., and Chowdrey, H. S., Substance P inhibits the release of anterior pituitary adrenocorticotropin via a central mechanism involving corticotropin-releasing factor-containing neurons in the hypothalamic paraventricular nucleus, *J. Neuroendocrinol.*, 5, 99, 1993.

26. Culman, J., Tschope, C., Jost, N., Itoi, K., and Unger, T., Substance P and neurokinin A induced desensitization to cardiovascular and behavioral effects: evidence for the involvement of different tachykinin receptors, *Brain Res.*, 625, 75, 1993.

27. Jessop, D. S., Chowdrey, H. H., Larsen, P. J., and Lightman, S. L., Substance P: multifunctional peptide in the hypothalamo-pituitary system?, *J. Endocrinol.*, 132, 331, 1992.

28. Abou-Samra, A.-B., Harwood, J. P., Catt, K. J., and Aguilera, G., Mechanisms of action of CRF and other regulators of ACTH release in pituitary corticotrophs, *Ann. NY Acad. Sci.*, 512, 67, 1987.

29. Gillies, G. E., Linton, E. A., and Lowry, P. J., Corticotropin releasing activity of the new CRF is potentiated several times by vasopressin, *Nature*, 299, 355, 1982.

30. Antoni, F. A., Vasopressinergic control of pituitary adrenocorticotropin secretion comes of age, *Front. Neuroendocrinol.*, 14, 76, 1993.

31. Engler, D., Pham, T., Fullerton, M. J. et al., Studies on the secretion of corticotropin releasing factor and arginine vasopressin into hypophyseal portal circulation of the conscious sheep, *Neuroendocrinology*, 49, 367, 1989.

32. Redekopp, C., Irvine, C. H. G., Donald, R. A. et al., Spontaneous and stimulated adrenocorticotropin and vasopressin pulsatile secretion in the pituitary venous effluent of the horse, *Endocrinology*, 118, 1410, 1986.

33. Horrocks, P. M., Jones, A. F., Ratclifee, W. A. et al., Patterns of ACTH and cortisol pulsatility over twenty-four hours in normal males and females, *Clin. Endocrinol.*, 32, 127, 1990.

34. Iranmanesh, A., Lizarralde, G., Short, D., and Veldhuis, J. D., Intensive venous sampling paradigms disclose high frequency adrenocorticotropin release episodes in normal men, *J. Clin. Endocrinol. Metab.*, 71, 1276, 1990.

35. Veldhuis, J. D., Iranmanesh, A., Johnson, M. L., and Lizarralde, G., Amplitude, but not frequency, modulation of adrenocorticotropin secretory bursts gives rise to the nyctohemeral rhythm of the corticotropic axis in man, *J. Clin. Endocrinol. Metab.*, 71, 452, 1990.

36. Aguilera, G., Factors controlling steroid biosynthesis in the zona glomerulosa of the adrenal, *J. Steroid Biochem. Mol. Biol.*, 45, 147, 1993.

37. Munck, A., Guyre, P. M., and Holbrook, N. J., Physiological functions of glucocorticoids in stress and their relation to pharmacological actions, *Endocr. Rev.*, 5, 25, 1984.

38. Smith, D. F. and Toft, D. O., Steroid receptors and their associated proteins, *Mol. Endocrinol.*, 7, 4, 1993.
39. Pratt, W. B., Glucocorticoid receptor structure and the initial events in signal transduction, *Prog. Clin. Biol. Res.*, 322, 119, 1990.
40. Jonat, C., Rahmsdorf, H. J., Park, K.-K. et al., Antitumor promotion and anti-inflammation: down modulation of AP-1 (fos/jun) activity by glucocorticoid hormone, *Cell*, 62, 1189, 1990.
41. Yang-Yen, H.-F., Chambard, J.-C., Sun, Y.-L. et al., Transcriptional interference between c-jun and the glucocorticoid receptor: mutual inhibition of DNA binding due to direct protein-protein interaction, *Cell*, 62, 1205, 1990.
42. Matsusaka, T., Fujikawa, K., Nishio, Y. et al., Transcription factors NF-IL6 and NF-KB synergistically activate transcription of the inflammatory cytokines, interleukin 6 and interleukin 8, *Proc. Natl. Acad. Sci. U.S.A.*, 90, 10193, 1993.
43. de Kloet, E. R., Brain corticosteroid receptor balance and homeostatic control, *Front. Neuroendocrinol.*, 12, 95, 1991.
44. Gilbey, M. and Spyer, K. M., Essential organization of the sympathetic nervous system, *Bailliere's Clin. Endocrinol. Metab.*, 7, 259, 1993.
45. Burnstock, G. and Miller, P., Structural and chemical organization of the autonomic nervous system with special reference to nor-adrenergic, non-cholinergic transmission, in *Autonomic Failure. A Textbook of Clinical Disorders of the Autonomic Nervous System*, Bannister, R. and Mathias, C. J., Eds., Oxford Medical Press, Oxford, 1989, 107.
46. Benarroch, E. E., Neuropeptides in the sympathetic system: presence, plasticity, modulation, and implications, *Ann. Neurol.*, 36, 6, 1994.
47. Elfvin, L.-G., Lindh, B., and Hokfelt, T., The chemical neuroanatomy of sympathetic ganglia, *Annu. Rev. Neurosci.*, 16, 471, 1993.
48. Nikolarakis, K. E., Almeida, O. F. X., and Herz, A., Stimulation of hypothalamic β-endorphin and dynorphin release by corticotropin-releasing factor, *Brain Res.*, 399, 152, 1986.
49. Roth, R. H., Tam, S. Y., Lda, Y. et al., Stress and the mesocorticolimbic dopamine systems, *Ann. NY Acad. Sci.*, 537, 138, 1988.
50. Gray, T. S., Amygdala, role in autonomic and neuroendocrine responses to stress, in *Stress, Neuropeptides and Systemic Disease*, McCubbin, J. A., Kaufman, P. G., and Nemeroff, C. B., Eds., Academic Press, New York, 1989, 37.
51. MacAdams, M. R., White, R. H., and Chipps, B. E., Reduction in serum testosterone levels during chronic glucocorticoid therapy, *Ann. Intern. Med.*, 140, 648, 1986.
52. Rabin, D., Schmidt, P., Gold, P. W., Rubinow, D., and Chrousos, G. P., Hypothalamic-pituitary-adrenal function in patients with the premenstrual syndrome, *J. Clin. Endocrinol. Metab.*, 71, 1158, 1990.
53. Rivier, C., Rivier, J., and Vale, W., Stress-induced inhibition of reproductive function: role of endogenous corticotropin releasing factor, *Science*, 231, 607, 1986.
54. Vamvakopoulos, N. C. and Chrousos, G. P., Evidence of direct estrogen regulation of human corticotropin releasing hormone gene expression: potential implications for the sexual dimorphism of the stress response and immune/inflammatory reaction, *J. Clin. Invest.*, 92, 1896, 1993.

55. Vamvakopoulos, N. C. and Chrousos, G. P., Hormonal regulation of human corticotropin releasing hormone expression. Implications for the stress response and the immune/inflammatory reaction, *Endocr. Rev.*, 15, 409, 1994.
56. Burguera, B., Muruais, C., Penalva, A., Diegeuz, C., and Casanueva, F., Dual and selective action of glucocorticoids upon basal and stimulated growth hormone release in man, *Neuroendocrinology*, 51, 51, 1990.
57. Dieguez, C., Page, M. D., and Scanlon, M. F., Growth hormone neuroregulation and its alterations in disease states, *Clin. Endocrinol.*, 28, 109, 1988.
58. Unterman, T. G. and Phillips, L. S., Glucocorticoid effects on somatomedins and somatomedin inhibitors, *J. Clin. Endocrinol. Metab.*, 61, 618, 1985.
59. Casanueva, F. F., Burguera, B., Muruais, C., and Dieguez, C., Acute administration of corticosteroids: a new and peculiar stimulus of growth hormone secretion in man, *J. Clin. Endocrinol. Metab.*, 70, 234, 1990.
60. Rivier, C. and Vale, W., Involvement of corticotropin releasing factor and somatostatin in stress-induced inhibition of growth hormone secretion in the rat, *Endocrinology*, 117, 2478, 1985.
61. Benker, G., Raida, M., Olbricht, T., Wagner, R., Reinhardt, W., and Reinwein, D., TSH secretion in Cushing's syndrome: relation to glucocorticoid excess, diabetes, goitre, and "the sick euthyroid syndrome", *Clin. Endocrinol.*, 33, 779, 1990.
62. Duick, D. S. and Wahner, H. W., Thyroid axis in patients with Cushing's syndrome, *Arch. Intern. Med.*, 139, 767, 1979.
63. Pasquali, R., Cantobelli, S., Casimiri, F. et al., The hypothalamic-pituitary-adrenal axis in obese women with different patterns of body fat distribution, *J. Clin. Endocrinol. Metab.*, 77, 341, 1993.
64. Gold, P. W., Loriaux, D. X., Roy, A. et al., Responses to the corticotropin-releasing hormone in the hypercortisolism of depression and Cushing's disease: pathophysiologic and diagnostic implications, *N. Engl. J. Med.*, 314, 1329, 1986.
65. Biorntorp, P., The associations between obesity, adipose tissue distribution and disease, *Acta. Med. Scand.*, 723, 121, 1988.
66. Streeten, D. H. P., Editorial: Is the hypothalamic-pituitary-adrenal hyperactivity important in the pathogenesis of excessive abdominal fat distribution?, *J. Clin. Endocrinol. Metab.*, 77, 339, 1993.
67. Monnikes, H., Schmidt, B. G., Tebbe, J., Bauer, C., and Tache, Y., Microinfusion of corticotropin releasing factor into the locus ceoruleus/subcoeruleus nuclei stimulates colonic motor function in rats, *Brain Res.*, 644, 101, 1994.
68. Suto, G., Kiraly, A., and Tache, Y., Interleukin 1 beta inhibits gastric emptying in rats: mediation through prostaglandin and corticotropin-releasing factor, *Gastroenterology*, 106, 1568, 1994.
69. Chrousos, G. P., The hypothalamic-pituitary-adrenal axis and immune-mediated inflammation, *N. Engl. J. Med.*, May 18, 1995.
70. Reichlin, S., Neuroendocrine-immune interactions, *N. Engl. J. Med.*, 329, 1246, 1993.
71. Akira, S., Hirano, T., Taga, T., and Kishimoto, T., Biology of multifunctional cytokines: IL-6 and related molecules (IL-1 and TNF), *FASEB J.*, 4, 2860, 1990.
72. Besedovsky, H. O. and del Rey, A., Immune-neuroendocrine circuits: integrative role of cytokines, *Front. Neuroendocrinol.*, 13, 61, 1992.

73. Bernardini, R., Kamilaris, T. C., Calogero, A. E. et al., Interactions between tumor necrosis factor-alpha, hypothalamic corticotropin-releasing hormone and adrenocorticotropin secretion in the rat, *Endocrinology*, 126, 2876, 1990.

74. Busbridge, N. J. and Grossman, A. B., Stress and the single cytokine: interleukin modulation of the pituitary-adrenal axis, *Mol. Cell. Endocrinol.*, 82, C209, 1991.

75. Sapolsky, R., Rivier, C., Yamamoto, G. et al., Interleukin-1 stimulates the secretion of hypothalamic corticotropin releasing factor, *Science*, 238, 522, 1987.

76. Mastorakos, G., Chrousos, G. P., and Weber, J., Recombinant interleukin-6 activates the hypothalamic-pituitary-adrenal axis in humans, *J. Clin. Endocrinol. Metab.*, 27, 2690, 1993.

77. Mastorakos, G., Weber, J. S., Magiakou, M. A., Gunn, H., and Chrousos, G. P., Hypothalamic-pituitary-adrenal axis activation and stimulation of systemic vasopressin secretion by recombinant interleukin-6 in humans, *J. Clin. Endocrinol. Metab.*, 79, 1191, 1994.

78. Reincke, M., Allolio, B., Arlt, W. et al., Impairment of adrenocortical function associated with increased tumor necrosis factor-alpha and interleukin-6 concentrations in African trypanosomiasis, *NeuroImmunoModulation*, 1, 14, 1994.

79. Bernardini, R., Calogero, A. E., Ehlich, Y. H. et al., The alkyl-ether phospholipid platelet-activating factor is a stimulator of the hypothalamic-pituitary-adrenal axis in the rat, *Endocrinology*, 125, 1067, 1989.

80. Bernardini, R., Chiarenza, A., Calogero, A. E. et al., Arachidonic acid metabolites modulate rat hypothalamic corticotropin releasing hormone in vitro, *Neuroendocrinology*, 50, 708, 1989.

81. Bernton, E. W., Beach, L. E., Holaday, J. W., Smallridge, R. C., and Fein, H. G., Release of multiple hormones by a direct effect of interleukin-1 on pituitary cells, *Science*, 238, 519, 1987.

82. Fukata, J., Usui, T., Naitoh, Y., Nakai, Y., and Imura, H., Effects of recombinant human interleukin-1α, -1β, -2 and -6 on ACTH synthesis and release in the mouse pituitary tumour cell line AtT-20, *J. Endocrinol.*, 122, 33, 1988.

83. Winter, J. S. D., Gow, K. W., Perry, Y. S., and Greenberg, A. H., A stimulatory effect of interleukin-1 on adrenocortical cortisol secretion mediated by prostaglandins, *Endocrinology*, 127, 1904, 1990.

84. Salas, M. A., Evans, S. W., Levell, M. J., and Whicher, J. T., Interleukin-6 and ACTH act synergistically to stimulate the release of corticosterone from adrenal gland cells, *Clin. Exp. Immunol.*, 79, 470, 1990.

85. Ottaway, C. A. and Husband, A. J., Central nervous system influences on lymphocyte migration, *Brain Behav. Immun.*, 6, 97, 1992.

86. Bellinger, D. L., Lorton, D., Felten, S. Y., and Felten, D. L., Innervation of lymphoid organs and implications in development, aging, and autoimmunity, *Int. J. Immunopharmacol.*, 14, 329, 1992.

87. Hirano, T., Akira, S., Taga, T., and Kishimoto, T., Biological and clinical aspects of interleukin-6, *Immunol. Today*, 11, 443, 1990.

88. Gold, P. W., Goowin, F., and Chrousos, G. P., Clinical and biochemical manifestations of depression: relationship to the neurobiology of stress, I, *N. Engl. J. Med.*, 319, 348, 1988.

89. Gold, P. W., Goodwin, F., and Chrousos, G. P., Clinical and biochemical manifestations of depression: relationship to the neurobiology of stress, II, *N. Engl. J. Med.*, 319, 413, 1988.

90. Raadsheer, F. C., Hoogendijk, W. J. G., Stam, F. S., Tilders, F. J. H., and Swaab, D. F., Increased numbers of corticotropin-releasing hormone expressing neurons in the hypothalamic paraventricular nucleus of depressed patients, *Neuroendocrinology*, 60, 436, 1994.

91. Gold, P. W., Gwirtsman, H., Avgerinos, P. et al., Abnormal hypothalamic-pituitary-adrenal function in anorexia nervosa: pathophysiologic mechanisms in underweight and weight-corrected patients, *N. Engl. J. Med.*, 314, 1335, 1986.

92. Kaye, W. H., Gwirtsman, H. E., George, D. T. et al., Elevated cerebrospinal fluid levels of immunoreactive corticotropin-releasing hormone in anorexia nervosa: relation to state of nutrition, adrenal function, and intensity of depression, *J. Clin. Endocrinol. Metab.*, 64, 203, 1987.

93. Malozowski, S., Muzzo, S., Burrows, R. et al., The hypothalamic-pituitary-adrenal axis in infantile malnutrition, *Clin. Endocrinol.*, 32, 461, 1990.

94. Insel, T. R., Kalin, N. H., Guttmacher, L. B., Cohen, R. M., and Murphy, D. L., The dexamethasone suppression test in obsessive-compulsive disorder, *Psychiatr. Res.*, 6, 153, 1982.

95. Gold, P. W., Pigott, T. A., Kling, M. K., Kalogeras, K., and Chrousos, G. P., Basic and clinical studies with corticotropin releasing hormone: implications for a possible role in panic disorder, *Psychiatr. Clin. North Am.*, 11, 327, 1988.

96. Luger, A., Deuster, P., Kyle, S. B. et al., Acute hypothalamic-pituitary-adrenal responses to the stress of treadmill excercise: physiologic adaptations to physical training, *N. Engl. J. Med.*, 316, 1309, 1987.

97. Wand, G. S. and Dobs, A. S., Alterations in the hypothalamic-pituitary-adrenal axis in actively drinking alcoholics, *J. Clin. Endocrinol. Metab.*, 72, 1290, 1991.

98. Bardeleben, V., Heuser, I., and Holsboer, F., Human CRH stimulation response during acute withdrawal and after medium-term abstention from alcohol abuse, *Psychoneuroendocrinology*, 14, 441, 1989.

99. Risher-Flowers, D., Adinoff, B., Ravitz, B. et al., Circadian rhythms of cortisol during alcohol withdrawal, *Adv. Alcohol Subst. Abuse*, 7, 37, 1988.

100. Roy, M. S., Roy, A., Gallucci, W. T. et al., The ovine corticotropin releasing hormone test in type I diabetic patients and controls: suggestion of mild chronic hypercortisolism, *Metabolism*, 42, 696, 1993.

101. Tsigos, C., Young, R. J., and White, A., Diabetic neuropathy is associated with increased activity of the hypothalamic-pituitary-adrenal axis, *J. Clin. Endocrinol. Metab.*, 76, 554, 1993.

102. DeBellis, M., Chrousos, G. P., Dorn, L. D. et al., Hypothalamic-pituitary-adrenal axis dysregulation in sexually abused girls, *J. Clin. Endocrinol. Metab.*, 78, 249, 1994.

103. Kamilaris, T. C., DeBold, R. C., Pavlou, S. N., Island, D. P., Hoursanidis, A., and Orth, D. N., Effect of altered thyroid hormone levels on hypothalamic-pituitary-adrenal function, *J. Clin. Endocrinol. Metab.*, 65, 994, 1987.

104. Rabin, D., Gold, P. W., Margioris, A., and Chrousos, G. P., Stress and repro-
     duction: interactions between the stress and reproductive axis, in
     Mechanisms of Physical and Emotional Stress, Chrousos, G. P., Loriaux, D. L.,
     and Gold, P. W., Eds., Plenum Press, New York, 1988, 377.
105. Margioris, A., Grino, M., Gold, P. W. et al., Human placenta and the hypo-
     thalamic-pituitary-adrenal axis, *Adv. Exp. Med. Biol.*, 245, 389, 1988.
106. Sasaki, A., Shinkawa, O., Margioris, A. N. et al., Immunoreactive corti-
     cotropin-releasing hormone in human plasma during pregnancy, labor and
     delivery, *J. Clin. Endocrinol. Metab.*, 64, 224, 1987.
107. Behan, D. P., Linton, E. A., and Lowry, P. J., Isolation of the human plasma
     corticotropin-releasing factor-binding protein, *J. Endocrinol.*, 122, 23, 1989.
108. Potter, E., Behan, D. P., Fischer, W. H., Linton, E. A., Lowry, P. J., and Vale,
     W., Cloning and characterization of the cDNAs for human and rat corti-
     cotropin-releasing factor-binding proteins, *Nature*, 349, 423, 1991.
109. Linton, E. A., Perkins, A. V., Woods, R. J. et al., Corticotropin releasing hor-
     mone-binding protein (CRH-BP): plasma levels decrease during the third
     trimester of normal human pregnancy, *J. Clin. Endocrinol. Metab.*, 76, 260,
     1993.
110. Demitrack, M., Dale, J., Straus, S. et al., Evidence of impaired activation of
     the hypothalamic-pituitary-adrenal axis in patients with chronic fatigue
     syndrome, *J. Clin. Endocrinol. Metab.*, 73, 1224, 1991.
111. Vanderpool, J., Rosenthal, N., Chrousos, G. P. et al., Evidence for hypo-
     thalamic CRH deficiency in patients with seasonal affective disorder, *J. Clin.
     Endocrinol. Metab.*, 72, 1382, 1991.
112. Griep, E. N., Boerdma, J. W., and de Kloet, E. R., Altered reactivity of the
     hypothalamic-pituitary-adrenal axis in the primary fibromyalgia syn-
     drome, *J. Rheumatol.*, 20, 469, 1993.
113. Elgerot, A., Psychological and physiological changes during tobacco-
     abstinence in habitual smokers, *J. Clin. Psychol.*, 34, 759, 1978.
114. Puddey, J. B., Vandongen, R., Neilin, L. J., and English, D., Haemodynamic
     and neuroendocrine consequences of stopping smoking—a controlled
     study, *Clin. Exp. Pharmacol. Physiol.*, 11, 423, 1984.
115. Kling, M. A., Doran, A., Rubinow, D. R. et al., CSF levels of CRH, ACTH,
     and SRIF in Cushing's syndrome, major depression, and normal volunteers:
     physiological and pathophysiological interrelationships, *J. Clin. Endocrinol.
     Metab.*, 72, 260, 1991.
116. Doherty, J. M., Nieman, L. K., Cutler, G. B., Jr., Chrousos, G. P., and Norton,
     J., Time to recovery of the hypothalamic-pituitary-adrenal axis following
     curative resection of adrenal tumors in patients with Cushing's syndrome,
     Surgery, 108, 1085, 1990.
117. Sternberg, E. M., Glowa, J., and Smith, M. A., Corticotropin releasing hor-
     mone related behavioral and neuroendocrine responses to stress in Lewis
     and Fischer rats, *Brain Res.*, 570, 54, 1992.
118. Sternberg, E. M., Chrousos, G. P., Wilder, R. L., and Gold, P. W., The stress
     response and the regulation of inflammatory disease: NIH combined clin-
     ical staff conference, *Ann. Intern. Med.*, 117, 854, 1992.
119. Sternberg, E. M., Hill, J. M., Chrousos, G. P. et al., Inflammatory mediator-
     induced hypothalamic-pituitary-adrenal axis activation is defective in strep-
     tococcal cell arthritis in Lewis rats, *Proc. Natl. Acad. Sci. U.S.A.*, 86, 2374, 1989.

120. Sternberg, E. M., Young, W. S., Jr., Bernardini, R. et al., A central nervous defect in the stress response is associated with susceptibiltiy to streptococcal cell wall arthritis in Lewis rats, *Proc. Natl. Acad. Sci. U.S.A.*, 86, 4771, 1989.
121. Chikanza, I. C., Petrou, P., Chrousos, G. P., Kingsley, G., and Panayi, G., Defective hypothalamic response to immune/inflammatory stimuli in patients with rheumatoid arthritis, *Arthritis Rheum.*, 35, 1281, 1992.
122. Chicanza, I. C., Chrousos, G. P., and Panayi, G. S., Abnormal neurendocrine-immune communications in patients with rheumatoid arthritis, *Eur. J. Clin. Invest.*, 22, 635, 1992.

chapter four

Stress and mental health

Kathleen A. Moore and Graham D. Burrows

Introduction

Stress is a ubiquitous term with no universally accepted definition (Norman and Malla, 1993a). Some researchers focus on the environment, describing stress as a stimulus, or stressor, that presumably gives rise to stress; others describe stress in terms of demands made upon the individual, whether these be psychological or somatic (Selye, 1982); while a third approach characterizes stress as a process that includes the interaction between the person and the demands of the environment in which the individual perceives a discrepancy between demand and resources (e.g., Lazarus and Folkman, 1984). How do these various definitions help in our understanding of the relationship, if any, between stress and mental health, or indeed, mental ill-health? This chapter does not attempt to review the total area of mental health, but will discuss some aspects of stress in relationship to the major psychiatric disorders.

Stress and/or anxiety?

What is meant when, as so often happens, the term anxiety is used either interchangeably with stress or, more particularly, to describe a reaction to a stressor? For instance, Spielberger (1976) noted that, historically, the construct of stress has been used to refer to negative situations or conditions that elicit anxiety reactions and to the stress reactions themselves. Lazarus (1966) also conceptualized anxiety as a stress emotion. What then is anxiety?

Burrows and Davies (1984) defined anxiety as a characteristic, unpleasant emotion induced by the anticipation of danger or frustration which threatens the security or homeostasis of the individual or the group to which he or she belongs (p.2). This challenge to the body's homeostasis is also seen in what Cannon (1929) called the "fight-or-flight" response to a stressor—here, the body's sympathetic nervous system is aroused to defend against a perceived threat and only returns to a homeostatic condition once the danger has passed.

0-8493-2908-6/96/$0.00+$.50
© 1996 by CRC Press, Inc.

Although in practice there is considerable interchange between the terms stress and anxiety as a reaction to an event, Endler and Parker (1990) suggest this frequently synonymous use is confusing and they provide an outline of the conceptual differences between the constructs. In terms of diagnostic distinctions between the terms it is important to consider criteria such as that provided by the *Diagnostic and Statistical Manual of Mental Disorders* (DSM) (American Psychiatric Association, APA, 1994).

Diagnostic criteria

Anxiety disorders, such as panic attack, agoraphobia, obsessive-compulsive disorder, have long-standing classifications and will not be discussed further here; however, stress per se has not been so well recognized. The DSM (APA, 1952) referred to "gross stress reactions", a reaction to extreme stress such as war, disasters, fires, earthquakes, or explosions. In the second edition (DSM-II APA, 1968), the term "transient situational disorder" was introduced and defined a reaction to unusual stress caused by a range of events from unwanted pregnancy to a death sentence. As Yehuda and colleagues (1993) pointed out, the underlying assumption of these disorders was that reactions to trauma would be characterized by quick recovery in normal individuals, whereas prolonged responses to the trauma would be regarded as secondary to preexisting personality traits or to constitutional vulnerability.

Post-traumatic stress disorder

DSM-111-R (APA, 1987) described "post-traumatic stress disorder" (PTSD) as a debilitating reaction to an event outside the range of normal human behavior with a duration of disturbance greater than 1 month. As Gersons and Carlier (1992) pointed out, experience of the traumatic event does not of itself elicit a diagnosis of PTSD, rather it is the reaction to the event. Apart from the condition that the event must be outside the range of normal human experience, PTSD reflects the definitional components of stress: there is an environmental stressor (event), placing demands upon the individual, where the individual perceives a discrepancy in resources to meet the demand. The potential chronicity of PTSD has been suggested by Davidson and Baum's (1986) study of subjects within a 5-mile radius of Three Mile Island. At 58 months after the event residents performed more poorly than controls in a proofreading task and exhibited symptoms of stress-related arousal.

There would be few who would dispute the causal link between a traumatic event and PTSD and, because PTSD is included as a diagnostic classification, no argument for causality will be developed. However, it remains unclear why between one quarter and one third of people experiencing traumatic events fail to develop clinical symptoms. Was the event not perceived as stressful enough? Did they have more resources available to meet the demand? Being cognizant that DSM-111-R (APA, 1987) has removed the suggestion of a preexisting condition underlying protracted reaction to a traumatic event, the question must be asked of those who fail to succumb: were they protected in some manner? If yes, does this suggest a vulnerability on the part of those who did experience the stress reaction? What is the nature of the vulnerability: biological, cognitive, or both?

Acute stress disorder

DSM-IV (APA, 1994) includes a new classification of acute stress disorder (ASD). The essential feature of this disorder is the development of characteristic anxiety, dissociative, and other symptoms that occur during or immediately after the trauma, last for at least 2 days and resolve within 1 month after exposure to the stressor or the diagnosis is changed (APA, 1994). If the symptoms are ongoing, it may be that a diagnosis of PTSD is warranted or, in some cases, it may be that symptoms of hopelessness and despair are such as to warrant a diagnosis of major depression.

Like PTSD, this diagnosis also involves a traumatic event (demand) with which the individual is expected to cope. As this diagnostic category is new, no empirical data exist on the prevalence of this disorder, although clinical experience certainly confirms its relevance. Neither is there any information on the course of patients with this disorder, nor the conversion from ASD to another diagnostic classification.

The deleterious effect of traumatic events on individuals experiencing them is clearly recognized by these two diagnostic classifications; however, no account is provided for the effect of life events where the experience is less menacing than "actual or threatened death" and/or where the emotional reaction to the threat was less intense.

It is also important to consider why those persons with a sustained post-trauma reaction may later become depressed, and why some life events may be associated with depression or other mental illnesses rather than an anxiety disorder. Brown (1993) suggested that life events can be categorized depicting a "loss" or "danger" (or both) and that the type of life event has implications for any ensuing illness. It is necessary to look to the literature for a discussion of these issues.

Life events

In their important work on the changes individuals need to make as a result of life events, Holmes and Rahe (1967) argued that such changes require a degree of psychological adaptation. They considered this adjustment to be stressful to the individual and developed their Social Readjustment Rating Scale (SRRS) to quantify that level of stress. The idea that life change produces stress is compatible with a definition of stress as

a condition of perceived imbalance between environmental (including social) demands and the capability of the individual to meet these demands
(McGrath, 1970) and with the more extreme circumstances that are now
recognized as PTSD or ASD (APA, 1994).

There are consistent significant correlations between life stress, measured on the SRRS, and illness. However, these are rarely greater then .30
(Dohrenwend and Dohrenwend, 1981; Rabkin and Struening, 1976) suggesting that stress accounts for less than 10% of the variance in illness. Of
course, people get sick for a number of reasons other than stress, but it is
also true that the SRRS has a number of weaknesses. Although the scale
lists a reasonably wide range of events and the ratings assigned to the
events were based upon a large sample, the items are subject to retrospective recall, some items appear to have less relevance in the 1980s and
1990s, and, although true to their original concept of "readjustment", the
scale does not always assess whether the event is a negative or positive
event: e.g., "change in work hours or conditions", yet these are rated
equally, with no allowance for the direction of the change to have a differential impact.

Subsequent researchers have focused on connection perspectives, using
such terms as "objective impact" (Paykel et al., 1971) and "contextual threat"
(Brown and Harris, 1978). Others have considered whether the events are
able to be dimensionalized, for instance, desirable versus undesirable
(Paykel et al., 1969; Vinokur and Selzer, 1975); still others are examining
possible mediating effects, such as personal lifestyle factors including diet,
sleep, and exercise (e.g., Coyne and Holyroyd, 1982; Moore, 1994).

Desirable versus undesirable

Vinokur and Selzer (1975) modified the SRRS to a 4-point Likert scale ranging from affected "a little to a great deal" and altered items so that they reflected a desirable versus an undesirable event. For example, "change in
working conditions" became (1) improvement in working conditions and (2)
deterioration in working conditions. They administered the modified scale
together with the Minnesota Multiphasic Personality Inventory (MMPI;
Hathaway and McKinley, 1970) and a series of questions related to behavioral indications of stress and anxiety to a sample of 1059 male drivers.

Negative life events were significantly correlated with self-report ratings of depression, suicidal ideation, paranoia, aggression, stress, and anxiety (range of r .25 to .38, r^2 6% to 14%, all $p < .01$). Many of the correlations
between these variables and the desirable life events were also statistically
significant but, as expected, the range of correlations was lower (r .07 to
.19, r^2 0% to 4%). Although the data support the proposed relationships between both negative and positive life events and feelings indicative of diminished psychological well-being, in neither case is the amount of shared
variance substantial.

Perceptions of life events: threats and losses

Parkes (1992) also used a sample of nonpsychiatric male workers, in this case control room operators for oil rigs, and compared those working and living "onshore" with those working and living "offshore". Whereas offshore workers were significantly more distressed on a measure of general mental health (General Health Questionnaire, GHQ-12) compared to those onshore, they were not different from normative data provided for 552 males working in an engineering plant. On particular subscales of the General Health Questionnaire (GHQ-60), offshore workers were significantly more anxious but there were no differences between the two groups for somatic symptoms or social dysfunction. As a consequence of the GHQ-60 subscale difference on anxiety, this variable was used as a covariate to again compare the two groups on the GHQ-12 and this reanalysis revealed no difference.

As expected from the group differences, discriminant function analysis revealed one function (k-1) with: "feeling constantly under strain"; "getting scared or panicky for no good reason"; "feeling strung up and nervous all the time"; "lose sleep over worry"; "found everything getting on top of you"; "getting edgy and bad tempered"; "difficulty remaining asleep"—all significant discriminators between offshore and onshore workers.

Parkes (1992) suggested that the offshore environment plays a causal role in the elevated anxiety levels. Interpreted in terms of life events, it may be that the constrained and artificial environment, close relations with others, concern over family left at home, and lack of perceived or actual support all contribute to levels of stress that are revealed on both the anxiety subscale of the GHQ-60 and the more generalized distress rating as suggested by the GHQ-12. It may also be that those workers living in the offshore environment reflected in their anxiety rating, a degree of concern related to the danger or threat to life associated with such an environment.

This hypothesis is consistent with the findings of Endler and colleagues (1962), who identified three anxiety dimensions (interpersonal threat, physical danger, and ambiguous threat) based on factor analysis of self-report anxiety responses to descriptions of 11 specific situations. Findlay-Jones and Brown (1981) demonstrated an association between the occurrence of a severe threat event and subsequent onset of an anxiety disorder, in a sample of 164 female attenders at a London general practice. When the life event was one of severe loss the resultant psychiatric disorder was more likely to be a depressive disorder.

It seems clear that there is an association between stress, especially undesirable life events, and reduced psychological well-being. Although the role of life events in the etiology of mental disorders remains controversial (Deadman et al., 1989), a review of the findings to date is presented in the following sections.

Panic disorder

Laraia and co-workers (1994) evaluated childhood influences on women diagnosed with panic disorder (PD) with agoraphobia. While they failed to find differences between patients and control groups in the number of deaths or divorces among significant others during childhood, the patient group reported a significantly higher percentage of non-illness-related parental separations than did control subjects. In relation to illness, results revealed that the patient group reported a higher mean number of members per household with chronic physical illness and alcohol/drug use problems. It was proposed that these early adverse environmental stressors, combined with Torgerson's (1988) suggestion of a genetic predisposition, or vulnerability, may interact to precipitate a later anxiety disorder. The relationship between these early stressors and subsequent negative affect may be more generalized than at first suggested. Stuart et al. (1990), using the Childhood Environment Questionnaire found that female patients suffering bulimia and depression also recalled significantly higher levels of childhood separation anxiety than did control subjects. Of course, the problems attendant to retrospective data prevail, as well as possible biases inherent in those who present for treatment and further, those who agree to participate in such studies.

Early parental separations and concomitant separation anxiety also discriminate between patients diagnosed as having panic disorder and those who met the DSM-111-R (APA, 1987) criteria for both panic disorder and borderline personality disorder (BPD) where the latter was considered the primary diagnosis (Friedman and Chernen, 1994). Both groups also reported multiple chronic stressors and elevated levels of acute stress, including a rating for medical emergency room visits. No suicide attempts were reported among the PD patients ($N = 72$); however, among the 69 patients diagnosed PD with BPD, there were 17 reported attempts. The authors warned that PD may be associated with severe psychopathology that may put patients at serious risk for suicide.

According to Burrows and Davies (1984) and Clark (1986), panic attacks can arise from the catastrophic misinterpretation of certain bodily sensations. For example, if physically healthy individuals misinterpret palpitations as an indication of an impending heart attack, they are likely to become anxious. This will increase or prolong the palpitations which, in turn, will lead to further anxiety. The person then has difficulty in reducing this state of arousal, which results in diminished coping and reduced functioning. Clinicians may also misinterpret the symptoms or fail to consider them outside their own area of speciality. For instance, Apfeldorf and colleagues (1994) suggested that cardiologists focus on atypical chest pain, pulmonologists on hyperventilation, and gastroenterologists on irritable bowel symptoms when, in fact, these various symptoms may actually be stress reactions or manifestations of panic disorder.

Depression

Based upon students' scores on the Centre for Epidemiological Studies Depression Scale, Hawkins et al. (1992) formed four groups: male, female, low and high levels of depression. Using depression level as the grouping variable, for females they found that: lower life satisfaction, higher levels of stress, perceived unattractiveness, and lower reported health were the most significant discriminators, whereas for males, less life satisfaction, lower feelings of attractiveness, higher stress, and more likely to use drugs prevailed. The overall classification rates were 84% for girls and 89% for boys. Applying Findlay-Jones and Brown's (1981) threat/loss model to these findings, these discriminators can be viewed in terms of losses: loss of life satisfaction, loss of attractiveness, and therefore those persons experiencing more loss would be expected to score higher on the depression rating scale.

Brown (1993) in a 3-year longitudinal study of women used the shortened form of Present State Examination to collate clinical material at a "caseness level", and a measure of life events and difficulties in order to categorize events occurring within the past 6 months as "loss" or "danger" or as both. The last category was limited to ratings of dual or multiple events: instances where an occurrence classified as danger, e.g., severe illness of partner, may have subsequently become a loss event, e.g., death of that partner, were treated solely as a loss. The authors found significant associations between loss and depression, danger and anxiety, and loss and danger combined in mixed-onset depression and anxiety. These findings replicated the earlier work of Finlay-Jones and Brown (1981). There is, however, no suggestion that these life events and difficulties always lead to depression or anxiety. For instance, 20% of women with a significant life event did not develop either anxiety or depression, versus 64% who did. It appears that some people may be more hardy to stress, whereas others have a vulnerability that, combined with the stressor, results in a psychopathology.

Fava et al. (1992) treated 60 depressed patients with fluoxetine using a cross-sectional comparison with nonpsychiatric controls. The pretreatment Hamilton Depression Ratings (M 21.5) and Perceived Stress Scale scores (M 38.8) were significantly higher for the depressed group compared to the control group (PSS: M 22.4), and there was a significant correlation between depression and stress scores. After treatment, the mean PSS score was significantly lower than at pretest and did not differ from the controls. Unfortunately, no gauge of maturation or historical effects is available, as the control group was not retested.

As perceived stress levels can be reduced by stress/type A cognitive-behavior modification programs in nonpsychiatric populations (e.g., Moore et al., 1992), it is interesting that here, a pharmacological intervention has produced similar results. Fava et al. (1992) suggested that serotonin dysregulations may be involved in stress reactions, and that the drug administered, fluoxetine, is a relatively selective serotonin uptake inhibitor. Data support the hypothesis that there may be neurobiological substrates for the relationship between stress and depression, which involve the hy-pothalamic-pituitary-adrenal (HPA) axis often activated in depression. The HPA axis activation would be evident in hypercortisolism, which has been found to be related to cognitive sequelae in depression (Sikes et al., 1989) (see also anorexia).

Anorexia nervosa

The importance and frequency of life events prior to the clinical onset of anorexia nervosa has been proposed by several authors (e.g., Donohoe, 1984; Schwabe et al., 1981). It has also been suggested that some of the psy-chosocial stressors that have been implicated in the onset of anorexia ner-vosa also increase the intrahypothalamic levels of corticotropin releasing hormone (CRH), a 41-amino-acid hypothalamic polypeptide, which could result in an anorectic action (Krahn et al., 1987).

CRH and hypothalamopituitary axis (HPA) activation: in the stress re-action, CRH has been shown to be directly involved in the glucocorticoid cascade, and determines an increase in corticotropin (ACTH) which, in turn, increases corticosteroids, i.e., cortisol (Sapolsky et al., 1986; Young and Akin, 1985). CRH appears to be involved in both adaptation to stress and the regulation of ingestive behavior and, therefore, indicates a link be-tween psychosocial stress and its neurobiological determinants, in this case, anorexia nervosa.

Support for this hypothesis is provided by Kahn and co-workers (1992), who compared anorectic patients with screened age- and sex-matched controls on a 40-minute memory task performed under pressure from extraneous and continuous "pink noise". Although the groups dis-played some heterogeneity, overall there was a significant increase in sali-vary cortisol level for the anorectic group and this remained so for up to 80 minutes after the task was completed. No such effect was present in the control group.

Schizophrenia

Empirical support for the importance of endogenous factors in the etiol-ogy of schizophrenia is increasing, e.g., genetic factors (Gottesman et al., 1987), as well as evidence for structural and neurophysiological abnor-malities (Buchsbaum, 1990; Meltzer, 1987). In conjunction with this increase in biological explanations, there has also been a growing interest in the possible role of stress in schizophrenia. This parallel pursuit of what some have previously considered incompatible etiologies represents a shift to-wards a more embracing biopsychosocial model which is influenced, not just by the research in this and other illnesses of demonstrated biological origin, but from clinical impressions which suggest that stress is implicated in relapse.

Early studies (e.g., Brown and Birley, 1968; Leff and Vaughn, 1980) have suggested that stressful life events that occur independently of the patient's behavior are more frequent in the weeks immediately before relapse. As with all studies of this nature, no matter the population under investigation, the assessed recall is for prior stressful events and may, therefore, be subject to a retrospective memory bias. Brown and Birley (1968) have named this the "search for meaning", suggesting that patients may enhance their level of stressors in order to accommodate their present state.

Nuechterlein and colleagues (1992) prospectively tracked 11 patients and found that life event frequencies, of sufficient magnitude to be considered life changes, occurred in the months immediately preceding psychotic exacerbations or relapse in these patients. The incidence of these life events was contrasted with life event frequencies for the same patients during other periods and with life event frequencies for 19 nonrelapsing patients. A significantly higher number of independent life events was reported in the month before relapse as against a comparable month that did not precede a relapse period for the same patients. The frequency of the life events in the month before the 11 patients experienced psychotic relapses was significantly higher than the 1-year average rate of life events for nonrelapsing patients. In order to reduce intergroup variance in studies of this kind, Norman and Malla (1993b) support the use of a repeated measures design whereby patients act as their own controls and the researcher looks for an association between stress and symptoms over different time frames.

If, as appears from these studies, many people with schizophrenia have strong aversive reactions to life stressors, Norman and Malla (1993b) suggested it is quite conceivable that they might adapt their lives to ensure minimum exposure to major stressors. This behavior would be expected on the basis of avoidance learning, and they posit that it also fits a common clinical impression that many patients with schizophrenia lead lives that do not include many of the acute, major life events (e.g., marriage, mortgages, pressure jobs) that are challenges to others; however, caution should be applied in attributing causality here without further evidence. Norman and Malla do not suggest that those suffering from schizophrenia have fewer stressors, rather these may be different in nature and include considerations such as loneliness or financial need.

A review by Norman and Malla (1993b) elicited studies in which the investigators stated they had made an explicit attempt to exclude from consideration those life events that are themselves likely to have been a result of changes in symptoms of schizophrenia. A summary of their report is presented.

Schizophrenia versus other psychiatric diagnostic groups—Seven of the eight studies reviewed compared patients with schizophrenia with depressed patients, while one study used patients suffering from schizophrenia, schizophreniform psychosis, and hypomania, and others used groups of chemically dependent patients, those diagnosed with personality disorder, adjustment and anxiety disorders. All studies report the use of inpatients and a retrospective design to assess the stressors for the period prior to admission or onset of illness. There were no significant differences on life event stress levels among the groups, indicating that the level of stress as an onset factor is no greater for patients with schizophrenia than those patients with other diagnoses.

Schizophrenia patients versus normal controls—Here they reviewed seven studies where life events were retrospectively assessed for periods of time from 3 to 12 months before admission, or before onset, relapse, or exacerbation of symptoms. The data were drawn from either structured interviews or checklists and 14 comparisons were available. In 5 of the 14 comparisons (36%), patients indicated significantly higher levels of stressors. None of the comparisons revealed higher stressors for the normal sample.

Life event stressors and symptoms within schizophrenia—Life stressors were assessed for (1) a period of time (3 weeks to 3 months) immediately before the worsening of symptoms, and (2) for the same people for comparison periods of time that did not immediately precede worsening of symptoms. Of the 30 comparisons relating level of stress to level of symptoms within groups of patients with schizophrenia, 23 (77%) yielded statistically significant findings of higher levels of antecedent life event stressors associated with time of worse symptoms. These findings are enhanced by the use of longitudinal design in three of the studies where the investigators assessed life stressors every 2 weeks over the course of a year; while another assessed stressor levels every month for a year.

Comparative results—In summary, this review shows that patients with schizophrenia were significantly higher in life stress in 36% of cases than normal controls; patients experiencing relapse experienced significantly higher levels of stress in 77% of cases than those not experiencing relapse; but there was no difference in the level of stressful life events for patients with schizophrenia versus patients with other diagnoses. It would seem that any rationale for expecting to find a significant difference between schizophrenia patients and patients with other diagnoses in their level of stress is problematic.

Although this review provides insight into the contribution of stress to mental ill-health, the authors caution that a wide range of assessment instruments and times were used in the various studies; there was no standard diagnostic criteria: DSM-1 through to DSM-111, also ICD or Kraepelinian criteria, all with their respective degrees of diagnostic stringency; and almost all studies included patients receiving medication. The exception to this last was Leff et al. (1973), whose findings, in conjunction with those of Birley and Brown (1970), suggest that patients without maintenance medication may be more likely to show worsening symptoms without major life events. It may be that medication protects against the neurochemistry of schizophrenia but cannot mediate against stressful life events. It may also be that patients with schizophrenia have fewer resources to successfully negotiate the demands posed by stressors, regardless of whether these resources are described in social, psychological, or neurological terms (e.g., Weinberger, 1987).

Vulnerability and mediators

Stress is clearly involved in the arousal of the sympathetic nervous system, preparing us for the "fight-or-flight" syndrome (Cannon, 1929), but it is important to understand that arousal only occurs if the event is perceived as a danger or a threat. The role of individual perceptions with regard to life events may partially explain why some people succumb to psychological distress more than others. The work of Beck, Ellis, and, in this area in particular, Endler, should be consulted for a full account of cognitive influences.

Although not clearly delineated, some researchers have suggested that genetic and biological factors are implicated in a vulnerability-stress or diathesis-stress model which increases the probability of mental disorder following significant stress for those persons (e.g., Norman and Malla, 1993b). Power and Champion (1986) posit a cognitive vulnerability. They suggest that some people may obtain much of their self-esteem from one, or few, areas of life and if this overinvested role is threatened or lost, the person is vulnerable to mental distress.

Conversely, Pearlin and co-workers (1981) showed that factors such as self-esteem, economic status, and a steady relationship, are influential in reducing the risks of depression. Kobasa et al. (1982) have even suggested a personality profile of those hardy to stress: control, committment, and challenge. It is interesting to observe that "challenge" can be viewed as the positive perception of "threat".

Conclusion

There is a considerable body of evidence to support the concept that stress, in the form of life events or demands upon the organism, is associated with impoverished mental health. The wide acceptance of this in severe forms is seen by the inclusion of PTSD and ASD in the DSM-1V (APA, 1994). It is also clear that not all people experiencing stress are moderately to severely affected. Factors such as social support, healthy lifestyle including diet and exercise, and a positive cognitive approach are all important in maintaining mental health.

Future researchers will need to continue investigations into the biological, environmental, and personal factors that mediate stress and its affects, for: "Medication [alone] cannot change aspects of the patient's environment which may be a source of anxiety" (Norman et al., 1988, p.366), rather, we must do it for ourselves and for others.

References

American Psychiatric Association (APA). (1952). *Diagnostic and Statistical Manual: Mental Disorders*. Washington, DC: APA.

American Psychiatric Association (APA). (1968). *Diagnostic and Statistical Manual of Mental Disorders* (2nd ed.). Washington, DC: APA.

American Psychiatric Association (APA). (1987). *Diagnostic and Statistical Manual of Mental Disorders* (3rd, rev. ed.). Washington, DC: APA.

American Psychiatric Association (APA). (1994). *Diagnostic and Statistical Manual of Mental Disorders* (4th ed.). Washington, DC: APA.

Apfeldorf, W. J., Shear, M. K., Leon, A. C., and Portera, L. (1994). A brief screen for panic disorder. *J. Anxiety Disorders*, 8, 71–78.

Birley, J. L. T. and Brown, G. W. (1970). Crisis and life changes preceding the onset or relapse of acute schizophrenia: clinical aspects. *Br. J. Psychiatry*, 116, 327–333.

Brown, G. W. (1993). Life events and affective disorders: replications and limitations. *Psychosom. Med.*, 55, 248–259.

Brown, G. W. and Birley, J. L. T. (1968). Crisis and life changes and the onset of schizophrenia. *J. Health Soc. Behav.*, 9, 203–214.

Brown, G. W. and Harris, T. (1978). *Social Origins of Depression: A Study of Psychiatric Disorders in Women*. London: Tavistock Publications.

Buchsbaum, M. S. (1990). Frontal lobes, basal ganglia, temporal lobes—three sites for schizophrenia? *Schizophrenia Bull.*, 16, 377–378.

Burrows, G. D. and Davies, B. (1984). Recognition and management of anxiety. In G. D. Burrows, T. R. Norman, and B. Davies (Eds.), *Antianxiety Agents*. pp. 1–11. Amsterdam: Elsevier Science Publishers.

Cannon, W. B. (1929). *Body Changes in Pain, Hunger, Fear and Rage*. (2nd ed.). New York: Appleton.

Clark, D. M. (1986). A cognitive approach to panic. *Behav. Res. Ther.*, 24, 461–470.

Coyne, J. and Holyroyd, K. (1982). Stress, coping, and illness: a transactional perspective. In T. Millon, C. Green, and R. Meagher (Eds.). *Handbook of Clinical Health Psychology*. pp. 103–127. New York: Plenum.

Davidson, L. M. and Baum, A. (1986). Chronic stress and posttraumatic stress disorders. *J. Consult. Clin. Psychol.*, 54, 303–308.

Deadman, J. M., Dewey, M. J., Owens, R. G., Leinster, S. J., and Slade, P. D. (1989). Threat and loss in breast cancer. *Psychol. Med.*, 19, 677–681.

Dohrenwend, B. S. and Dohrenwend, B. P. (Eds.). (1981). *Stressful Life Events and Their Contexts*. New York: Rutgers University Press.

Donohoe, T. P. (1984). Stress-induced anorexia: implications for anorexia nervosa. *Life Sci.*, 34, 203–218.

Endler, N. S. and Parker, J. D. A. (1990). Stress and anxiety: conceptual and assessment issues. *Stress Med.*, 6, 243–248.

Endler, N. S., Hunt, J. McV., and Rosenstein, A. J. (1962). An S-R inventory of anxiousness. *Psychol. Monogr.*, 76 (17, Whole No. 536), 1–31.

Fava, M., Rosenbaum, J. F., McCarthy, M., Pava, J. A., Steingard, R., and Fox, R. (1992). Correlations between perceived stress and depressive symptoms among depressive outpatients. *Stress Med.*, 8, 73–76.

Findlay-Jones, R. A. and Brown, G. W. (1981). Types of stressful life event and the onset of anxiety and depressive disorders. *Pychol. Med.*, 11, 803–815.

Friedman, S. and Chernen, L. (1994). Discriminating the panic disorder patient from patients with borderline personality disorder. *J. Anxiety Disorders*, 8, 49–61.

Gersons, B. P. R. and Carlier, I. V. E. (1992). Post-traumatic stress disorder: the history of a recent concept. *Br. J. Psychiatry*, 161, 742–748.

Gottesman, I. I., McGuffin, P., and Farmer, A. E. (1987). Clinical genetics as clues to the "real" genetics of schizophrenia. *Schizophrenia Bull.*, 13, 23–47.

Hathaway, S. R. and McKinley, J. C. (1970). *Minnesota Multiphasic Personality Inventory, Revised*. Minneapolis, MN: University of Minnesota.

Hawkins, W. E., Hawkins, M. J., and Seeley, J. (1992). Stress, health-related behavior and quality of life on depressive symptomatology in a sample of adolescents. *Psychol. Rep.*, 71, 183–186.

Holmes, T. H. and Rahe, R. H. (1967). The Social Readjustment Rating Scale. *J. Psychosom. Res.*, 11, 213–218.

Kahn, J. P., Gross, M. J., Mejean, L., Burlet, C., and Laxenaire, M. (1992). Could stress help understand the pathophysiology of anorexia nervosa? *Stress Med.*, 8, 199–205.

Kobasa, S. C., Maddi, S. R., and Kahn, S. (1982). Hardiness and health: a prospective study. *J. Personality Soc. Psychol.*, 42, 168–177.

Krahn, D. D., Morley, J. E., and Levine, A. S. (1987). In P. J. V. Beumont, G. D. Burrows, and R. C. Casper (Eds.), *Handbook of Eating Disorders, Part 1. Anorexia and Bulimia Nervosa*. pp.23–43. Amsterdam: Elsevier.

Laraia, M. T., Stuart, G. W., Frye, L. H., Lydiard, R. B., and Ballenger, J. C. (1994). Childhood environment of women having panic disorder with agoraphobia. *J. Anxiety Disorders*, 8, 1–17.

Lazarus, R. S. (1966). *Patterns of Adjustment* (3rd ed.). New York: McGraw Hill.

Lazarus, R. S. and Folkman, S. (1984). *Stress, Appraisal, and Coping*. New York: Springer.

Leff, J. and Vaughn, C. (1980). The interaction of life events and relatives' expressed emotion in schizophrenia and depressive neurosis. *Br. J. Psychiatry*, 136, 146–153.

Leff, J., Hirsch, S., and Gaind, R. (1973). Life events and maintenance therapy in schizophrenic relapse. *Br. J. Psychiatry*, 123, 659–660.

McGrath, J. E. (1970). *Social and Psychological Factors in Stress*. New York: Holt, Reinhart & Winston.

Meltzer, H. Y. (1987). Biological studies in schizophrenia. *Schizophrenia Bull.*, 13, 77–111.

Moore, K. A. (1994). The effect of exercise on body image, self-esteem and mood. *Mental Health Aust.*, 5, 38–41.

Moore, K., Dalziel, J., and Burrows, G. D. (1992). Stress: how to define and challenge it. *J. Mental Health Found.*, 3(4), 33–40.

Norman, R. M. G. and Malla, A. K. (1993a). Stressful life events and schizophrenia. I. A review of the research. *Br. J. Psychiatry*, 162, 161–166.

Norman, R. M. G. and Malla, A. K. (1993b). Stressful life events and schizophrenia. II. Conceptual and methodological issues. *Br. J. Psychiatry*, 162, 166–174.

Norman, T. R., Judd, F. K., Marriott, P. F., and Burrows, G. D. (1988). Physical treatment of anxiety: the benzodiazepines. In M. Roth, R. Noyes, Jr., and G. D. Burrows (Eds.), *Handbook of Anxiety, Vol. 1. Biological, Clinical and Cultural Perspectives*. pp.355–384. Amsterdam: Elsevier Science Publishers.

Nuechterlein, K. H., Dawson, M. E., Gitlin, M., Ventura, J., Goldstein, M. J., Snyder, K. S., Yee, C. M., and Mintz, J. (1992). Developmental processes in schizo-phrenic disorders: longitudinal studies of vulnerability and stress. *Schizophrenia Bull.*, 18, 387–424.

Parkes, K. R. (1992). Mental health in the oil industry: a comparative study of on-shore and offshore employees. *Psychol. Med.*, 22, 997–1009.

Paykel, E. S., Myers, J. K., Dienelt, M. N., Klerman, G. L., Lindenthal, J. J., and Pepper, M. P. (1969). Life events and depression: a controlled study. *Arch. Gen. Psychiatry*, 21, 753–760.

Paykel, E. S., Prusoff, B. A., and Uhlenhuth, E. H. (1971). Scaling of life events. *Arch. Gen. Psychiatry*, 25, 340–347.

Pearlin, L. I., Lieberman, M. A., Menaghan, E. G., and Mullan, J. T. (1981). The stress process. *J. Health Soc. Behav.*, 22, 337–356.

Power, M. J. and Champion, L. A. (1986). Cognitive approaches to depression: a theoretical critique. *Br. J. Clin. Psychol.*, 25, 201–212.

Rabkin, J. G. and Struening, E. L. (1976). Life events, stress, and illness. *Science*, 194, 1031–1040.

Sapolsky, R. M., Krey, L. C., and McEwen, B. S. (1986). The neuroendocrinology of stress and ageing: the glucocorticoid cascade hypothesis. *Endocrinol. Rev.*, 7, 284–301.

Schwabe, A. D., Lippe, B. M., Chang, R. J., Pops, M. A., and Yager, J. (1981). Anorexia nervosa. *Ann. Intern. Med.*, 94, 371–381.

Selye, H. (1982). History and present status of the stress concept. In L. Goldberger and S. Breznitz (Eds.), *Handbook of Stress: Theoretical and Clinical Aspects.* pp.7–17. New York: The Free Press.

Sikes, C. R., Stokes, P. E., and Lasley, B. J. (1989). Cognitive sequelae of hypothala-mic-pituitary-adrenal (HPA) dysregulation in depression (abstract). *Biol. Psychiatry*, 25, 148A–149A.

Spielberger, C. D. (1976). The nature and measurement of anxiety. In C. D. Spielberger and R. Diaz-Guerrero (Eds.), *Cross Cultural Anxiety*, pp 237–250. New York: Wiley.

Stuart, G. W., Laraia, M. T., Ballenger, J. C., and Lydiard, R. B. (1990). Early family experiences of women with bulimina and depression. *Arch. Psychiatric Nurs.*, 4, 43–52.

Torgerson, S. (1988). Genetic. In C. G. Last and M. Hersen (Eds.), *Handbook of Anxiety Disorders.* pp. 159–170. New York: Pergamon Press.

Vinokur, A. and Selzer, M. L. (1975). Desirable versus undesirable life events: their relationship to stress and mental distress. *J. Personality Soc. Psychol.*, 2, 329–337.

Weinberger, D. R. (1987). Implications of normal brain development for the patho-genesis of schizophrenia. *Arch. Gen. Psychiatry*, 44, 660–669.

Yehuda, R., Resnick, H., Kahana, B., and Giller, E. L. (1993). Long-lasting hormonal alterations to extreme stress in humans: normative or maladaptive? *Psychosom. Med.*, 55, 287–297.

Young, E. A. and Akin, H. (1985). Corticotropin releasing factor stimulation of adreno-corticotropin and beta-endorphin release: effects of acute and chronic stress. *Endrocrinology*, 117, 23–30.

chapter five

Stress, burnout, and health

Ronald J. Burke and Astrid M. Richardsen

Introduction

The concepts of stress and burnout are closely related. Burnout has been associated with a variety of job stressors, and recent writing on burnout reflects attempts to integrate burnout into larger conceptual frameworks, such as general stress theory (Hobfoll and Freedy, 1993) and occupational stress theory (Cox et al., 1993). The broadest definitions (Freudenberger and Richelson, 1980) equate burnout with stress, connect burnout with a long list of adverse health and well-being variables, and suggest it is caused by the relentless pursuit of success. Other definitions are narrower, relating burnout to human service professions with interpersonal stress as its cause (Maslach and Jackson, 1981). Burnout appears to be a unique type of stress syndrome that can be distinguished from other forms of stress (Cordes and Dougherty, 1993). There is little agreement among consultants, clinicians, researchers, managers, and administrators about what burnout is and, consequently, our understanding of the concept, what produces it and what results from it, is still far from complete (Maslach, 1982). There is a need to clarify the position of burnout in a network of variables included in the study of organizational behavior (Cordes and Dougherty, 1993).

This chapter reviews recent research on work stressors and burnout, and consequences of prolonged work stress. We also present some intervention studies in order to show that it is possible both to prevent and to alleviate burnout in professional workers. Burnout seems to be related to important individual, organizational, and client outcomes (Cherniss, 1980a; Maslach and Jackson, 1981). It may also be widespread; that is, it may be a large problem among helping professionals. Over the past 20 years our society has become increasingly professionalized, and a growing number of individuals are being helped by professionals. The latter include social workers, teachers, police officers, nurses, physicians, psychotherapists, counselors, psychiatrists, ministers, child care workers, mental health workers, prison personnel, legal services attorneys, psychiatric nurses, probation officers, and agency administrators, among others.

0-8493-2908-6/96/$0.00+$.50
© 1996 by CRC Press, Inc.

Thus, if these individuals are prone to burnout, it may be a widespread problem. Well-designed individual and organizationally based interventions to prevent prolonged job stress are in demand, and it is important to provide a framework within which interventions are both possible and effective.

Burnout can be considered prolonged job stress (Maslach and Schaufeli, 1993). In terms of Selye's definition of the stress process, i.e., alarm, resistance, and exhaustion, burnout may be likened to the third stage, exhaustion. Thus, burnout can be distinguished from stress in terms of time, since normally all three stages in Selye's model are considered stress. However, stress and burnout cannot be distinguished on the basis of symptoms, only in terms of process. Recent work presents how burnout has been clearly distinguished from other forms of stress, both conceptually and empirically (Cordes and Dougherty, 1993).

One of the challenges in burnout research is to integrate research findings into a coherent and comprehensive framework that consistently and reliably reflects the dynamics of the burnout process in a variety of work settings. A comprehensive model of burnout must incorporate various individual and organizational variables that constitute sources of stress and demands leading to the development of burnout, consequences of burnout in terms of personal, work-related, and organizational outcomes, and be able to provide a framework for multilevel interventions to alleviate burnout.

Relationships between job stressors and burnout

The stressors that contribute to burnout are generally well defined (Shinn, 1982). However, patterns of causality are difficult to determine, partly because studies have assessed variables at only one point in time, and partly because many of these variables are interdependent. Even when multivariate models are used, the results are ambiguous when the predictor variables are highly intercorrelated (Shinn, 1982). This creates problems at both theoretical and practical levels. The future of burnout research depends on the use of more sophisticated research designs to facilitate the development of comprehensive approaches (Kahill, 1988).

There are some major themes in different theories of what produces burnout and what results from it (Maslach, 1982, 1993; Maslach and Schaufeli, 1993). Most causal analyses have emphasized difficult interpersonal relationships at work, job demands, and characteristics of the organizational setting. There has been less emphasis on individual aspects (e.g., expectations, personality traits). However, recent studies suggest that the primary sources of burnout are related to both organizational conditions and personal characteristics of the helping professional (Burke et al., 1984; Dolan and Renaud, 1992; Richardsen et al., 1992; Schwab et al., 1986).

Organizational variables

Two different emphases have dominated the study of organizational variables related to burnout (Maslach and Jackson, 1984a). One focus has been the nature of the employee's personal relationship with clients. The second emphasis has been on the employee-organization relationship, studying feedback, control and role clarity, social support, and expectation.

Interpersonal relationships. Studies generally find that the more stressful the contact with clients is, the higher the burnout scores. According to Maslach (1978), client factors that may be stressful include type of client problems (e.g., the seriousness of illness, and the probability of change or cure); personal relevance of client problems (e.g., staff person may over-identify with client); the rules governing the staff-client relationship (both implicit and explicit); and client stance (e.g., being passive and dependent). In addition, negative feedback, complaints and criticisms, and anger and frustration from clients about the staff or the institution may be stressful for staff to hear. Other studies have found the same effects of client negativity in a number of populations outside the medical profession, e.g., teachers reacting to student misbehavior (Punch and Tuttleman, 1991).

Studies have also found negative effects stemming from interpersonal relationships with other colleagues. It seems that the nature of interaction with supervisors is related to a number of work stress measures, including burnout (Bacharach et al., 1990). Additional data have indicated that stress from conflicts between job and family responsibilities in managerial women was related to higher incidence of irritation, anxiety, and depression (Greenglass, 1985).

Job demands. Several measures of quantitative workload have been related to burnout. Leiter (1988b, 1991a, 1991b) has consistently found that work overload is significantly related to emotional exhaustion, but does not contribute to depersonalization or personal accomplishment. Similar findings have been reported by several other researchers (Jackson et al., 1986, 1987). Work overload may constitute the sheer number of clients seen, i.e., large caseloads (Jackson et al., 1986: Maslach and Jackson, 1984b), high workload demands with low decision latitude (Landsbergis, 1988); or just overall work stress (Friesen and Sarros, 1986; Kaufman and Beehr, 1989). Burnout scores are always higher in work settings characterized by overload.

Other organizational variables. Role conflict and role ambiguity have been identified as important contributors to the development of burnout (Schwab et al., 1986). Role conflict is the simultaneous occurrence of two or more sets of inconsistent, expected role behaviors (Farber, 1983) representing multiple sources of demand (Jackson et al., 1987). Role ambiguity is the lack of clear, consistent information regarding the rights, duties, and responsibilities of the job, and how these duties and responsibilities can best be performed. Studies have found that where high levels of role conflict are present, professionals experience high levels of emotional exhaustion and fatigue as well as negative attitudes toward recipients, but not a reduction in personal accomplishment (Friesen and Sarros, 1986; Jackson et al., 1987; Schwab and Iwanicki, 1982; Schwab et al., 1986).

Lack of control or autonomy in one's job may also contribute to burnout (Jackson, 1983; Pines et al., 1981; Schwab et al., 1986). In several studies, participation in decision making contributed significantly to depersonalization, but not to the other two burnout components (Jackson et al., 1987; Schwab et al., 1986). Autonomy in terms of job content was related to personal accomplishment among teachers (Jackson et al., 1986). However, Landsbergis (1988) found, among health care workers, that job decision latitude contributed to all three components of burnout. Jobs that combined high workload demands with low decision authority were associated with higher burnout and more job strain.

Lack of social support may lead to burnout (Pines et al., 1981; Leiter and Maslach, 1988). An effective support group includes people who can provide emotional comfort, confront people when behavior is inappropriate, provide technical support in work-related areas, encourage individual growth, serve as active listeners, and share similar values, beliefs, and perceptions of reality (Pines et al., 1981). Support may come from various sources, from administration, co-workers, or others outside the work environment. Social support in relation to burnout has focused on social support both at work from co-workers and supervisors, and social support outside of work, primarily from family.

Social support from colleagues, in the form of friendship and help, may be an important element in a worker's satisfaction with the job and experience of burnout. Interactions with co-workers may not always be supportive; however, sometimes interpersonal contacts at work are negative due to conflicts and disagreements among people (Leiter and Maslach, 1988). A number of studies have shown that lack of peer support is correlated with burnout (Burke et al., 1984; Dignam and West, 1988; Leiter, 1988a, 1991a; Ross et al., 1989). For example, Leiter (1991a) has consistently found that workers who are experiencing emotional exhaustion are more likely to depersonalize perceptions of clients or diminish feelings of accomplishment if they lack supportive relationships with co-workers as well as with their immediate supervisors.

There is evidence that social support has a direct effect on burnout (Cummins, 1990; Jayaratne et al., 1988; Ross et al., 1989), rather than functioning as a buffer or a moderating variable between job stressors and work strain such as burnout (Fusilier et al., 1987; Russell et al., 1987), i.e., lack of supportive relationships contributes directly to higher burnout. However, the existence of support may help the worker cope with stress and burnout better. Social support was found to have important main effects in reducing the level of unmet-expectations stress and facilitating positive adjustment outcomes in newcomers to the nursing profession (Fisher, 1985).

The evidence for the role of extra-work supports in developing or alleviating burnout is not clear. Several studies have indicated that lack of home and family supports is associated with increased burnout in the helping professions (Burke et al., 1984; Leiter, 1990; Zedeck et al., 1988). However, other studies have found no relationships between burnout and family support or support from friends and relatives (Constable and Russell, 1986; Golembiewski et al., 1991). However, different measures were used to assess family supports and may have affected the results.

Individual and personality variables

There is general agreement that burnout-prone individuals are empathic, sensitive, dedicated, idealistic, and people-oriented, but also anxious, obsessional, overenthusiastic, and susceptible to overidentification with others (Cherniss, 1980b; Farber, 1983; Freudenberger and Richelson, 1980). Most researchers have emphasized the central role of work-related stresses in the etiology of burnout (Farber, 1983). However, several studies have found relationships between various personality characteristics and burnout. McCranie and Brandsma (1988) found that higher burnout scores among physicians were significantly correlated with a number of Minnesota Multiphasic Personality Inventory (MMPI) scales measuring low self-esteem, feelings of inadequacy, dysphoria, and obsessive worry, passivity, social anxiety, and withdrawal from others (Hathaway and McKinley, 1989). Studies have also found relationships between various stress outcomes and type A personality characteristics (Farber, 1983; Kirchmeyer, 1988), as well as hardiness and neuroticism (Hills and Norvell, 1991). Significant relationships have also been found between all the burnout scales and reports of anxiety (Gold and Michael, 1985; Morgan and Krehbiel, 1985). Some studies have indicated that a high anxiety trait may make a person more susceptible to burnout (Cherniss, 1980a; Goodman, 1991; Richardsen et al., 1992).

Consequences of burnout

Burnout has been linked to various work-related behaviors and attitudes, e.g., absenteeism, job turnover, reduced effort, and reduced job satisfaction (Pierce and Molloy, 1990; Schwab et al., 1986; Wolpin et al., 1991), as well as to several individual health variables, e.g., psychosomatic symptoms, lower quality of personal life (Burke et al., 1984b; Greller and Parsons, 1988; Schwab et al., 1986). It is important to establish the objective consequences of burnout for both individuals and organizations, in order to stimulate commitment to implementation and long-term evaluation of both individual coping efforts and organizational-level interventions.

Absenteeism—The evidence linking burnout to absenteeism is not consistent (Kahill, 1988). Several authors have found measures of burnout to be related to tardiness, frequency of breaks, and absenteeism (Maslach and Jackson, 1981; Pines et al., 1981; Schwab et al., 1986). However, the relationships rarely account for large amounts of variance in absenteeism (Lazaro et al., 1985). For example, emotional exhaustion accounted for only 3% of the variance in self-reported absence among teachers (Schwab et al., 1986). Other studies have found no relationship between absenteeism and burnout (Lazaro et al., 1985; Quattrochi-Tubin et al., 1982). For example, Lazaro et al. (1985) found that absenteeism was not correlated with any burnout measure after controlling for age and sex, which they concluded was surprising in light of previous research.

Turnover—Firth and Britton (1989) conducted a predictive study of absence and turnover among 106 nursing staff. Burnout measures, role ambiguity, and support from supervisor were assessed, then absence through sickness and job turnover were measured over the subsequent 2 years. Role ambiguity predicted frequency of short absences in the subsequent 12 months. Perceived lack of support predicted absences of more than 4 days, while emotional exhaustion predicted absences of more than 7 days, in the subsequent 12 months. Feelings of depersonalization were correlated with departure from the job during the subsequent 2 years. This indicates that absenteeism and turnover are related behaviors that may be influenced by different stressors in the work environment.

Work attitudes—It seems clear from the research evidence that burnout is associated with a number of work-related behaviors and attitudes, but studies have also shown that occupational burnout also influences workers' functioning outside work (Maslach and Jackson, 1986; Zedeck et al., 1988). For example, Wolpin et al. (1991) found that both negative work setting characteristics and marital dissatisfaction were associated with greater work stressors, which in turn were associated with increased burnout, which in turn resulted in decreased job satisfaction.

Health—Evidence indicates that burnout is related to poor health, e.g., fatigue and physical depletion or exhaustion, sleep difficulties, and specific somatic problems such as headaches, gastrointestinal disturbances, colds, and flu (Kahill, 1988). Burnout may also lead to health-related problems, e.g., insomnia, increased use of medications and alcohol. In a study of men and women in police work (Burke et al., 1984), individuals scoring higher on two burnout measures reported more psychosomatic symptoms (e.g., poor appetite, headaches, heart pains); more negative feeling states (e.g., anger, depression, insomnia); and less job satisfaction. High burnout scores were also related to lifestyle practices associated with poorer health (e.g., consuming alcohol, smoking), and tangible signs of poorer health (e.g., high blood pressure). Similar results have been found in other studies of police officers (Burke, 1987), and in several studies of teachers (Burke and Greenglass, 1989; Pierce and Molloy, 1990). In addition, burnout has been linked to a number of emotional symptoms, e.g., depression (Firth et al., 1987; Schonfeld, 1989), guilt (Pines et al., 1981), and anxiety and tension (Fimian and Cross, 1986; Gold and Michael, 1985; Morgan and Krehbiel, 1985). Chronic job stress may be more strongly related to psychological distress than episodic stressful events (Schonfeld, 1989, 1990). In a longitudinal study of teachers, Greenglass and Burke (1990) found that burnout contributed significantly to subsequent depression for both men and women.

Quality of life—Finally, there is evidence that burnout may affect workers' home life. All three burnout components contributed significantly to lowered quality of personal life among teachers (Schwab et al., 1986), although, combined, the three aspects accounted for only 12% of the variance. Among police officers, emotional exhaustion has been linked to coming home tense, anxious, and angry; complaining about work problems; and being more withdrawn at home (Jackson and Maslach, 1982). Studies have indicated that workers experiencing burnout are more likely to have unsatisfactory marriages (Burke and Greenglass, 1989; Jackson and Maslach, 1982), and that they indicate a greater negative impact of the job on home and family than workers who are not burned out (Burke, 1987; Burke et al., 1984; Zedeck et al., 1988).

Burnout as a process

The most commonly used definition of burnout has been proposed by Maslach (1978). Maslach (1982) with Jackson et al. (1986) defined burnout as a syndrome of emotional exhaustion, depersonalization, and reduced personal accomplishment that occurs among individuals who work with people in some capacity. Emotional exhaustion refers to feelings of being emotionally overextended and drained by one's contact with other people. Depersonalization refers to an unfeeling and callous response toward these people, who are usually the recipients of one's service or care. This feeling state is usually thought of as a coping mechanism to deal with emotional exhaustion. Reduced personal accomplishment refers to a decline in one's feeling of competence and successful achievement in one's work with people. Leiter and Maslach (1988) propose a developmental model in which emotional exhaustion develops first, then depersonalization and reduced personal accomplishment.

One of the advantages of viewing burnout as a process over time is that it allows us to track burnout's antecedents, particularly those features of the organization that contribute to the development of stress and then burnout. This has both theoretical and practical implications. By being able to specify more precisely those factors that contribute to burnout at a given point in time, we elaborate on the theoretical underpinnings of burnout and its development. From a practical perspective, it is of great value to the organization and its managers to be able to specify just what the causes of burnout are at a given time. Assuming that there is access to, and means of, implementing appropriate intervention procedures, it is possible not only to improve the worker's morale but also to prevent physical and emotional harm. In recent years, several developmental models viewing burnout as a process have been proposed and have generated research activity which has contributed to our knowledge.

Cherniss (1980b) defined burnout as a transactional process consisting of job stress, worker strain, and psychological accommodation. More specifically, the development of burnout was conceptualized as consisting of three stages. The first stage involves an imbalance between work demands and an individual's resources to deal with these demands (stress). The second stage, an immediate, short-term emotional response to this imbalance, is characterized by feelings of anxiety, tension, fatigue, and exhaustion (strain). The third stage of burnout is marked by a number of changes in attitude and behavior. These include a tendency to treat clients in a detached or mechanical fashion, or a cynical preoccupation with gratification of one's own needs (defensive coping). Burnout, then, is defined as a process in which workers disengage from their work in response to stress and strain experienced on the job. The process begins when the helper experiences stress and strain that cannot be alleviated through active problem-solving. The changes in attitude and behavior associated with burnout provide a psychological escape. Burnout occurs over time—it is a process—and represents one way of adapting to, or coping with, particular sources of stress. Two studies have provided considerable empirical support for the model (Burke et al., 1984; Burke and Greenglass, 1989). Correlations indicated that proposed work setting and stress antecedents were significantly correlated with a measure of negative attitude change (or burnout) proposed by Cherniss, and burnout was also found to be associated with undesirable personal and organizational outcomes.

Leiter (1989, 1991a,b) has proposed and researched a process model of burnout based on two assumptions. The first is that components of burnout influence one another over time, as proposed by Leiter and Maslach (1988), and the second is that the three components have distinct relationships with environmental conditions and individual difference characteristics (Leiter, 1991b). The model defines emotional exhaustion as a reaction to occupational stressors; the impact of these on various outcomes is mediated through emotional exhaustion. The principal stressors he has considered are work overload and conflict with people in the work setting. These will have impact on depersonalization, accomplishment, and other outcomes to the extent that they have an impact on emotional exhaustion. Effective skill utilization and coping efforts are proposed to have a buffering effect on exhaustion and personal accomplishment. Supervisor and co-worker support, positive client relationships, and autonomy are proposed to buffer other aspects of burnout.

Leiter found considerable support for his model in several studies. However, in some studies (Leiter, 1989, 1991a) the hypothesized direct link between depersonalization and personal accomplishment was not supported. This has been confirmed by recent work by Lee and Ashforth (1993). It seems that the relationship of personal accomplishment with the other two Maslach Burnout Inventory (MBI) subscales could be better explained by their shared association with other measures, especially social support (Leiter, 1991b).

Interventions to reduce burnout

Many researchers and workers have considered burnout a serious and pervasive work-force problem (Golembiewski, 1984). There is a growing awareness that stress is a costly problem, frequently associated with declining productivity and significant health consequences, yet reviews of the literature note that there are few scientific studies evaluating stress reduction and management procedures (Bruning and Frew, 1986; Farber, 1983; Matteson and Ivancevich, 1986). Farber (1983) also noted that efforts to formulate and validate treatment approaches to burnout have been hindered by factors such as the lack of clear distinctions between the concepts of stress and burnout, the lack of a commonly accepted etiological model, and the tendency to focus interventions on a limited number of variables.

Golembiewski's work, and that of others (e.g., Burke and Greenglass, 1991), have provided some indications of incidence and of stability of burnout scores. If such estimates of stability and persistence are valid, alleviating burnout through interventions may be a considerable but necessary challenge. Cherniss (1992) has argued that human service professionals *can* recover from early career burnout. Interestingly, he found that some of the conditions that helped these professionals recover from burnout were the same ones that helped to prevent burnout. These were new work situations that provided more autonomy, organizational support, and interesting work. In most cases these changes came about through turnover or promotion.

Over the years writers have suggested a number of interventions that can be used to reduce burnout in the workplace. Most of these interventions were aimed at reducing burnout at the source, i.e., changing the work environment in order to reduce the potential for burnout among workers. Specific examples include staff development and counseling (Cherniss, 1980b), increasing worker involvement and participation in decision making (Schwab et al., 1986), improving supervision through clarification of work goals (Maslach and Jackson, 1984b; Schwab et al., 1986), and facilitating the development of social support (Schwab et al., 1986), among others. Other studies have looked at individual coping efforts and styles and have attempted to evaluate the effects of these on stress reactions (Leiter, 1990; Parkes, 1990; Schonfeld, 1990).

Several studies have indicated the effectiveness of individual level interventions in reducing stress and burnout (Bruning and Frew, 1986; Golembiewski and Rountree, 1991; Higgins, 1986). Bruning and Frew (1986) evaluated three intervention strategies in a longitudinal study of supervisors, managers, engineers, and support personnel in a manufacturing facility. The strategies were cognitive skills training, relaxation/meditation training, and exercise training. Results indicated that four of seven attitudinal measures showed significant change due to treatments; these were self-esteem, satisfaction with supervisor, co-worker, and with promotion. Tests to determine if any treatment or treatments were superior in improving attitudes showed that improvements in self-esteem were apparent for all the treatment groups, and that the meditation/relaxation group showed the greatest improvements in the satisfaction measures. Higgins (1986) also found no significant differences between two treatment groups in a stress reduction program, but both treatment groups were significantly different from the control group. Emotional exhaustion and personal strain scores decreased significantly from pre- to post-test in both treatment groups, but both scores increased in the control group. The results from these studies suggest that relatively brief programs can produce significant reductions in self-reported stress, and also that improvements in attitudes may be directly related to broad-based stress intervention strategies in longitudinal field settings.

Other individual intervention strategies have also been successful in reducing burnout. Golembiewski and Rountree (1991) studied an intervention strategy derived from organization development theory, which consisted of an off-site training session combining group work and collaborating in pairs on how to build an ideal team. Results indicated a sharp shift in the burnout phase distribution of the participants, and reaction to supervision scores were significantly different between treatment and control groups after the intervention, but not prior to it. The authors concluded that the success rate of interaction-centered interventions was quite impressive, and suggested further use of regenerative interaction designs in ameliorating burnout.

The importance of organizational-level interventions aimed at environmental sources of professional and managerial stress, rather than individual-level interventions, emerges from a field experiment conducted by Ganster et al. (1982). They evaluated a stress management training program in a field experiment with 99 public agency employees randomly assigned to treatment and control groups. The training program consisted of 16 hours of training spread over 8 weeks. Treatment participants exhibited significantly lower epinephrine and depression levels than did controls at the post-test, and 4-month follow-up levels did not regress to initial pre-test levels. However, the treatment effects were not found in a subsequent intervention on the original control group.

Research conducted by Shinn and co-workers (1984) leads to similar conclusions. Coping efforts to reduce stressors and strain were assessed at three levels: by individual workers, by groups of workers to help one another (social support), and by their employing human service agencies. Although many more individual coping responses were mentioned than group or agency-initiated responses, only the group responses were associated with low levels of strain. Thus, it appears that in the work setting, individual coping responses may be less useful than higher-level strategies involving groups of workers or entire units or organizations. Other researchers (Leiter, 1991b) also conclude that chronic, organizationally generated stressors may be resistant to reduction through individual coping efforts.

Ivancevich and Matteson (1987) made the point that organization-based stress management intervention programs incorporating well-designed evaluations have rarely been undertaken. They (along with Murphy, 1987) offer suggestions for increasing researcher interest to scientifically designing, implementing, and evaluating organizational-level stress management intervention programs. Murphy (1988) found few well-designed evaluations of interventions aimed at reducing work stressors. Of those he identified, all were found to consistently show benefits. Yet stressor reduction represents the most direct way to reduce stress, since it deals with the source (Golembiewski et al., 1987). This has been termed "primary prevention" in the stress management literature.

Conclusions

Burnout is a serious stress problem in many work settings. Efforts need to be devoted to exploring and understanding how to reduce stress levels in organizations (Kyriacou, 1987). In order to understand fully sources and consequences of burnout, and individual differences that may exist, we may have to include cognitive variables (e.g., Leiter, 1990, 1991a; Meier, 1983, 1984) such as how work environments are appraised, and how coping resources are assessed and used. Cherniss (1992) also suggests that researchers devote more attention to the problem of tedium. After a few years, much professional work becomes routine and predictable. What are some ways of alleviating the tedium that exists in professional workplaces? How can the workplace be kept vibrant?

The quantity of psychological burnout research has grown markedly in recent years, as has general interest in the subject. Yet in spite of this larger volume, our understanding of the burnout phenomenon remains limited. This results from the complexity of the burnout process itself, as well as a variety of dilemmas and ambiguities facing burnout researchers. The latter involve issues of definition, measurement, references from data collected at one point in time, small and often nonrepresentative samples, the absence of integrated models, and overly simplistic research design and data analysis approaches.

A continuing commitment to psychological burnout research will almost certainly be the case over the next decade. Burnout is now beginning to be examined in cross-cultural setting with findings consistent with those found previously in North America (Shirom, 1989; Richardsen et al., 1992). The magnitude and complexity of the problem warrants this attention and investment. The number of researchers now interested in psychological burnout has grown, as can be evidenced from recent publications in the area (Cordes and Dougherty, 1993; Schaufeli et al., 1993). Some advances in conceptualization have already taken place (Buunk and Schaufeli, 1993; Cherniss, 1980a; Cordes and Dougherty, 1993; Cox et al., 1993; Golembiewski and Munzenrider, 1988; Hobfoll and Freedy, 1993; Leiter 1991b). But much more systematic research is needed to elucidate the factors involved in the experience and manifestations of psychological burnout, and to test the theoretical propositions that have been proposed in recent works. It appears that increase in our understanding of psychological burnout will only come slowly.

Acknowledgment

Preparation of this manuscript was supported in part by the Faculty of Administrative Studies, York University and the Department of Psychology, University of Tromsø, Norway.

References

Bacharach, S. B., Bainberger, P., and Mitchell, S. (1990). Work design, role conflict, and role ambiguity: the case of elementary and secondary schools. *Educ. Evaluation Policy Anal.*, 12, 415–432.

Bruning, N. S. and Frew, D. R. (1986). Can stress intervention strategies improve self-esteem, manifest anxiety, and job satisfaction? A longitudinal field experiment. *J. Health Hum. Resources Admin.*, 9, 110–124.

Burke, R. J. (1987). Burnout in police work: an examination of the Cherniss model. *Group Organization Studies*, 12, 174–188.

Burke, R. J. and Greenglass, E. R. (1989). Psychological burnout among men and women in teaching: an examination of the Cherniss model. *Hum. Relations*, 42, 261–273.

Burke, R. J. and Greenglass, E. R. (1991). A longitudinal study of progressive phases of psychological burnout. *J. Health Hum. Resources Admin.*, 13, 390–408.

Burke, R. J., Shearer, J., and Deszca, G. (1984). Burnout among men and women in police work: an examination of the Cherniss model. *J. Health Hum. Resources Admin.*, 7, 162–188.

Buunk, B. P. and Schaufeli, W. B. (1993). Burnout: a perspective from social comparison theory. In W. B. Schaufeli, C. Maslach, and T. Marek (Eds.), *Professional Burnout: Recent Developments in Theory and Research.* (pp. 53–73). Washington, DC: Taylor and Francis.

Capel, S. A. (1991). A longitudinal study of burnout in teachers. *Br. J. of Educ. Psychol.*, 61, 36–45.

Cherniss, C. (1980a). *Professional Burnout in Human Service Organizations*. New York: Praeger.

Cherniss, C. (1980b). *Staff Burnout: Job Stress in the Human Services*. Beverly Hills, CA: Sage.

Cherniss, C. (1990). Natural recovery from burnout: results of a 10-year follow-up study. *J. Health Hum. Resources Admin.*, 13, 132–154.

Cherniss, C. (1992). Long-term consequences of burnout: an exploratory study. *J. of Organizational Behav.*, 13, 1–11.

Constable, J. F. and Russel, D. W. (1986). The effects of social support and the work environment upon burnout among nurses. *J. Hum. Stress*, 12, 20–26.

Cordes, C. L. and Dougherty, T. W. (1993). A review and an integration of research on job burnout. *Acad. of Manage. Rev.*, 18, 621–656.

Cox, T., Kuk, G., and Leiter, M. P. (1993). Burnout, health, work stress, and organizational healthiness. In W. B. Schaufeli, C. Maslach, and T. Marek (Eds.), *Professional Burnout: Recent Developments in Theory and Research*. (pp. 177–193). Washington, DC: Taylor and Francis.

Cummins, R. C. (1990). Job stress and the buffering effect of supervisory support. *Group Organization Studies*, 15, 92–104.

Dignam, J. T. and West, S. G. (1988). Social support in the workplace: tests of six theoretical models. *Am. J. Community Psychol.*, 16, 701–724.

Dolan, S. L. and Renaud, S. (1992). Individual, organizational and social determinants of managerial burnout: a multivariate approach. *J. Soc. Behav. Personality*, 7, 95–100.

Farber, B. A. (1983). Introduction: a critical perspective on burnout. In B. A. Farber (Ed.), *Stress and Burnout in the Human Service Professions*. (pp. 1–22). New York: Pergamon.

Fimian, M. J. and Cross, A. H. (1986). Stress and burnout among preadolescent and early adolescent gifted students: a preliminary investigation. *J. Early Adolescence*, 6, 247–267.

Firth, H. and Britton, P. (1989). Burnout; absence and turnover amongst British nursing staff. *J. Occup. Psychol.*, 62, 55–59.

Firth, H., McKeown, P., McIntee, J., and Britton, P. (1987). Professional depression, "burnout" and personality in longstay nursing. *Int. J. Nurs. Studies*, 24, 227–237.

Fisher, C. D. (1985). Social support and adjustment to work: a longitudinal study. *J. Manage.*, 11, 39–53.

Freudenberger, H. J. and Richelson, G. (1980). *Burn-Out: The High Cost of High Achievement*. New York: Anchor Press.

Friesen, D. and Sarros, J. (1986). Sources of burnout among educators. *J. Organizational Behav.*, 10, 179–188.

Fusilier, M. R., Ganster, D. C., and Mayes, B. T. (1987). Effects of social support, role stress; and locus of control on health. *J. Manage.*, 13, 517–528.

Ganster, D. C., Mayes, B. T., Sime, W. E., and Tharp, G. D. (1982). Managing occupational stress: a field experiment. *J. Appl. Psychol.*, 67, 533–542.

Gold, Y. and Michael, W. B. (1985). Academic self-concept correlates of potential burnout in a sample of first-semester elementary school practice teachers: a concurrent validity study. *Educ. Psychol. Meas.*, 45, 909–914.

Golembiewski, R. T. (1984). An orientation to psychological burnout: probably something old, definitely something new. *J. Health Hum. Resources Admin.*, 7, 153–161.

Golembiewski, R. T. and Munzenrider, R. F. (1988). *Phases of Burnout: Developments in Concepts and Applications.* New York: Praeger.

Golembiewski, R. T. and Rountree, B. (1991). Releasing human potential for collaboration: a social intervention targeting supervisory relationships and stress. *Public Admin. Q.*, 15, 32–45.

Golembiewski, R. T., Bower, D., and Kim, B. S. (1991). Family features, performance at work, and phases of burnout. Unpublished manuscript.

Golembiewski, R. T., Hilles, R., and Daly, R. (1987). Some effects of multiple OD interventions on burnout and work site features. *J. Appl. Behav. Sci.*, 23, 295–313.

Goodman, A. M. (1991). A model for police officer burnout. *J. Business Psychol.*, 5, 85–99.

Greenglass, E. R. (1985). Psychological implications of sex bias in the work place. *Acad. Psychol. Bull.*, 7, 227–240.

Greenglass, E. R. and Burke, R. J. (1990). Burnout over time. *J. Health Hum. Resources Admin.*, 13, 192–204.

Greller, M. and Parsons, C. K. (1988). Psychosomatic complaints scale of stress: measure development and psychometric properties. *Educ. Psychol. Meas.*, 48, 1051–1065.

Hathaway, S. R. and McKinley, J. C. (1989). *Minnesota Multiphasic Personality Inventory—2.* Minneapolis, MN: University of Minnesota.

Higgins, N. C. (1986). Occupational stress and working women: the effectiveness of two stress reduction programs. *J. Vocational Behav.*, 29, 66–78.

Hills, H. and Norvell, N. (1991). An examination of hardiness and neuroticism as potential moderators of stress outcomes. *Behav. Med.*, 19, 31–38.

Hobfoll, S. E. and Freedy, J. (1993). Conservation of resources: a general stress theory applied to burnout. In W. B. Schaufeli, C. Maslach, and T. Marek (Eds.), *Professional Burnout: Recent Developments in Theory and Research.* (pp. 115–129). Washington, DC: Taylor and Francis.

Ivancevich, J. M. and Matteson, M. T. (1987). Organizational level stress management interventions: a review and recommendations. In J. M. Ivancevich and D. C. Ganster, (Eds.), *Job Stress: From Theory to Suggestion.* (pp. 229–248). New York: Howarth Press.

Jackson, S. E. (1983). Participation in decision making as a strategy for reducing job-related strain. *J. Appl. Psychol.*, 68, 3–19.

Jackson, S. E. and Maslach, C. (1982). After-effects of job related stress: families as victims. *J. Occup. Behav.*, 3, 63–77.

Jackson, S. E., Schwab, R. L., and Schuler, R. S. (1986). Toward an understanding of the burnout phenomenon. *J. Appl. Psychol.*, 71, 630–640.

Jackson, S. E., Turner, J. A., and Brief, A. P. (1987). Correlates of burnout among public service lawyers. *J. Occup. Behav.*, 8, 39–49.

Jayaratne, S., Himle, D., and Chess, W. A. (1988). Dealing with work stress and strain: is the perception of support more important than its use? *J. Appl. Behav. Sci.*, 24, 191–202.

Kahill, S. (1988). Symptoms of professional burnout: a review of the empirical evidence. *Can. Psychol.*, 29, 284–297.

Kaufman, G. M. and Beehr, T. A. (1989). Occupational stressors, individual strains, and social supports among police officers. *Hum. Relations*, 42, 185–197.

Kirchmeyer, S. L. (1988). Coping with competing demands: interruption and the type A pattern. *J. Appl. Psychol.*, 73, 621–629.

Kyriacou, C. (1987). Teacher stress and burnout: an international review. *Educ. Res.*, 29, 146–152.

Landsbergis, P. (1988). Occupational stress among health care workers: a test of the job demands control model. *J. Appl. Behav. Sci.*, 25, 131–144.

Lazaro, L., Shinn, M., and Robinson, P. E. (1985). Burnout, performance, and job withdrawal behavior. *J. Health Hum. Resources Admin.*, 7, 213–234.

Lee, R. T. and Ashforth, B. E. (1993). A longitudinal study of burnout among supervisors and managers: comparisons between the Leiter and Maslach (1988) and Golembiewski et al. (1986) models. *Organizational Behavior and Human Decision Processes*, 54, 241–256.

Leiter, M. P. (1988a). Burnout as a function of communication patterns. A study of multidisciplinary mental health team. *Group Organization Studies*, 13, 111–128.

Leiter, M. P. (1988b). Commitment as a function of stress reactions among nurses: a model of psychological evaluations of work settings. *Can. J. Community Mental Health*, 7, 115–132.

Leiter, M. P. (1989). Conceptual implications of two models of burnout: a response to Golembiewski. *Group Organization Studies*, 14, 15–22.

Leiter, M. P. (1990). The impact of family resources, control coping, and skill utilization on the development of burnout: a longitudinal study. *Hum. Relations*, 43, 1067–1083.

Leiter, M. P. (1991a). Coping patterns as predictors of burnout: the function of control and escapist coping. *J. Occup. Behav.*, 12, 123–144.

Leiter, M. P. (1991b). The dream denied: professional burnout and the constraints of human service organizations. *Can. Psychol.*, 32, 547–555.

Leiter, M. P. and Maslach, C. (1988). The impact of interpersonal environment on burnout and organizational commitment. *J. Occup. Behav.*, 9, 297–308.

Maslach, C. (1978). The client role in staff burnout. *J. Soc. Issues*, 34, 111–124.

Maslach C. (1982). Understanding burnout: definitional issues in analyzing a complex phenomenon. In W. S. Paine (Ed.), *Job Stress and Burnout: Research, Theory and Intervention Perspectives*, (pp. 29–40). Beverly Hills, CA: Sage.

Maslach, C. (1993). Burnout: a multidimensional perspective. In W. B. Schaufeli, C. Maslach, and T. Marek (Eds.), *Professional Burnout: Recent Developments in Theory and Research.* (pp. 19–42). Washington, DC: Taylor and Francis.

Maslach, C. and Jackson, S. (1981). The measurement of experienced burnout. *J. Occup. Behav.*, 2, 99–115.

Maslach, C. and Jackson, S. E. (1984a). Burnout in organizational settings. In S. Oskamp (Ed.), *Applied Social Psychology Annual*, Vol. 5. pp. 133–153. Beverly Hills, CA: Sage.

Maslach, C. and Jackson, S. E. (1984b). Patterns of burnout among a national sample of public contact workers. *J. Health Hum. Resource Admin.*, 7, 189–212.

Maslach, C. and Jackson, S. E. (1986). *Maslach Burnout Inventory Manual* (2nd ed.). Palo Alto, CA: Consulting Psychologists Press, Inc.

Maslach, C. and Schaufeli, W. B. (1993). Historical and conceptual development of burnout. In W. B. Schaufeli, C. Maslach, and T. Marek (Eds.), *Professional Burnout: Recent Developments in Theory and Research.* (pp. 1–17). Washington, DC: Taylor and Francis.

Matteson, M. T. and Ivancevich, J. M. (1986). An exploratory investigation of CES as an employee stress management procedure. *J. Health Hum. Resource Admin.*, 9, 93–109.

McCranie, E. W. and Brandsma, J. M. (1988). Personality antecedents of burnout among middle-aged physicians. *Behav. Med.*, 36, 889–910.

Meier, S. T. (1983). Toward a theory of burnout. *Hum. Relations*, 36, 899–910.

Meier, S. T. (1984). The construct validity of burnout. *J. Occup. Psychol.*, 57, 211–219.

Morgan, S. R. and Krehbiel, R. (1985). The psychological condition of burned-out teachers with a nonhumanistic orientation. *J. Hum. Educ. Dev.*, 24, 59–67.

Murphy, L. R. (1987). A review of organizational stress management research: methodological considerations. In J. M. Ivancevich and D. C. Ganster (Eds.), *Job Stress: From Theory to Suggestion*, (pp. 215–227). Howarth Press, New York.

Murphy, L. R. (1988). Workplace interventions for stress reduction and prevention. In C. L. Cooper and R. Payne (Eds.), *Causes, Coping and Consequences of Stress at Work.* (pp. 301–339). New York, Wiley.

Parkes, K. R. (1990). Coping, negative affectivity, and the work environment: additive and interactive predictors of mental health. *J. Appl. Psychol.*, 75, 399–409.

Pierce, C. M. B. and Molloy, G. N. (1990). Psychological and biographical differences between secondary school teachers experiencing high and low levels of burnout. *Br. J. Educ. Psychol.*, 60, 37–51.

Pines, A., Aronson, E., and Kafry, D. (1981). *Burnout: From Tedium to Personal Growth.* New York: The Free Press.

Punch, K. F. and Tuttlemann, E. (1991). Stressful factors and the likelihood of psychological distress among classroom teachers. *Educ. Res.*, 33, 65–69.

Quattrochi-Tubin, S., Jones, J. W., and Breedlove, V. (1982). The burnout syndrome in geriatric counselors and service workers. *Activities Adaptation Aging*, 3, 65–76.

Richardsen, A. M., Burke, R. J., and Leiter, M. P. (1992). Occupational demands, psychological burnout and anxiety among hospital personnel in Norway. *Anxiety, Stress Coping*, 5, 55–68.

Ross, R. R., Altmaier, E. M., and Russel, D. W. (1989). Job stress, social support, and burnout among counseling center staff. *J. Counseling Psychol.*, 36, 464–470.

Russell, D. W., Altmaier, E., and van Velzen, D. (1987). Job-related stress, social support, and burnout among classroom teachers. *J. Appl. Psychol.*, 72, 269–274.

Schaufeli, W. B., Maslach, C., and Marek, T. (1993). The future of burnout. In W. B. Schaufeli, C. Maslach, and T. Marek (Eds.), *Professional Burnout: Recent Developments in Theory and Research.* (pp. 253–260). Washington, DC: Taylor and Francis.

Schonfeld, I. S. (1989). Psychological distress in a sample of teachers. *J. Psychol.*, 124, 321–338.

Schonfeld, I. S. (1990). Coping with job-related stress: the case of teachers. *J. Occup. Psychol.*, 63, 141–149.

Schwab, R. L. and Iwanicki, E. F. (1982). Perceived role conflict, role ambiguity and teacher burnout. *Educ. Admin. Q.*, 18, 60–74.

Schwab, R. L., Jackson, S. E., and Schuler, R. S. (1986). Educator burnout: sources and consequences. *Educ. Res. Q.*, 10, 15–30.

Selye, H. (1956). *The Stress of Life.* New York: McGraw Hill.

Shinn, M. (1982). Methodological issues: evaluating and using information. In W. S. Paine (Ed.), *Job Stress and Burnout: Research, Theory and Intervention Perspectives.* (pp. 61–82). Beverly Hills, CA: Sage.

Shinn, M., Rosario, M., March, H., and Chestnut, D. E. (1984). Coping with job stress and burnout in the human services. *J. Personality Soc. Psychol.*, 46, 864–876.

Shirom, A. (1989). Burnout in work organizations. In C. L. Cooper and I. T. Robertson (Eds.), *International Review of Industrial and Organizational Psychology*, (pp. 25–48). New York: Wiley.

Wade, D. C., Cooley, E., and Savicki, V. (1986). A longitudinal study of burnout. *Child. Youth Services Rev.*, 8, 161–173.

Wolpin, J., Burke, R. J., and Greenglass, E. R. (1991). Is job satisfaction an antecedent or a consequence of psychological burnout? *Hum. Relations*, 44, 193–209.

Zedeck, S., Maslach, C., Mosier, K., and Skitka, L. (1988). Affective response to work and quality of family life: employee and spouse perspectives. In E. Goldsmith (Ed.), Work and Family: Theory, Research, and Applications [Special Issue]. *J. Soc. Behav. Personality*, 3, 135–157.

Section 2

Life events, stress, and illness

chapter six

Life stress, personal control, and the risk of disease

Shirley Fisher

Introduction

The notion that there is a relationship between life stresses and the risk of disease has been an implicit part of folklore and psychosomatic medicine for a considerable time. Burton (1977) noted a number of precipitants for depression, which included loneliness, poverty, and difficult marital states. Later, similar observations by Holmes and Rahe (1967) led to the suggestion that life stress experiences might play a role in physical disease.

Wyler and co-workers (1971) assigned values representing seriousness of 42 diseases in 232 patients. The correlation with magnitude of life change in the preceding 2 years was .648 for chronic disease. However, no significant relationship was found with infectious disease of acute onset. The data suggested that constant adaptive requirement lowers the threshold to chronic disease. Life change was argued to be relevant to causation time of onset and severity of disease.

Holmes and Rahe tested the hypothesis by developing a questionnaire, the schedule of recent experiences (SRE), which catalogued self-reported life events and provided a quantitative index of the level of impact caused by particular life stresses. The resulting scale provided an index of life change units (LCUs). It was found that high cumulative scores across a period of time raised the risk of disease. However, predictions concerning specific forms of illness were found to be unreliable, and it is argued that predictive power for chronic disease is low (see Connolly, 1975).

Retrospective studies (e.g., Holmes and Rahe, 1967) showed that there was an increase in LCUs in the first 2 years prior to illness. Studies suggested that below LCU values of 150, there was no reason to expect ill health; between 150 and 300 LCU, approximately half the individuals reported an illness in the following year. For 300 LCU the risk was 70%. A later study involving 2500 U.S. Navy officers (see Rahe, 1972) identified a buildup of LCUs prior to illness.

0-8493-2908-6/96/$0.00+$.50

Dohrenwend et al. (1978) emphasized some of the methodological difficulties in independently assessing life events and argued that life events could be categorized into three aspects. There were life events confounded with general distress and maladjustment and those that were confounded with existing psychological problems. Research that confounds these factors weakens the possibility of obtaining valid associations. There are a number of related issues: the time of onset of physical illness may be unknown and it may be cause or consequence of a critical life event. Thus, the time locking of life events and illness remains a major problem. Even if the causal association could be established, the interpretation is difficult. For example, more car drivers wearing seat belts are involved in car accidents, but this should not be taken to imply that wearing seat belts causes car accidents.

More recent research by Rahe (1989) demonstrated that in the case of sudden cardiac death the cumulative life events score for the previous 3 years was high. Life change units predicted both prospectively and retrospectively the risk of cardiac death.

Epidemiological evidence

Figure 1 (Fisher, 1984) illustrates a selection of epidemiological data on the role of gender and marital status in morbidity and mortality. The data indicate that females have better health expectancies than males. The role of genetic as well as lifestyle factors may be important.

The data provide considerable emphasis on the role of psychological status and disease. They indicate that those who are single or divorced have a greater risk of poor health, relative to married aged-matched controls. This is especially true for males. These findings underline the importance of psychological factors in mediating disease, but the reasons remain equivocal. One possibility is self-selection into marriage; perhaps the physically robust individuals have a better chance of selecting the right partner or surviving the rigors of marriage. A second possibility is that female partners offer in marriage the social support that reduces life stress on males.

Migration and health

Detailed insight into the impact of life events on individuals has been produced by research concerned with major moves either away from home or of the complete home. The research also provides some indication of vulnerability factors.

In historical perspective, studies on relocation and migration have provided strong indications of relationships with poor mental and physical health. The difficulty of attributing causation remains important; although there is a tendency to attribute the causes of ill health to the geographical transition, self-selection factors may be operative: those who move away

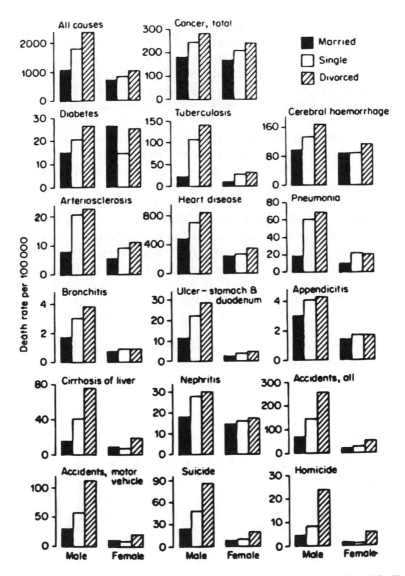

Figure 1 Standardized death rates for different causes of death in the U.S. (From Fisher, S., *Handbook of Life Stress Cognition and Health*, Reason, J., Ed., John Wiley & Sons, Ltd., Chichester, U.K., 1989. With permission.)

may be poor or discontented with a previous environment, or may relish the excitement of moving.

A number of early studies focused on the health of migrant communities as compared with that of the indigenous population. For example, Odegaard (1932) reported greater rates of hospital admissions for mental disorder among Norwegian immigrants to Minnesota than for either the native-born of Minnesota or Norway. Malzberg and Lee (1940) reported a similar result for populations in New York when age, color, and sex were taken into account. These studies, although not devoid of the above-stated methodological difficulties, point to the vulnerability of the migrant group. The reasons for the effect remain unclear; there may have been exposure to adverse environments, mediating behaviors may increase the risk of ill health, general poverty factors may weaken resources through poor nutrition, etc.

There is also evidence that moves within a country may also affect the risk of mental disorder. Kleiner and Parker (1963) demonstrated the prevalence of psychoneurotic and psychosomatic symptoms in native-born Americans migrating within the U.S.

The most quoted work that focuses on the confounding of circumstantial factors with the effects of mobility, is that of Faris and Dunham (1939) who, using home ownership as an index of stability and rental status as an index of mobility in the city of Chicago, found a negative association with mobility and mental health. However, since the mobile areas of cities were also most socially disorganized and associated with poverty, the effect of general living stress could not be ruled out. Also, those with poor mental health may become incompetent and drift down to ghetto areas of cities.

The studies underline the close association with poverty, social class, and lack of educational and social mobility in such cases. Thus, moves may reflect or create underlying conditions associated with psychopathology, and are inextricably linked.

Specific response to moves

Work by Fried (1963) was useful in establishing that there are effects in the detail of activity following moves that might raise the risk of psychopathology. Fried was concerned with relocation to new and better housing within the city, so the impact should be less devastating than a geographical move or migration. Nevertheless, the impact on individuals was very high. Fried classified the reaction as a "grief like" response. Parts of the former home were revisited and many remaining objects acquired a symbolic significance in the minds of the previous occupants. Status defined by occupational, situational, or personal factors was a major factor in adjustment.

An interesting outcome of a longitudinal study on the effects of relocation by Stokols and colleagues (1983) was an indication that, even though mobility might be the fashion for a vigorous, modern economic nation, moving may have negative implications. The study involved 242 adult employees, 121 of whom completed a follow-up study of emotional and physical well-being 3 months after a move to a new job in a new location. The authors obtained self-report data on mobility history and reported that frequent relocation was associated with a greater number of illness-related symptoms and reduced satisfaction. The study indicated the adverse effect of moves on those with "low exploratory tendency", described in terms of lack of exploration of various aspects of the psychosocial environment.

Work on homesickness by Fisher and Hood (1987) as a response to the move from home into residence at either boarding school (secondary education) or university (tertiary education) has provided more information about the impact of a discrete, potentially positive life event. Students, interviewed in the first term at university and asked to describe the features of their new experience, reported a variety of cognitive, emotional, and motivational symptoms associated with missing home, wanting to go home, and feeling lost or distressed in the current environment.

Table 1 shows the meanings that students give to the term homesickness and provides some indication of the range of perceptions and symptoms involved. Neither homesick nor non-homesick students differed in the meanings given to the term (see Fisher and Elder, 1990).

When given a questionnaire that required respondents to say whether or not homesickness had been or was experienced, over 70% of first-year students said that it was. Of those, about 10 to 15% had severe symptoms involving depression, tearfulness, obsessionality, sleeping and eating disorders.

In a prospective study in which students were assessed 2 months before leaving home to take up a university place and then later when they were in their sixth term at university, the evidence suggested a major change for new resident students in terms of psychoneurotic symptoms, particularly with respect to depression, anxiety, and obsessionality, and somatic symptoms (symptoms related to physical health) (see Table 2).

Less expected, was the finding that the effect of increased depression was true for nonresident or home-based students as well as residents. It seemed that attendance at a university, even without the insecurity of taking up a place in residence, has a major negative effect on students (see Fisher and Elder, 1990).

The relationship between stress and disease

Social disruption and anxiety

One emphasis taken by those seeking to understand the relationship between stress and ill health is that of social disruption. There are a number of slightly different focuses, but the general argument is that the individual exists in a social context and life events create changes within this context that lead to and maintain raised anxiety.

Wolff (1953) formulated four main postulates that he argued could provide the basis for understanding the increased risk of illness as a response to change: (1) changes affect the folklore and taboos of a culture; (2) the threats created by these taboos often become overexaggerated and create

Table 1 Features Utilized in Definitions of Homesickness for Homesick and Non-Homesick First-Year Students

Feature categories from definitions provided	Frequently reported features and percentage of subjects reporting feature	
	Homesick (n = 60) f(%)	Non-homesick (n = 60) f(%)
'Missing home environment'; 'Missing house, home, area, etc.'	18 (30.0)	16 (40.0)
'Missing parents/family'; 'Longing for people at home'	20 (33.3)	12 (30.0)
'Wanting to go home'; 'Feeling a need to return home'	14 (23.3)	11 (27.5)
'Missing friends'; 'Longing for friends'	18 (30.0)	5 (12.5)
'Feeling of loneliness'	3 (5.0)	7 (17.5)
'Feeling depressed'	3 (5.0)	3 (7.5)
'Missing someone close to talk to'	4 (6.7)	1 (2.5)
'Feeling insecure'	3 (5.0)	2 (5.0)
'Obsession with thoughts of home'; 'Thoughts about home'	3 (5.0)	3 (7.5)
'Feeling unhappy'	1 (1.7)	3 (7.5)
'Feeling unloved'	2 (3.3)	1 (2.5)
'Disorientation'; 'Feeling lost in new environment'	2 (3.3)	1 (2.5)
'A longing for familiar company and places'	1 (1.7)	1 (2.5)
'Thinking of the past'	1 (1.7)	2 (5.0)
'Feeling of not belonging'	1 (1.7)	1 (2.5)
'Regret that life had changed'; 'A feeling of regret'	3 (5.0)	0 (0.0)
'Feeling isolated'; 'Cut off from the world'	2 (3.3)	1 (2.5)
'Feeling uneasy'	0 (0.0)	2 (5.0)
'Feeling ill'	1 (1.7)	0 (0.0)
'Dissatisfaction with present situation'	1 (1.7)	0 (0.0)
'Unable to cope'	1 (1.7)	0 (0.0)
'Unable to do anything'	1 (1.7)	0 (0.0)
'Hating the present place'	0 (0.0)	1 (2.5)

Note: The following features were endorsed by only one person in the following groups. Homesick: 'Thinking that home was better than here'; 'Feeling of making a mistake'; 'Sinking feeling in stomach'; 'Loss of appetite'; 'Feeling of desperation' and 'Crying'. Non-homesick: 'New self-reliance'; 'Feeling of desolation' and 'Feeling unsettled'.

Adapted from Fisher, Murray, and Frazer, 1985.

Table 2   Cognitive Failure, Mental Health, and Adjustment Profiles Before and
After the Transition in Homesick and Non-Homesick Residents[a]

	Not Homesick (n = 42)		Homesick (n = 22)	
	$\bar{\chi}$	SD	$\bar{\chi}$	SD
At home				
MHQ1	22.81	(8.6)	29.2[b]	(12.5)
Obsessional (personality)	2.61	(2.2)	3.72[c]	(2.7)
Somatic	3.21	(2.5)	4.54[c]	(2.7)
Depression	1.89	(1.6)	3.82[b]	(2.8)
CFQ1	32.64	(10.66)	36.9NS	(12.3)
Sixth Week at University				
MHQ2	23.0	(11.54)	33.04[b]	(14.1)
Anxiety	3.78	(3.1)	6.48[b]	(3.7)
Somatic	2.63	(2.1)	5.17[d]	(2.9)
Depression	2.56	(2.3)	4.48[b]	(3.2)
Obsessional (symptoms)	2.54	(1.6)	3.35[c]	(2.1)
CFQ2	38.21	(11.88)	42.78NS	(13.5)
CAQ	100.69	(17.7)	84.31[d]	(18.2)
DRI	4.0	(3.2)	8.50[d]	(4.2)

[a] As designed by "not homesick" versus three other categories of "homesick" on self-rating scale (from Fisher and Hood, 1987).
[b] p < .01.
[c] p < .05.
[d] p < .001.

anxiety; (3) formalized methods for dealing with those threats are part of the culture; and (4) cultural change reduces the possibility of the use of familiar methods for dealing with threat.

Wolff argued that situations of rapid cultural change create cultural pressures but remove anxiety-reduction techniques: "The participant mistrusts habits and intuitions, and social experience no longer leads to a common sense of values" (p.15). Industrialization and family destabilization are regarded as sources of threat in modern society.

Social status and chronic disease

Research by Dodge and Martin (1970) was stimulated by interest in the rise in chronic disease levels in the U.S. by within-state differences in chronic disease levels, and also by differences in subpopulations as a function of age, race, and marital status.

Infectious disease rates have decreased and chronic disease rates have increased in the U.S. from 1900 to 1953. At least one explanation is that improved medical services have reduced the mortalities from infectious diseases and prolonged the lifespan. However, it remains plausible that stress factors are partially responsible for the increase, especially in view of sub-population vulnerabilities and because chronic disease levels show a general upward trend and not just a step-function rise following the control of infectious disease by inoculation and antibacterial treatments.

Dodge and Martin (1970) founded a social stress theory to account for within- and between-state differences in the incidence of chronic diseases such as heart disease and malignant neoplasms. For example, 1951 mortality rates for New York were 938.5 (per 100 000) for heart disease and 238.9 (per 100 000) for malignant disease, whereas in Mississippi rates were 488.4 and 163.3, respectively.

The result of comparing chronic disease levels per state with levels of infant mortality suggested that differing health care resource levels were not responsible for the interstate differences. In contrast, comparison with suicide rates yields positive evidence of the role of stress factor. The role of marital status was further identified as a mediating factor in that even in states where chronic disease levels were high, those who were male and married were less at risk.

Status incongruity

Totman (1979) proposed a theory that assumes that the individual becomes at risk for illness when social mobility or status incongruity occurs. Totman proposes a structural theory which assumes that people make sense of each other's actions in terms of social rules and conventions. Thus, each individual is equipped with a set of prescriptive rules. For these rules to exist they must be resistant to change, although some clarification or refinement can occur as the result of social interactions. Social change creates a situation of rule breakdown. Exits, losses, marital schism could all be seen in terms of the breakdown of rules. For example, a bereaved person, in addition to grieving for a lost loved one, may also lose an aspect of his or her identity and has to evolve a new life and new status in the community.

The details of how social disharmony creates increased risk of illness need to be explored. One possibility is that anxiety levels increase and that there is long-term damage to health mediated by persistent states of mental preoccupation which are linked with distress and unhappiness.

Social status

Loss of social status is argued to be important by Gilbert (1989). He proposes a "go-stop" model of the reaction to situations of failure and loss, including loss of status. The "go" phase involves active searching, accompanied by raised anxiety, whereas the "stop" phase involves giving up and helplessness.

The control model

Fisher (1986) developed a "control" model of the reaction to life events, level of demand of control over various aspects of the new lifestyle. Change is assumed to create discrepancies because of novelty and decreases the level of control a person experiences in relation to the new environment. Laboratory studies of animals and people suggest that power or mastery over the environment is likely to have an ameliorating effect on threat: animals provided with the instrumental means for avoiding punishment generally show fewer signs of physical lesion and disease than those who do not. Research indicates that human beings are more likely to choose to have control over noxious stimulation and are more likely to be tolerant of unpleasant stimulation if it is self-delivered. For those who do not choose direct control, more complex strategies may be operating (see Fisher, 1986, Chapter 2).

Karasek (1979) reported that job strain in working environments can be defined with respect to two dimensions—demand (or work load) and discretion (control). Job strain is reported when demand is high and control is low. Perceived challenge is more likely when demand and control are both high. In this analysis, a major life event might be argued to create a "job strain" environment. The bereaved person has to cope with the strain of living a life without the help and protection of the partner; the relocated have to find out how to cope with life in a new place.

Agendas for control

However, the assumption that in human subjects there is a total preference for control is undermined by early experiments on shock in experimental settings. In a study by Pervin (1963), subjects were given electric shock that was externally determined or self-delivered. There was a preference for the latter, but not for all subjects, and the biological differences in response to shock were minimal. The effect was greatest in terms of tolerance of shock and willingness to take part in the study.

However, experiments by Ball and Vogler (1971) showed that there may be different motives for accepting apparent low control. Subjects were asked to indicate reasons for choosing either machine shock or self-delivered shock. Those in the former situation gave explanations that indicated a wish for different kinds of control. There were obviously different agendas operating. Some subjects reported trying to foil the experimenter, or being religious and wanting to accept delivered punishment. In nearly all cases, a motive for apparently accepting low control could be identified. Perhaps the private agenda determines what is perceived as high control. Apparent lack of control may be a false appraisal by observers.

Stress and the biological basis of disease

In order to understand how psychological states of the individual might influence the risk of antigens becoming established or chronic diseases developing, there needs to be some attempt to link psychological states with biological states. We might begin to imagine that psychological states are rich and varied and link with biological activity in such a way as to raise the risk of particular diseases. Biological states are now known to be highly complex, and it is possible that ways of thinking about the world might create patterns that are associated with particular illnesses.

The effect of stress on biological activity was first described in terms of a unitary state of increased arousal, implying that any number of different kinds of stressful experience (e.g., bereavement, failure, surgical operations, public speaking, illness, job loss) would be associated with nonspecific arousal effects (Selye, 1956). Cannon (1932, 1936) was one of the first to make sense of the biological state that accompanied the experience of stress in terms of the need to restore equilibrium. The biological response to the disequilibrium produced by stress was assumed to provide the power to restore the balance. However, this did not change the basic assumption of the nonspecificity of the biological state. The question of why one man reacts to stress with ulcers and another with heart disease (Malmo and Shagass, 1949) provided an early challenge to this assumption.

Perhaps the attempt to link even physiological states to disease proclivities will remain undefinable. Weiner (1982) points out that in any population some individuals are at risk for disease but the illness never materializes. One example is the presence of elevated levels of pepsinogen isoenzymes, which is a biological marker for peptic duodenal ulcer. Such a marker can occur in persons who remain well. Weiner concludes that the individual is programmed for disease by a multitude of predisposing markers and psychological sensitivities. However, it might be possible to begin to probe the medium in which markers exist. Perhaps the person with a biological marker favoring a peptic ulcer remains well unless creating or encountering stresses that produce changes in gastric activity. A risk model based on *compatibility* and *synchrony* of biological and psychological patterns might be the answer. Also, existing biological markers that should predispose towards illness might be created and sustained by stressful life experiences. It then requires a further life event to create the synchronous existence of sufficient risk factors for a particular kind of illness.

Hormone characteristics and disease susceptibility

Disease and the overriding of autoregulatory devices

The main effects of the hormones that are released in stressful conditions are to mobilize and activate a number of bodily resources. The side effects that occur may result directly from these changes and may be interpreted as illnesses. Thus, dizziness, tension, stomach cramps, palpitations, and respiratory problems may be part of the state of hyperarousal created by stress. The individual who is uninformed about the effects of stress on bodily systems may label the symptoms as being part of some more profound disease or disorder and there may be self-confirming aspects.

Adverse long-term effects on biological function could be encouraged by factors that increase the level and duration of stress hormones. Moderate levels of catecholamine are characteristic of daily life. However, chronic circulation of these elevated hormone levels increases risk of structural disorder. Experience of threatening but intractable problems or events characterized by low control should provide ideal conditions in this respect. Life stresses often tend to provide such conditions.

The human capacity to re-experience unpleasant events in reflective thinking or to anticipate and hence experience much of the threat of an impending event in advance, provides a major means of driving and maintaining states of pathological arousal. One consequence is persistent functional abuse of bodily systems. Sterling and Eyer (1981) describe a number of autonomous regulatory controls that act to self-limit the physiological response. For example, a rise in the concentration of glucose in the blood stimulates the pancreas to secrete insulin. Insulin encourages the uptake of sugar by muscle fat and liver cells, thus creating a negative feedback loop, which results in a drop in the level of glucose in the blood. Such autoregulatory systems should, if correctly functioning, protect against functional abuse of bodily mechanisms. Unfortunately, as Sterling and Eyer point out, the neural system can override these self-regulatory systems. The authors argue that the facility for the overriding of autonomous systems enables adaptive and anticipatory response to fluctuating circumstances to occur.

In addition, wear and tear take some toll on bodily activity. Sterling and Eyer (1989) review evidence to suggest that the hormones suppressed during high arousal are those that promote synthetic or anabolic processes requiring energy. Thus, there is reduced capacity for cell repair and maintenance of immunological systems. Equally, catabolic activity rises, resulting in more free cholesterol and fatty acids, raised blood sugar levels, drop in cellular activity, shrinkage of the thymus, and swelling of the adrenal glands to maintain hormone production. Thus, if human decision overrides the autoregulatory loops that prevent persistent high levels of catabolic activity, the risk of "somatization", of functional abuse leading to structural change increases.

They have the potential to increase the risk of illness. First, the period of elevated arousal may be driven and maintained, resulting in a protracted stress experience. Second, a preoccupied person is likely to be rendered incompetent and thus may inadvertently create more stresses as well as being unable to cope effectively with the initial threat. Fisher (1984) argued that stresses create a demand for accurate, productive activity, while simultaneously creating mental states in which competence levels are often reduced. A number of feedback loops resulting in progressive loss of control were identified, which lead towards a state of complete incompetence or crisis. The failure to act competently may increase the threatening properties of the life event unless it is self-limiting. Moreover, the individual may become aware of his own inabilities to cope and this could result in further self-focused preoccupation.

Decision and specific hormonal consequences

Decisions about control in specific situations may directly determine hormone balance and hence the propensity to different categories of illness. As will be apparent from the previous section, although catecholamines and corticoid hormones do not have mutually exclusive jurisdiction over aspects of bodily function in stress, there is some evidence of "division of labor". Raised cortisol has a more immediate influence on the immune response system, whereas catecholamine levels have a predominant effect on biological arousal.

From studies involving catecholamines in stressful environments, there is both direct and indirect evidence to suggest that the balance of adrenaline and noradrenaline is a variable influenced by human decision. Ax (1953) distinguished anger- and fear-producing situations in terms of adrenaline-noradrenaline characteristics; the anger profile was linked with increases in both hormones, whereas the fear profile was associated with raised adrenaline.

Funkenstein et al. (1957) examined the effects of contrived public failure on competitive college students and reported two distinguishable response patterns that could be predicted with great accuracy by a close associate of each student. The first response style, termed "anger-in", was a self-blaming style associated with a physiological pattern typical of raised adrenaline. The second response style, termed "anger-out", was associated with changes symptomatic of raised noradrenaline.

Work involving direct catecholamine measurement by Frankenhaeuser and colleagues has identified different balances of adrenaline and noradrenaline as a function of work context. For example, Frankenhaeuser and Gardell (1976) investigated jobs in a sawmill and showed that conditions of repetition and short-cycle operations are more likely to be associated with lack of subjective well-being and raised adrenaline, whereas conditions of restricted work posture are more likely to be associated with increased irritation and raised levels of noradrenaline.

Frankenhaeuser and Rissler (1970) showed that increasing situational control was accompanied by a preponderance of noradrenaline to adrenaline. Weiss (1968) demonstrated increased noradrenaline levels in rats provided with the means to avoid shock, but not in yoked controls. Mason et al. (1968) confirmed that novelty and uncertainty were more likely to be associated with raised adrenaline, whereas stereotyped situations were more likely to be accompanied by raised noradrenaline.

The implications of different ratios of adrenaline-noradrenaline balance for the risk of illness have yet to be worked out. Collectively, chronic elevated levels of catecholamines increase the risk of cardiovascular and gastrointestinal changes. In the former case, hormone balance may be influential: noradrenaline is more likely to raise blood pressure through vasoconstriction, whereas adrenaline is more likely to act via increased cardiac output.

A recent analysis by Fisher (1986), based on physiological evidence from Frankenhaeuser and Johansson (1982) suggested that decisions about whether control is possible have implications for the ratio of circulating catecholamines and corticoid hormones. When there is high control, the individual should experience challenge, whereas when there is no control, there is risk of helplessness accompanied by distress if there are punishing consequences. In ambiguous situations, decisions about control may involve protracted worry, as the individual seeks to explore the consequences of possible courses of action. Life stresses may create states of "mental chess", in which the individual rehearses possible moves and countermoves in order to decide on a course of action.

Psychophysiological research (Frankenhaeuser and Johansson, 1982) has provided support for the importance of decision in stressful environments, although unfortunately based on comparisons afforded by different laboratory tasks. A 1-hour vigilance task involving changes in intensity of a weak light was stated to be designed so as to involve low control over outcome. Performance was accompanied by raised subjective effort and perceived distress. The predominant hormone was raised cortisol. By comparison, a choice reaction time task with a high degree of personal control over stimulus rate was associated with raised self-reported effort but no distress. The predominant hormones were catecholamines.

A field study by Johansson and Sanden (1982) involved a group of operators engaged in planning production and control where there was a high degree of control over the work. By contrast, process controllers in the same industry worked under monotonous conditions, remained passive, but were required to detect critical signals associated with disturbances in the process. The study showed that the active planning task was associated with primarily positive feelings and raised catecholamine levels, whereas the passive, understimulating process-monitoring task was associated with unease, with some small increase in adrenaline and cortisol levels.

The above studies do not provide proof that perceived control is the direct determinant of hormone pattern, but the reported relationship between effortful situations and raised catecholamines and distressing situations with elevated cortisol and catecholamines is supported. The implications are that differential decision about controllability may turn out to be a major factor influencing prevailing hormone states and hence the proclivity to certain illnesses.

Control strategies and the risk of disease

The basis of the control model

It is assumed that change and novelty evoke decision-making responses, especially if threat or danger is implied. Contexts associated with negative situations need to be appraised to determine level of response.

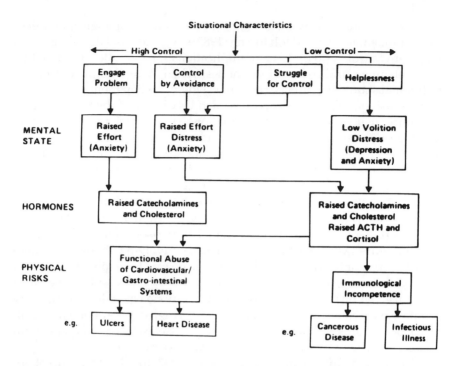

Figure 2 Map of possible routes from cognitive factors in perception of control to mental disorder and physical illness. (From Fisher, S., *Handbook of Life Stress Cognition and Health*, Reason, J., Ed., John Wiley & Sons, Ltd., Chichester, U.K., 1989. With permission.)

Figure 2 illustrates that a series of decisions is needed to determine whether effective control is possible, except in situations where the likelihood of control is represented in knowledge (e.g., untrained people cannot fly aircraft). The decisions identified in Figure 2 have implications for hormone balance and, in prolonged or recurrent scenarios, have implications for health outcome.

The fruit machine analogy

The risk model developed by Fisher (1988) is based on an analogy with a gambling machine that is known in the U.K. as a "fruit machine". The individual is assumed to have basic biological and psychological risk factors determined genetically. In terms of the "fruit machine", there is thus a built-in probability of achieving four lemons. The number of times the handle is pulled determines the probability of acquiring lemons in a fixed period of time. This is like saying that the experience of work might increase the wear and tear on bodily systems and increases the risk of gastroenteric or cardiovascular disease.

However, we must also add the role of perceived personal control. Whether a person perceives that he or she has control determines the way in which the lever is pulled. Low control situations may result in more anxiety (more lever pulls). In addition, we have to consider control styles and ability to avoid a secondary problem or create a solution. The nature of the risk is aided by the particular balance of hormones such as adrenalin, noradrenaline, and cortisol, although in general most levels will contribute to wear and tear.

References

Ax, A. I. (1953). The physiological differentiation between fear and anger in humans. *Psychol. Med.*, 15, 433–442.

Ball, T. S. and Vogler, R. E. (1971). Uncertain pain and the pain of uncertainty. *Perceptual Motor Skills*, 33, 1195–1203.

Burton, R. (1977). *The Anatomy of Melancholy: What It Is, with All The Kinds, Causes, Symptoms, Prognostics and Several Cures of It*. H. Jackson (Ed.). New York: Random House.

Cannon, W. B. (1932). *The Wisdom of the Body*. New York: Norton.

Cannon, W. B. (1936). *Bodily Changes in Pain, Hunger, Fear and Rage*. New York: Appleton-Century-Crofts.

Connolly, J. (1975). Circumstances, events and illness. *Medicine*, 2(10), 454–458.

Dodge, D. L. and Martin, W. T. (1970). *Social Stress and Chronic Illness*. Indiana: Notre Dame Press.

Dohrenwend, B. S., Krasnoff, L., Askenasy, A. R., and Dohrenwend, B. P. (1978). Exemplification of a method for scaling life events: the PERI Life Events Scale. *J. Health Soc. Behav.*, 19, 205–229.

Faris, R. E. L. and Dunham, H. W. (1939). *Mental Disorders in Urban Areas*. Chicago: University of Chicago Press.

Fisher, S. (1984). Stress, In P. Kuper and M. Kuper (Eds.). *The Encyclopedia of the Social Sciences*. London: Routledge and Kegan Paul.

Fisher, S. (1986). The perception of performance in stress: the utilisation of cognitive facts by non-depressed and depressed students. *Perception*, 14, 501–510.

Fisher, S. (1988). *Homesickness and the Psychological effects of Transition and Change*. London: Lawrence Erlbaum Associates.

Fisher, S. and Elder, L. (1990). Epidemiological problem analysis: a new approach to the measurement of stress. *Stress Med.* (Special Edition), 10, 1–16.

Fisher, S. and Hood, B. (1987). The stress of the transition to university: a longitudinal study of psychological disturbances, absent-mindedness and vulnerability to homesickness. *Br. J. Psychol.*, 78, 425–441.

Frankenhaeuser, M. and Gardell, B. (1976). Underload and overload in working life: outline of a multidisciplinary approach. *J. Hum. Stress*, 2, 35–46.

Frankenhaeuser, M. and Johansson, J. (1982). Stress at Work: Psychogiological and Psychosocial Aspects. Paper presented at the 20th International Congress of Applied Psychology, Edinburgh, July 25–31.

Frankenhaeuser, M. and Rissler, A. (1970). Effects of punishment on catecholamine release and the efficiency of performance. *Psychopharmacologia (Bol)*, 17, 378–390.

Fried, M. (1963). Transitional functions of working class communities: implications for forced relocation. In M. B. Kantor, (Ed.). *Mobility and Mental Health*. Springfield, IL: Charles C. Thomas.

Funkenstein, D. H., King, S. H., and Drolette, M. E. (1957). *Mastery of Stress*. Cambridge, MA: Harvard University Press.

Gilbert, P. (1989). Psychobiological interaction in depression. In S. Fisher and J. Reason (Eds.). *Handbook of Life Stress, Cognition and Health*. London: John Wiley & Sons.

Holmes, T. H. and Rahe, R. H. (1967). The social readjustment rating scale. *J. Psychosom. Res.*, 11, 213–218.

Johannsson, G. and Sanden, P. (1982). Mental load and job satisfaction of control room operators. *Rapporter* (Department of Psychology, University of Stockholm), No. 40.

Karasek, R. A. (1979). Job demands, job decision latitude and mental strain: implication for job redesign. *Admin. Sci. Q.*, 24, 43–48.

Kleiner, R. J. and Parker, S. (1963). Goal striving and psychosomatic symptoms in a migrant and non-migrant population. In M. B. Kantor (Ed.). *Mobility and Mental Health*. Springfield, IL: Charles C. Thomas.

Malmo, R. B. and Shagass, C. (1949). Physiologic study of symptom mechanisms in psychiatric patients under stress. *Psychosom. Med.*, 11, 25.

Malzberg, B. and Lee, E. S. (1940). *Migration and Mental Disease: a Study of First Admissions to Hospital for Mental Disease*. New York: Social Science Research Council.

Mason, J. W., Brady, J. V., and Tolliver, G. A. (1968). Plasma and urinary 17-hydrocorticosteroid responses to 72 hour avoidance sessions in the monkey. *Psychosom. Med.*, 30, 608–630.

Odegaard, O. (1932). Emigration and insanity: a study of mental disease among the Norwegian born population of Minnesota. *Acta Psychiatr. Neurol. Suppl.*, 1–4.

Pervin, L. A. (1963). The need to predict and control under conditions of threat. *J. Personality*, 31, 570–587.

Rahe, R. H. (1972). Subjects' recent life changes and their near future illness reports. *Ann. Clin. Res.*, 4, 250–265.

Rahe, R. (1989). Recent life changes and coronary heart disease: 10 years' research. In S. Fisher and J. Reason (Eds.). *Handbook of Life Stress, Cognition and Health*. London: John Wiley & Sons.

Selye, H. (1956). *The Stress of Life*. London: Longmans Green and Company.

Sterling, P. and Eyer, J. (1981). Biological basis of stress related mortality. *Soc. Sci. Med.*, 15E, 3–42.

Sterling, P. and Eyer, J. (1989). Allostasis: a new paradigm to explain arousal pathology. In S. Fisher and J. Reason (Eds.). *Handbook of Life Stress, Cognition and Health*. London: John Wiley & Sons.

Stokols, D., Shumaker, S. A., and Martinez, J. (1983). Residential mobility and personal well being. *J. Environ. Psychol.*, 3, 5–19.

Totman, R. (1979). *Social Causes of Illness*. London: Souvenir Press.

Weiner, H. (1982). The prospects for psychosomatic medicine: selected topics. *Psychosom. Med.*, 44, 491–517.

Weiss, J. M. (1968). Effects of coping responses on stress. *J. Comp. Physiol. Psychol.*, 65, 251–266.

Wolff, H. G. (1953). *Stress and Disease*. Springfield, IL: Charles C. Thomas.

Wyler, A. R., Masuda, M., and Holmes, T. H. (1971). Magnitude of life events and seriousness of illness. *Psychosom. Med.*, 33, 115–122.

chapter seven

Critical life changes and cardiovascular disease

Töres Theorell

"Broken hearts" occurring in relation to critical life changes have been frequently recorded in literature for a long time. In *scientific* literature, "life changes" in relation to cardiovascular disease have mostly been conceptualized as changes in the psychosocial environment of the individual. They are identified accordingly as environmental processes that are clearly defined in time and distinguishable from "chronic difficulties". Cardiovascular disease is often distinct from the temporal aspect—everyone knows when cardiovascular death has occurred, and a myocardial infarction is a disease that mostly has dramatic symptoms. There are exceptions to the rule that cardiovascular disease is well defined in time, however. Myocardial infarction does not always give rise to symptoms, and the early stages of hypertension are mostly asymptomatic. In the cardiovascular literature critical life changes have also been distinct from their own consequences— life changes are seen as stressors and not responses to environmental conditions.

The following chapter will be confined to "normal" life changes that could occur to most people. Thus, only occasionally reference will be made to the effects of natural catastrophes, nuclear disasters, war conditions, and similar large-scale traumatic events. Furthermore, there will be little discussion regarding the small events of the daily round of life; hassles and uplifts as they have been labeled in the scientific literature.

Psychological and physiological reactions to life changes are grounded in the interplay between individual and environment. Figure 1 (after Kagan and Levi, 1971) illustrates this interplay. The individual's way of reacting (individual program) is constituted both by genetic factors and by previous experiences of life changes. It changes throughout life due to the constant flow of experiences. Modern twin research has tried to explore these relationships (Lichtenstein, 1993); the results indicate that neither environment nor genetic factors separately can explain individual program. The components of type A behavior (one of which, for instance, hostility, has been observed to be of particular importance to the risk of developing

0-8493-2908-6/96/$0.00+$.50
© 1996 by CRC Press, Inc.

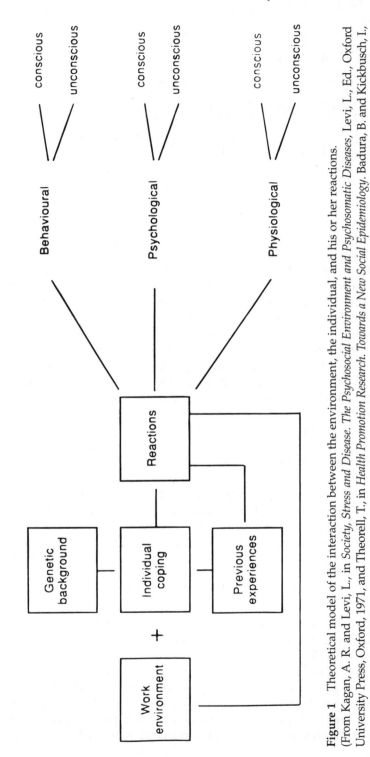

Figure 1 Theoretical model of the interaction between the environment, the individual, and his or her reactions. (From Kagan, A. R. and Levi, L., in *Society, Stress and Disease. The Psychosocial Environment and Psychosomatic Diseases*, Levi, L., Ed., Oxford University Press, Oxford, 1971, and Theorell, T., in *Health Promotion Research. Towards a New Social Epidemiology*. Badura, B. and Kickbusch, I., Eds., WHO Regional Publications, European Series No. 37, Copenhagen, 1991. With permission.)

cardiovascular disease at an early age), have been shown to be determined partly by genetic factors, partly by childhood experiences, and partly by the experiences of adult life.

A sociological and a psychological approach to life changes

In the 1960s two American psychiatrists, Holmes and Rahe (1967), presented a list of life changes that human beings could be exposed to. Randomly selected men and women had been asked to judge how much adaptation would be required in these different situations. Averages were calculated from these ratings and used as "life change scores" (LCU). This list was labeled the Schedule of Recent Experiences, SRE. Corresponding schedules were produced in several other countries. This had a marked effect on research regarding the effects of life changes on cardiovascular disease risk.

The basic idea underlying the SRE research was nonspecific—it was assumed according to Selye's stress theory (the general adaptation syndrome) that a nonspecific accumulation of life changes during a short period of time would increase vulnerability to illness. Another important assumption was that it would make no difference whether the life change was positive or negative—the required adaptation was the important component in illness etiology. According to Selye, a massive effort to adapt to a dramatic change would arouse the sympatho-adreno-cortical system.

The general theory regarding effects of nonspecific accumulation of life changes during a short period of time has been verified in a number of epidemiological studies. It is also clear, however, that the nonspecific effect of change, as it has been measured so far, is of low magnitude. In the case of cardiovascular disease, several retrospective studies, initially published in Sweden and Finland by Rahe, Theorell, and colleagues (summarized by Rahe, 1990), showed that patients who had a first myocardial infarction reported a nonspecific accumulation of critical life changes during the months preceding the disease onset. In a similar way, close relatives of patients who had died a sudden cardiac death reported that the patient had an accumulation of critical life changes during the months preceding the death. When these results were repeated in prospective studies (Hollis et al., 1990; Theorell et al., 1975) the findings were not significant, however (see below). The negative findings in the prospective studies may be partly explained by insensitive methods. Another explanation, which has been emphasized by Rahe (1990), is that the retrospective studies have related the amount of life change going on during the period immediately preceding the onset of myocardial infarction to the subject's habitual level of life change during the preceding years. The relevant dimension to the individual may be the amount of life change during a given period in relation to the level that he/she has become used to. Furthermore, the prospective studies mostly lack information about the period immediately preceding the myocardioal infarction. Still, the absence of statistically significant effects of nonspecific change in the individual on the risk of developing cardiovascular disease points out that nonspecific life change may be hard to relate to cardiovascular disease unless previous experiences and way of coping are taken into account.

Holmes' and Rahe's work soon elicited several competing theories regarding the study of nonspecific life change. Very soon two opposite schools could be recognized, a sociological and a psychological. The sociological tradition stresses the importance of the characteristics of the life change and the circumstances around it. Death of spouse, for instance, is very different depending on whether the spouse dies unexpectedly and suddenly or whether he/she dies after a long period of illness. A pregnancy has different significance depending on whether the woman is single and lacks good social context or whether she is married and has good social conditions. According to this theory it is possible to classify the life change by means of a systematic interview and a standardized classification system. This classification (according to Brown and Harris, 1978) also makes it possible to rate the degree of social threat inherent in the change. The classification requires a rather extensive interview. The subject's opinion about the life change is of no importance to the classification, according to this perspective. This method was also used in a retrospective study of amount of life change preceding myocardial infarction, and a clear relationship was found (Connolly, 1976).

By contrast, the psychological tradition stresses the importance of the subject's own opinion. According to this line of reasoning the objective characteristics of the life change itself are of no significance. The psychological meaning to the individual and his/her interpretation of it are the only significant factors. Different aspects of the subject's interpretation could be described, such as (see Dohrenwend and Dohrenwend, 1974):

Possibility of predicting the life change
Positive or negative experience
Gain or loss
Desirability
Controllability

To the clinician, neglect of either sociological or psychological perspectives is erroneous. If we disregard the interpretation of the individual we might run the risk of supporting individuals who do not need any support in a life change that we have categorized as important according to the sociological tradition. Furthermore, we might disregard the need for support to a sensitive individual whose life change we have categorized as unimportant. Conversely, if our actions are based upon the individual's interpretation only, we might disregard individuals who need support but deny this need or are not even aware of it. Furthermore, a purely psychological attitude may also lead to the acceptance of unbearable external conditions simply because the belief is spread that the only important factor is the individual's way of coping—"external conditions are unimportant anyway".

During periods of peace, society has time to organize support for its citizens. Sweden has had this situation for a long time. This may partly explain why there has been such a strong interest in support structures aimed at helping citizens to manage critical life changes. In such a social climate the sociological tradition becomes the most important one, and this is also the situation in which the measurement and analysis of the life change itself were stimulated.

During periods of war and crisis, on the other hand, when many citizens are exposed to strongly threatening situations, the individual may feel that his own method of dealing with distressing critical life changes is the only relevant factor. This was the climate in which the scientific interest in the individual's way of coping with problems started growing. For instance, Ben Shalit, who was a military psychologist at the time, created his "coping wheel", a method for recording strategies for coping with critical life changes during war situations in Israel during the 1960s. He did this in order to be able to predict which soldiers would be more likely than others to cope with difficult war situations. Antonovsky's interest in "sense of coherence", a theory that is the basis of a questionnaire for measuring coping strategies, was aroused when he studied long-term consequences of having been exposed to and having survived a period in a concentration camp during the second world war (Antonovsky, 1987).

The conclusion is that the group of cardiovascular patients to focus on with regard to support in critical life changes has to be identified both sociologically and psychologically. This is of importance particularly in cardiovascular rehabilitation. The systematic method has not been used sufficiently in this field so far.

Positive and negative

To the clinician it is important that the information about a life change that the patient is going through is structured in such a way that it is easily interpreted. It may be meaningful to ask the patient to fill out a short questionnaire in which he/she is asked to record not only which life changes have occurred and when they occurred but also the extent to which the event has had positive or negative significance.

In a recent study we could show that blood pressure and, in parallel, serum triglycerides changed in different directions while subjects were going through important life changes that they rated themselves as positive and negative, respectively (Theorell and Emlund, 1993). In this case the individuals were followed on four occasions during a year. On every occasion blood pressure and triglycerides were measured. When the year had passed the individuals were asked whether they had experienced important life changes during the past year and, if so, when. They were also asked to rate on a visual analogue scale (from most negative = personal catastrophe to most positive = total happiness) the emotional significance that the life change had. Those who rated the life change as moderately positive or moderately negative were regarded as individuals who had had insignificant life changes. Three groups were compared with one another, a positive, a negative, and a non-event group with either no recorded or insignificant life changes. Figure 2 shows changes in diastolic blood pressure and serum triglycerides from before to after the life changes (beginning and end of the year in the non-event group) in the three groups. The positive life change group showed an improved cardiovascular risk pattern, whereas the negative life change group showed the opposite pattern. Other authors have also pointed out that the distinction between positive and negative life changes may be important (see Dohrenwend and Dohrenwend, 1974 as well as Edwards and Cooper, 1988). However, it seems to be important also to distinguish between different types of outcome. For instance, as pointed out by Brown and collaborators, any life change, positive or negative, may trigger the onset of a schizophrenic episode, while clinical depression is preceded, in the typical case, by serious negative life changes.

In the small study of positive and negative life changes referred to above it was observed that some types of life changes could have either clearly negative or clearly positive emotional significance; divorce, for instance, was rated as negative by some subjects and positive by other subjects. A person who has gone through a certain life change may also change his opinion about it after some time.

If we disregard that a given life change may have different significance to different subjects depending on previous experiences, it is also true that different groups in society are exposed to different amounts of positive and negative life changes. It has been pointed out that there may be systematic differences between social groups, for instance, from this point of view. This could even contribute to differences in the prevalence of cardiovascular disorder in different social groups—higher prevalence in low social groups than in high (see Dohrenwend and Dohrenwend, 1974). In our own research we have noticed that young men with low blood pressure levels report retrospectively that they have experienced more positive life changes during their adolescence than men of the same age with high blood pressure (Svensson and Theorell, 1983). In another study we observed (Isaksson et al., 1993) that middle-aged persons who were treated for high blood pressure in a specialized outclinic and who did not show the expected normalization of blood pressure despite adequate medication (which may be due to more advanced secondary complications arising from the hypertension)—so-called therapy-resistant patients—reported retrospectively for the most recent 10-year period in their lives that they had experienced fewer positive life changes during that period than had those who had the expected normalization of blood pressure. In this study it was observed that there was a complicated interplay between chronic

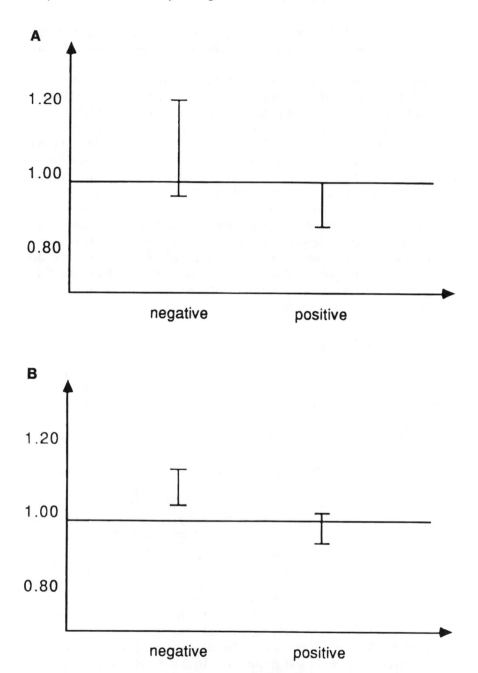

Figure 2   (A) Change in diastolic blood pressure at rest before and after "negative" and "positive" major life change (ratio after/before). Means and 95% confidence limits. (B) Change in serum triglycerides (logarithmic transformation) before and after "negative" and "positive" major life change (ration after/before). Means and 95% confidence limits. (Adapted from Theorell and Emlund, 1993.)

pathophysiological condition, life changes, social group, and lack of ability to describe emotional feelings in the web of causation behind resistance to treatment.

Although it is important to make a distinction between positive and negative life changes, it is also important to state that the original Holmes and Rahe hypothesis regarding the nonspecific effects on health risk of an accumulation of life changes that require adaptation may still be valid regardless of positive or negative loading. The example of schizophrenic episodes is described above, but there are also other examples of relevant health outcomes that may be triggered by an accumulation of life changes in general. A positive life change may also lead to complications. Promotion at work is usually regarded as a positive life change, but it may also induce unexpected demands for adaptation, both for the individual and for his/her family—in some situations of this kind, illness risks may increase. Angina pectoris, for example, is due to a shortage of oxygen in the heart muscle—narrowing of coronary arteries constitutes the basis for this. Shortage of oxygen arises in physically or emotionally demanding situations that may be both positive and negative.

Specific relationships

In a study of 7000 middle-aged building construction workers (Theorell et al., 1975), every man was asked to report life changes that he had exerienced during the past year. Subsequently all subjects were followed in official registers for 2 years. Although high life change scores were not predictive, per se, of increased risk of developing a myocardial infarction, during follow-up there were specific associations between certain kinds of life changes and the subsequent onset of a long-lasting medical disorder. Thus, subjects who reported that their wife had become seriously ill during the past year were more likely than other subjects to develop long-lasting new episodes of disorders in the locomotor system. Those who reported increased responsibility at work were more likely than others to develop a myocardial infarction during follow-up, and a general index of work change and load was associated with 60% excess risk of developing a myocardial infarction during 2 years of follow-up (Theorell and Floderus-Myrhed, 1977), even when biomedical risk factors had been taken into account (Theorell et al., 1977). A high index of nonspecific change, however, was associated with increased risk of developing long-lasting psychiatric disorder. Accordingly, in this study the nonspecific effects of critical life changes seemed to be of less importance to the development of cardiovascular disease than to psychiatric conditions.

However, when the interaction between nonspecific change and long-lasting difficulties was taken into account, significant relationships were observed. Thus, men who reported both a high score for "life discord"—with components of hostility and chronic life difficulties—and a high score for life change during the past year were more likely to have a markedly elevated blood pressure, whereas those who reported neither many life changes nor many chronic difficulties, or those reporting either many life changes with little discord or few life changes with plenty of discord, did not have elevated blood pressure (Theorell, 1976). These results were not adjusted for other risk factors, however.

Low prevalence of life changes

In the discussion regarding nonspecific and more specific effects of life changes it should also be pointed out that there are conditions that seem to be more prevalent in subjects who report few life changes. One example of this may be the early stages of hypertension. In a retrospective study of young men with asymptomatic elevation of blood pressure (Theorell et al., 1986), it was shown that these subjects reported fewer life changes in general (positive and negative) during the year preceding the examination than did a comparable group of young men without blood pressure elevation. There was even an inverse relationship between the number of reported life changes during that year and adrenaline concentration in blood at rest—the fewer reported life changes, the higher the adrenaline concentration at rest. It is plausible that subjects with propensity for blood pressure elevation have increasing blood pressure levels during periods with an accumulation of critical life changes but that they have few such life changes during ordinary conditions. A high habitual level of life changes would serve as the equivalent of "vaccination" against adverse health effects of an accumulation of critical life changes.

Physiological correlates of life changes

Not only the general sympathoadrenal activation level, but also other physiological processes, may change as a result of life changes. Specific constellations of physiological changes may take place during life changes. This may be used in order to increase our understanding of what occurs to a group of persons who go through a specific life change. In some critical life changes persons may deny the importance of the event, and when there is pronounced alexithymia (inability to interpret and discriminate between different emotions) there may be a tendency not to describe any psychological reactions to the event, despite the fact that the physiological reactions to it may even be stronger than in other subjects.

That an accumulation of life change units during a given week is associated with the amount of adrenaline excreted in the urine during the same week has been shown in a study of men who had suffered a myocardial infarction and who had returned to daily activities at work and at home. During weeks with many life changes with high demands for adaptation nonspecifically the adrenaline excretion was elevated, and vice versa (Theorell et al., 1972). It was shown that the effect on adrenaline excretion of a high accumulated score in real life was comparable to the effects that have been observed during pronounced experimental stress situations in the laboratory. Our calculations showed that a doubling of the total life change score during 1 week compared to the previous one was associated with a 50% increase in urinary adrenaline excretion during the active day hours. On the other hand, the individual variation in responses was pronounced; in one third of the subjects there was a strong correlation, in another third only a moderate one, and in the last third of the subjects there was no correlation at all. It is also quite possible that the variations in adrenaline excretion were more pronounced and the correlations possibly more evident in this kind of patients than in others. In a later study, Chadwick et al. (1979) found that a high life change score correlated positively with high urinary excretion of catecholamines but only in subjects with type A behavior, not in those with type B behavior. In several of the cases studied we could also show that there was a temporal association between the onset of a life change with concomitant increase in adrenaline excretion and the subsequent onset of increase in number of angina pectoris attacks.

Many studies have shown that one way of mirroring what the meaning of a life change has been for a person is to do an interview while physiological reactions are being recorded. This could be seen as a method aimed at making the person re-experience that life change symbolically. Two examples will be described from my own experiences. Both were patients who had been cared for in the hospital because they had suffered from myocardial infarctions, and life changes that occurred during the months preceding the onset of the myocardial infarction were discussed.

The first patient was a 39-year-old researcher who described an unusual accumulation of life changes during the 3 months preceding the myocardial infarction. He had problems with his boss; difficulties in achieving funding for his research was the reason. Furthermore, he had gone through a sudden, unexpected marital separation during this period. When these life changes were discussed increased heart rate, stroke volume (the volume of blood that is expelled with each heart stroke), and decreased finger pulse volume (which could be evidence of constriction in the peripheral vessels, which could lead to increasing resistance for the heart to work against). All of these changes per se could induce elevated blood pressure, and the patient's blood pressure increased strikingly—the systolic blood pressure from 135 to 180 mmHg. The patient clearly showed during the interview that he was bothered by the topics being discussed—he felt that he had been humiliated in several ways.

The second patient was a 40-year-old clerk. During the months preceding the myocardial infarction, he had been forced to work overtime to a considerable extent. Furthermore, his son had been in a traffic accident. He showed less pronounced physiological reactions to the conversation. The heart rate decreased and the finger pulse volume increased. The stroke volume increased. Altogether these changes resulted in very small changes in blood pressure—the systolic blood pressure only increased from 125 to 130 mmHg. The patient's attitude to the life changes that he had gone through differed from the attitude that the first patient had during the interview. The second patient blamed the onset of the myocardial infarction on his supervisor, who had forced him to do excessive overtime work ("I warned him before and even told him that if you force me to do this, I shall probably have a heart attack"). One interpretation of this is that this man's self-esteem had not been threatened by the reported life changes. The same was true of the traffic accident—the blame was on his son, and nothing really dangerous had actually happened (see de Faire and Theorell, 1984).

These two cases illustrate the fact that different attitudes to the life changes during the interview, which may possibly also reflect different coping strategies to the life changes when they occurred in real life, may have been associated with different physiological reactions. In the first case psychological support was more important during the rehabilitation after the myocardial infarction than it was in the second case.

Cardiac arrhythmias

There are several individual case reports in the literature describing the importance of critical life changes to bouts of arrhythmias. Three cases may illustrate that re-experiencing, in the form of merely thinking about, critical life changes could be of importance to the development of clinically important arrhythmias.

The first patient was a 35-year-old businessman who had been traveling extensively. He consulted me because he had had bouts of tachyarrhythmias. Medical examination showed that he had no signs of thyrotoxicosis, pre-excitation syndrome, or other common causes of bouts of cardiac arrhythmia. His arrhythmia episodes—fast tachycardia—usually started and ended suddenly, without advance warning, and he had no idea about triggering factors. Interviews merely showed that he was hardworking but that he had a happy family life. After several consultations, we decided that he should try to explore himself the possibilities of what might trigger his attacks. After several weeks he called. He thought that he had found the triggering factor. During a vacation trip he was traveling with his family through a city that he had visited for his work several months before. During this visit he had had an extramarital affair with a woman who lived on a street that he now passed with his family. When his car passed the woman's house, a dramatic bout of tachycardia started, and the patient realized that the bouts had always been triggered by reminders of the extramarital affair. With this new insight the bouts gradually disappeared. This case is of interest because the man had denied the extramarital affair psychologically to the extent that he had been unable to see the relationship with the arrhythmia episodes. However, when he was reminded in a very concrete way of the event and actually also had a tachycardia attack, he was able to gain insight. It illustrates that the clinician may often get the relevant information but that self-exploration is necessary and that strong denial mechanisms may make it necessary to wait for a long time.

The second patient was serving as a sales clerk. He was 45 years old and responsible for one small department in a department store and had suffered a myocardial infarction several months before. While he was being interviewed in my office, three potentially dangerous tachyarrhythmias were recorded on an electrocardiogram (Figure 3). The first occurred during talk about the acute life-threatening onset of his heart disease. The other two episodes, however, occurred during discussion of a specific work matter. There had recently been some thefts, and it was suspected that someone in his department was responsible. The patient was under strong pressure to find the thief but he had no way of controlling the situation or finding out what was going on. Discussions about other important matters, such as the death of his first wife and his present sex life, were not associated with dangerous arrhythmias in this case. During the discussions with this man it became evident that it was very threatening to him to have the responsibility of revealing that one of his own work mates was a thief.

The third patient was an immigrant clerk, 45 years old. He had suffered a large myocardial infarction and had occasional bouts of angina pectoris but was back at work. Two years after the initial myocardial infarction, he drove his car despite too high a blood concentration of alcohol. A minor accident occurred—he hit the car in front of him while waiting in a traffic line. During discussions with the other drivers, the patient became very aggressive and violent. This led to prosecution and the patient was sentenced to jail. I tried to plead medical reasons for pardon. I even explained to the court that this man would lose everything in his social situation and that he was likely to die a cardiovascular death if they would take him to jail. The negotiations took half a year. Finally they decided to force him to go to jail. The same day he had a large myocardial septal infarct and died the following day. It is interesting in this case that the dramatic incident itself did not elicit a myocardial infarction—the jail term meant a very serious social threat to him, and as long as he thought he could avoid this, nothing serious happened to his cardiovascular health.

Unemployment

During a period of rising unemployment in the whole industrialized world the life change "becoming unemployed" has grown in importance to caregivers because of the large numbers of people who run the risk of

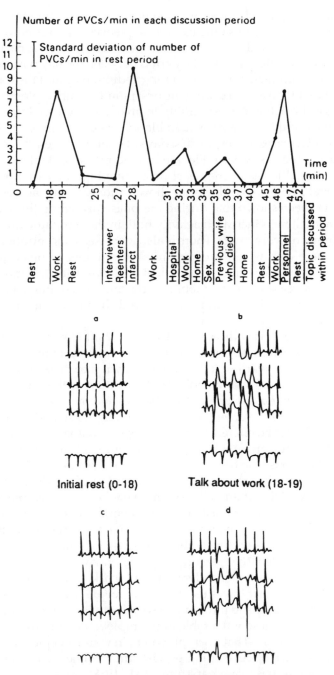

Figure 3   Electrocardiographic recordings during a stressful interview with a patient. (Adapted from Theorell et al., 1981.)

becoming unemployed. Some research was done regarding the medical, psychological, and physiological consequences of becoming unemployed. It was shown that strong anxiety reactions may arise particularly during the anticipatory phase (the period between the day when the subject becomes informed about the coming redundancy and the day when unemployment starts) and during the first months of unemployment. The physiological reaction corresponding to anxiety—increased urinary catecholamine excretion as well as high blood concentration of cortisol and prolactin—decreases during the first days of unemployment but increases again during the first weeks. Elevated blood pressure (Janlert, 1991), as well as lowered levels of the heart protective high density lipoprotein (Arnetz et al., 1991), have also been shown after long-lasting unemployment. It has been shown that during the phase preceding the actual unemployment there is increased activity both in the sympathoadrenal and in the adrenocortical activity. There is also increased concentration of prolactin in the blood, which is of potential importance to blood pressure regulation, at least in women (Theorell et al., 1993). These reactions could be due to increased energy mobilization and concomitant protection against uneasy bodily sensations during a difficult situation inducing a profound feeling of powerlessness.

Research has also indicated that a significant elevation of the total serum cholesterol may be observed after some months of unemployment. In one study of shipyard workers it was shown that those men who had the most pronounced serum cholesterol elevation in this situation were those who had marked sleeping disturbances and those who were threatened financially by the unemployment—namely, those under 58 years of age who could not be offered a special pension (Mattiasson et al., 1990).

Psychiatric research regarding consequences of unemployment has shown that persons who become unemployed often have feelings of guilt and shame, even when this is not at all relevant, such as when a whole industry has been laid off and all workers have become unemployed. The social network may be seriously hurt by unemployment. In one study of unemployed people in southern Sweden during the 1980s, one of the findings was that contacts with neighbors decreased among unemployed individuals. It is evident that persons who do not have easy access to social contacts are particularly dependent on paid work, since paid work is the only social activity that forces us to be with people whom we would otherwise not choose to spend time with in social activity. Certain groups with latent problems are also vulnerable in unemployment; for instance, those with latent alcoholism. That unemployment in young people is associated with increased risk of developing psychosomatic illness has been shown in prospective studies (Hammarström, et al., 1988).

Another important result from research is the finding that rising unemployment rates affect not only those who become redundant but also those who stay in the working force. The remaining employees are hit by fluctuations in work intensity. These may be hard to predict and can be associated with periods of peak load with excessive overtime work intermingled with periods of low intensity and renewed threats of redundancy. Threats of redundancy may lead to tense relationships and deteriorating social climate in the worksite. This generalized effect—on many groups—of rising unemployment rates may explain why years of high unemployement has been associated with higher cardiovascular mortality than in other years. In some studies a delayed effect of several years has been observed, although this has been debated in the literature (see Brenner and Mooney, 1983; Janlert, 1991).

The relative importance of life changes in triggering illness episodes

The answer to this is very difficult to obtain, partly because the definitions are vague. There is, however, literature regarding the magnitude of associations between life changes and onset of illness. A substantial part of this literature deals with specific life changes in relationship to specific disorders. One example is that during the Israeli-Arab wars, a rising incidence of "pregnancy toxicosis" resulting in high blood pressure was recorded in those areas that were hit most extensively by the war. Another example is the increased prevalence of high blood pressure in populations who migrate from one country to another (Beaglehole et al., 1979; Cassel, 1975). A third example is the increase in cardiovascular mortality that has been observed in some studies (but not all) in newly bereaved subjects (Parkes et al., 1969).

Another part of the literature describes the effects of life changes in general on illness in general—a test of the ideas originally presented by Holmes and Rahe. One difficulty has been that in many of the studies that have been published self-administered questionnaires have been utilized both for recording the life changes and the subsequent illness episodes. The results of such studies could be hard to interpret, since it is not known what precedes what. This is particularly true when there has been concomitant recording of life changes and illness experience. Some associations have been established, however. There is agreement that there is a relationship between nonspecific life changes and deteriorated health conditions, although the associations are weak. In the study of 7000 middle-aged building construction workers the relative risk of developing a myocardial infarction associated with change and load at work was 1.6. This risk was unaffected by known biomedical risk factors. In middle-aged men it has been shown that the association between an accumulation of critical life changes during one period and the subsequent years may be modified by social support. When the social support is good the association between life changes and subsequent myocardial infarction risk is small, but when the social support is bad, the relationship is strong (Rosengren et al., 1993).

Post-traumatic stress syndrome

It has been suspected for a long time that difficult life changes during childhood, for instance incest and physical abuse, could influence morbidity
later in adult life. It has been suspected that patients with chronic pain syndromes may have had more such experiences than others. Such a hypothesis is very difficult to examine scientifically, since subjects do not willingly
report such life changes and may even suppress them. In an ongoing study
of the effects of art psychotherapy, it has been shown that during art psychotherapy patients with long-lasting psychosomatic illness start telling
about this kind of experiences but that it may take a long time—several
months—before they do so. The expressive arts may help the patient with
associations that enable him/her to remember. In this study symptoms of
depression and anxiety were common and pronounced during the first
whole year of treatment but decreased significantly after a year. During
the first months the patients have to establish trust and after this, pro-
cessing of previous experiences may start. What the role of these early traumatic experiences may be on cardiovascular morbidity is unknown and
remains a future field for research.

Interventions

In the clinical situation it is obvious that the clinician can do many things
to improve his/her patients' ability to cope with critical life changes. This
is particularly relevant in cardiac rehabilitation and in long-term follow-
up of patients with chronic cardiovascular conditions, such as angina pectoris and arrhythmias. Some of these are outlined in the clinical examples
presented above and could be summarized as follows:

1. Systematic interest in the patient's ongoing life changes; questions
   should not be too vague ("Is there anything going on in your life?").
   More specific questions are preferable, for instance regarding
   changes in work responsibilities, working hours, conflicts at work
   or at home, changes in the health of family members or close friends,
   etc. This enables the patient to analyze more specifically his/her
   own life changes. Life change scores can be used. Excellent questionnaires have been constructed (see, for instance, Rahe, 1990). If
   such questionnaires are used, it is important that they form the basis
   for a clinical conversation.
2. Physiological monitoring—as outlined above, it is possible to monitor relevant physiological parameters in the patient in relation to
   ongoing life changes. This may serve as a kind of "biofeedback".
   Parameters of relevance may be serum lipids, carbohydrate metabolism, blood pressure (preferably measured during activity at work
   and at home), 24-hour recording of electrocardiogram for the recording of arrthythmias and ST-segment depression.

3. Physiological monitoring during conversation about critical life changes that the patient has gone through, as outlined above. This may be of great help to the patient in increasing his/her understanding of the relationship between life situation and clinical course.

What has been published regarding support to people going through critical life changes? Most of the literature could be divided into reports describing family psychotherapy during family crises and reports describing changes in the work situation. Very little of this has been related specifically to cardiovascular disease, and I have therefore selected some examples that are potentially of relevance to cardiovascular disease. Some of these are useful in the clinical setting and others, although this has to be proved, could be of relevance to primary prevention.

According to the psychological and sociological frameworks described above, an important distinction could also be made between interventions aiming at the improvement of individual coping strategies in difficult situations and interventions improving the framework surrounding critical life changes. Another distinct group of publications deals with factors of importance to successful coping with critical life changes, for instance, "stamina", positive vitality helping subjects to cope (Colerick, 1985). It has been pointed out that an emotional coping style (to react with feelings and not with cognitive coping, logical reasoning, in crisis) is associated with increased illness risk. This is a complicated area, however, because long-lasting suppression of emotions may increase the risk of illness development according to other research results. Our own research results in the field of hypertension point in this direction (see above).

On the other hand, the published number of critical evaluations of the effects of improved framework in critical life changes is small. An evaluation of the effects of psychological support to newly bereaved widows has been published (Parkes, 1980). According to the results of this study, the incidence and severity of psychiatric disorder was lower after the first year of follow-up in the support group than it was in a similarly selected comparison group of widows who did not receive any offer of improved support. Another study has been published in which ten 2-hour lessons were given regarding coping with critical life changes (Marx et al., 1984). The participants were North American students. During the first lessons the group leader actively showed how to solve crisis situations. During the following lessons the participants were active in role plays and other exercises practicing how to solve problems in crisis. During the follow-up period the participants in the intervention groups showed a decrease in number of illness episodes and number of sick leave days—an improvement that was not observed in the comparison group, who had not been trained in this way. These approaches have not been evaluated in relation to cardiovascular disease.

Examples of changes in the framework

In a cancer ward a special support program was designed for relatives (Häggmark, 1989). It was reasoned that the needs of the relatives had been seriously neglected and that the staff could play a key role in improved support by means of increased information to, and participation of, relatives in the practical care of the patient. It was hypothesized that the offer of such a program would result in decreased suffering in the relatives. A support program was started in one of the wards. This program had several components—increased possibility for relatives to spend time in the ward and to receive information in specially designed group meetings and, finally, in selected cases, education in practical care. Which of these components could be of importance is impossible to deduce from the results of the evaluation. There were parts in the program that were not appreciated by all relatives. Several relatives felt a pressure to take the patient home for home care and found that this was unfair. The staff regarded the program in a very positive way, but follow-up showed that they also may have perceived difficulties; they may not have thought of relatives so much previously and now there were demands on them to provide service to this new group without special education.

The program was evaluated in relatives who were offered increased participation (although all who were offered this did not participate in it), as well as in a comparison group of relatives who were comparable with regard to gender and age, as well as the type and severity of the cancer in the patient. Neuroendocrine measurements, psychiatric standardized assessments of depression, anxiety, and mental exhaustion, social activity/coping and attitudes to taking the patient home for home care were made once a month in both groups. Whenever a patient died, his/her relative was followed with the same measurements 1 month, 2 months, and 1 year after the death of the patient. The results showed that the relatives who were offered the special program were much more prepared mentally for the death of the patient. They also showed much less mental exhaustion than relatives in the comparison group during the terminal stage of the patient's illness, as well as after the first month following the patient's death (Häggmark et al., 1991). After one whole year of follow-up there were significantly fewer signs of depression in the experimental group than in the comparison group. Interestingly, it was in the "activated group" (i.e., those who had been offered the special program for relatives) that a marked and statistically significant rise in plasma cortisol concentration was observed during the terminal phase of the patient's illness (Theorell et al., 1987). In the comparison group there was no such clear tendency. During the active care period the plasma concentration of prolactin tended to be lower in the experimental group. This could be explained by a more active coping pattern in this group.

The example seems to illustrate that it is possible to create active programs for the prevention of depression after the cancer death of a relative.

As expected the relative who had been offered the program became more aware of the risk of near-future death of the patient, which may be one reason why relatives who had been offered the program had less severe and also fewer long-lasting illness episodes during follow-up. In a more general sense it could be stated that increased ability to predict and control may improve the relative's ability to predict the illness course and also decrease the late psychological complications. Increased ability to predict and to have control over the psychological course has decreased the adverse consequences of this critical life change. This example may be of significance to the prevention of cardiovascular disorder, since depression is an important factor in the prediction of death in patients who have suffered a myocardial infarction, for instance.

One other example involves subway train drivers who have been exposed to the Person Under Train (PUT) situation (Theorell et al., 1992, 1994). In this situation the drivers have been in control when their trains have ridden as a person. A recently published study showed drivers who have been exposed to this situation and who are followed during 1 year are more likely than comparable drivers who have not gone through this experience to be on long-term sick leave during the year following the event. The percentage on sick leave for at least 1 month during the period 3 to 12 months after the event was 25% higher than expected. Three weeks after the PUT event, increased sleep disturbance and elevated plasma concentration of prolactin were observed—this acute psychophysiological "normal" reaction, however, had no relationship with long-term sick leave later during the year of follow-up.

Two other factors recorded 3 weeks after PUT did have a statistically significant and mutually independent predictive relationship with long-term sick leave, namely, degree of depression (as reported by the subject in a self-administered questionnaire) and plasma concentration of cortisol. This may indicate that those who were already in bad psychic health when the accident occurred were those who were most likely to suffer from PUT for a long time. The circumstances were also of significance in the prediction; if the person under train either died or was only mildly injured, the likelihood was small that the driver would be on long-term sick leave. When the person under train had been seriously injured, on the other hand, the likelihood was much greater that the driver would be absent from work for a long time. Another observation was that those drivers who had gone through the PUT experience perceived their psychosocial working environment as good during the first months but later reported serious deterioration. No similar observation was made in the comparison group of drivers.

In summary, social support in this situation (and perhaps in other similar situations as well, such as those occurring in health care in which deaths of patients who have become emotionally important to the caregiver and whose death may partly be due to the care, are frequent) is needed most urgently several months after the event. According to the drivers who were interviewed in this study, the best source of support is probably drivers who have experienced the same situation. Support should be organized from this source for a long time after the PUT situation. A smaller subgroup of drivers need professional help from psychologists who have been trained in trauma psychology. These may perhaps be identified according to the observations reported—by means of self-reported depression and a high plasma cortisol level. The results may also indicate that it could be of help for the driver to receive information regarding the person who had been seriously injured—how the rehabilitation is proceeding, etc. Merely doing the study increased the awareness in the employer (the Stockholm county) that this is an important event and that rehabilitation of the drivers has to start during an early phase. The potential importance of these observations for the prevention of cardiovascular disorder is indirect—lack of social support is a known risk factor in relation to myocardial infarction risk, and in this case, the provision of long-lasting social support in a crisis situation may be crucial in the prevention of depression in many cases (which increases the risk of developing cardiovascular disorder).

Summary

Critical life changes are undoubtedly important potential stressors to patients and others and seem to have both specific and nonspecific importance to the cardiovascular disorders. Merely discussing critical life changes with patients may be therapeutically meaningful, since such a discussion may help the patient to obtain an improved perspective. The individual's previous experiences, social support, and individual characteristics are important in the prediction of health consequences of critical life changes. The characteristics of the life change itself are also important—different types of critical life changes are of significance to different types of health outcome. For instance, changes in the working situation may be of particular importance to the development of myocardial infarction in middle-aged men, and, according to many researchers, unemployment may influence both cardiovascular risk factors and the risk of cardiovascular disorders in the population adversely. In some situations life changes that are perceived as positive may be associated with improved health. A supportive framework as well as interventions aiming at improved individual coping may be useful in the prevention of adverse health outcomes.

References

Antonovsky, A. (1987). *Unraveling the Mystery of Health*. San Francisco: Jossey-Bass.
Arnetz, B. B., Brenner, S-O., Levi, L. et al. (1991). Neuroendocrine and immunologic effects of unemployment and job insecurity. *Psychother. Psychosom.*, 55, 76–80.
Beaglehole, R., Eyles, E., and Prior, I. (1979). Blood pressure and migration in children. *Int. J. Epidemiol.*, 8, 5–10.
Brenner, M. H. and Mooney, A. (1983). Unemployment and health in the context of economic change. *Soc. Sci. Med.*, 17, 1125–1138.

Brown, G. W. and Harris, T. (1978). *Social Origins of Depression—A Study of Psychiatric Disorders in Women*. London: Tavistock.

Cassel, J. (1975). Studies of hypertension in migrants. In Oglesby, P. (Ed). *Epidemiology and Control of Hypertension*. pp. 41–58. New York: Stratton.

Chadwick, J., Chesney, M., Black, G. W., Rosenman, R. M., and Sevelius, G. G. (1979). *Psychological Job Stress and Coronary Heart Disease*. Menlo Park: Stanford Research Institute.

Colerick, E. J. (1985). Stamina in later life. *Soc. Sci. Med.*, 21, 997–1006.

Connolly, J. (1976). Life events before myocardial infarction. *J. Hum. Stress*, 2, 3–17.

Dohrenwend, B. S. and Dohrenwend, B. P. (Eds). (1974). *Stressful Life Events, Their Nature and Effects*. New York: Wiley.

Edwards, J. R. and Cooper, C. I. (1988). The impacts of positive psychological states and physical health: a review and theoretical framework. *Soc. Sci. Med.*, 27, 1447–1459.

de Faire, U. and Theorell, T. (1984). *Life Stress and Coronary Heart Disease*. St. Louis: Warren H. Green.

Häggmark, C. (1989). Invitation to relatives to participate in the care of the cancer patient at the hospital. Effects of an activation programme. Academic thesis. Karolinska Institute, Stockholm, Sweden.

Häggmark, C., Bachner, M., and Theorell, T. (1991). A follow-up of psychological state in relatives of cancer patients one year after the patient's death. Effects of an activation programme. *Acta Oncol.*, 30, 677–684.

Hammarström, A., Janlert, U., and Theorell, T. (1988). Youth unemployment and ill health: results from a 2-year follow-up study. *Soc. Sci. Med.*, 26, 1025–1033.

Hollis, J. F., Connett, J. E., Stevens, V. J., and Greenlick, M. R. (1990). Stressful life events, type A behavior, and the prediction of cardiovascular and total mortality over six years. *J. Behav. Med.*, 13, 263–280.

Holmes, T. H. and Rahe, R. H. (1967). The social readjustment rating scale. *J. Psychosom. Res.*, 11, 213–218.

Isaksson, H., Konarski, K., and Theorell, T. (1992). The psychological and social condition of hypertensives resistant to pharmacological treatment. *Soc. Sci. Med.* 35(7), 869–875.

Janlert, U. (1991). Work deprivation and health. Consequences of job loss and unemployment. Academic thesis. Department of Social Medicine, Karolinska Institute, Stockholm, Sweden.

Kagan, A. R. and Levi, L. (1971). Adaptation of the psychosocial environment to man's abilities and needs. In L. Levi (Ed) *Society, Stress and Disease. The Psychosocial Environment and Psychosomatic Diseases*. pp. 399–404. London: Oxford University Press.

Lichtenstein, P. (1993). Genetic and environmental mediation of the association between psychosocial factors and health. Academic thesis. Karolinska Institute, Stockholm, Sweden.

Marx, M. B., Somes, G. W., Garrity, T. F., Reeb, A. C., Jr., and Maffeo, P. A. (1984). The influence of a supportive, problemsolving group intervention on the health status of students with great recent life change. *J. Psychosom. Res.*, 28, 275–278.

Mattiasson, I., Lindgärde, F., Nilsson, J. Å., and Theorell, T. (1990). Threat of unemployment and cardiovascular risk factors: longitudinal study of quality of sleep and serum cholesterol concentrations in men threatened with redundancy. *Br. Med. J.*, 301, 461–466.

Parkes, C. M. (1980). Bereavement counselling: does it work? *Br. Med. J.*, iii, 281.

Parkes, C. M., Benjamin, B., and Fitzgerald, R. G. (1969). Broken heart: a statistical study of increased mortality among widowers. *Br. Med. J.*, 1, 740.

Rahe, R. H. (1990). Life change, stress responsivity, and captivity research. Presidential address. *Psychosom. Med.*, 52, 373–396.

Rosengren, A., Orth-Gomér, K., Wedel, H., and Wilhelmsen, L. (1993). Stressful life events, social support, and mortality in men born in 1933. *Br. Med. J.*, 307, 1102–1105.

Shalit, B. (1978). Report number 1: the instrument, design, administration and scoring. *FOA Rep.*, 2, 10450.

Svensson, J. and Theorell, T. (1983). Life events and elevated blood pressure in young men. *J. Psychosom. Med.*, 27, 445–455.

Theorell, T. (1976). Selected illnesses and somatic risk factors in relation to two psychosocial stress indices—a prospective study of middle-aged construction building workers. *J. Psychosom. Res.*, 20, 7–20.

Theorell, T. (1991). Health promotion in the workplace. In B. Badura and I. Kickbusch (Eds). *Health Promotion Research. Towards a New Social Epidemiology.* WHO Regional Publications European Series No. 37. Copenhagen: World Health Organization.

Theorell, T. and Emlund, N. (1993). On physiological effects of positive and negative life changes—a longitudinal study. *J. Psychosom. Res.*, 37, 653–659.

Theorell, T. and Floderus-Myrhed, B. (1977). `Work-load' and risk of myocardial infarction: a prospective psychosocial analysis. *Int. J. Epidemiol.*, 6, 17–21.

Theorell, T., Lind, E., Fröberg, J., Karlsson, C. G., and Levi, L. (1972). A longitudinal study of 21 coronary subjects—life changes, catecholamines and related biochemical variables. *Psychosom. Med.* 34, 505–516.

Theorell, T., Floderus, B., and Lind, E. (1975). The relationship of disturbing life-changes and emotions to the early development of myocardial infarction and other serious illnesses. *Int. J. Epidemiol.*, 4, 281–293.

Theorell, T., Olsson, A., and Engholm, G. (1977). Concrete work and myocardial infarction. *Scand. J. Work Environ. Health*, 3, 144–153.

Theorell, T., Svensson, J., Knox, S., Waller, D., and Alvarez, M. (1986). Young men with high blood pressure report *few* recent life events. *J. Psychosom. Res.*, 30, 243–249.

Theorell, T., Häggmark, C., and Eneroth, P. (1987). Psycho-endocrinological reactions in female relatives of cancer patients. Effects of an activation programme. *Acta Oncol.*, 26, 419–424.

Theorell, T., Leymann, H., Jodko, M., Konarski, K., Norbeck, H. E., and Eneroth, P. (1992). "Person under train" incidents: medical consequences for subway drivers. *Psychosom. Med.*, 54, 480–488.

Theorell, T., Ahlberg-Hultén, G., Jodko, M., Sigala, F., and de la Torre, B. (1993). Influence of job strain and emotion on blood pressure levels in female hospital personnel during work hours. *Scand. J. Work Environ. Health*, 19, 264–269.

Theorell, T., Leymann, H., Jodko, M., Konarski, K., and Norbeck, H. E. (1994). "Person under train" incidents from the subway driver's point of view—a prospective 1-year follow-up study: the design, and medical and psychiatric data. *Soc. Sci. Med.*, 38, 471–475.

Theorell, T., Lind, E., Lundberg, U., Christensson, T., and Edhag, O. (1981). The individual and his work in relation to a myocardial infarction. In *Society, Stress and Disease*, L. Levi (Ed.), Vol. 4, pp. 191–199. London: Oxford University Press.

chapter eight

Life events, coping, and cancer

E. Brian Faragher

Introduction

The possibility of a direct, and potentially causal, relationship between psychological factors and all forms of cancer has been hypothesized for centuries. Nevertheless, this premise remains controversial, the published evidence having failed so far to produce either a cumulative acceptance or rejection of the hypothesis. Arguably, the very earliest advocate of such a link was Galen[1] who, in his treatise on tumors *De Tumoribus*, observed a connection between cancer and personality, reporting that malignancies seemed to occur more frequently in "*melancholic*" than in "*sanguine*" women. More contemporarily, supportive anecdotal evidence was furnished during the 18th and 19th centuries by such eminent physicians as Guy and Paget.[2]

The first known empirical evidence of a relationship between psychosocial stress and cancer was provided by the publication in 1893 of Herbert Snow's book *Cancer and the Cancer Process*.[3] He reported a study of 250 successive patients treated at the London Cancer Hospital between 1883 and 1893. Some form of "immediate antecedent trouble" was identified for 156 (63%) of these individuals, thus forging the first definite empirical link connecting emotional stress with cancer. This publication also marked the early stages of serious research during the latter part of the 19th and early part of the 20 centuries into the exact nature of any association between these entities, culminating in the book *A Psychological Study of Cancer*.[4] Based on her work with cancer sufferers, Evans noticed that the loss of a love object or important emotional relationship was a frequent precursor to the diagnosis of the disease. This led her to believe that some people, when experiencing grief, direct their psychic energy inwards against their own natural body defences. In a more recent historical review, LeShan[5] also observed that the loss of a major emotional relationship was commonly reported as preceding the detection of a malignancy.

Interest in the overall relationship between antecedent psychosocial stress (as measured by the occurrence of adverse, stress-inducing life events) and many different forms of illness has increased since Evans published her work, although the greatest attention has only been directed at this problem over the last three decades.[6] Most research has been concentrated into the cardiovascular field; the relationship between stress and heart disease, particularly myocardial infarction and hypertension, has been well documented and is now widely recognized.[7-9] An association between maternal stress and low birthweight has been reported by Newton and Hunt.[10] Apparent correlations between several forms of malignancy and antecedent stress have been published by Lehrer[11] (gastric carcinoma), Jacobs and Charles[12] (pediatric carcinoma), Eysenck[13] (lung cancer), and Cooper[14] (breast cancer).

In more recent years, a considerable amount of attention has been directed at a possible association between breast cancer and psychosocial stress (Cooper,[15] Cooper and Watson[16]). However, "given the absence of any known major environmental precursors to breast cancer, it is perhaps surprising to discover how little research has been done on the link with psychosocial stress" (Cooper, et al.[17]). The few studies that have been published tend to be methodologically flawed, producing findings that are, at best, both contradictory and confusing. Even among those studies that report a relationship between psychosocial stress and breast cancer, there is no definite consensus as to the form and strength of the association. At present, the only inference that can be drawn with any degree of confidence is that any relationship between psychosocial factors and breast cancer is likely to be a complex interrelationship involving a combination of potentially predisposing stressful events, coping abilities, personality, and personal support systems.

Published studies in this field can be subdivided broadly into two categories. In the first, attention has been focused primarily on the possibility of a link between the pathogenesis of breast cancer and emotional history or adverse life events. In the second, studies have tended to concentrate on examining the relationship between various psychometric predispositions and breast cancer. These latter studies can themselves be further divided into two subgroups; those which address the role of behavioral traits (personality) in the disease process, and those which examine the types and effectiveness of coping skills employed by individuals when dealing with stressful situations.

Life events and cancer

In terms of the empirical epidemiological research available, most attention has been directed towards life events research. In LeShan's[5] early review of 75 studies on psychological factors thought to be associated with the development of malignant disease, he concluded that "the most consistently reported, relevant psychological factor has been the loss of a major emotional relationship prior to the first-noted symptoms of neoplasm". He later carried out a large-scale epidemiological study[18] into mortality rates among groups of people likely to be affected by the loss of a close emotional relationship. He predicted that cancer mortality rates should be highest for widowed, next highest for divorced, and lowest for married and then single persons, if the theory of loss of emotional relationships was valid. He analyzed epidemiological data from a number of studies, age-adjusting the mortality rates, and found that the data were consistent with this hypothesis.

Muslin and colleagues[19] carried out an investigation of 165 women who were about to have a breast biopsy. The women were interviewed and given a life events questionnaire prior to diagnosis, from which 37 matched pairs of malignant and benign subjects were produced. Twice as many diagnosed cancer patients were found to have had "a permanent loss of a first degree relative or other person whom the subject specifically stated was emotionally important to her" than did the benign group. Concurrently, Schmale and Iker[20] reported a study exploring the same phenomenon among a group of women who were reporting for a cone biopsy as a result of a positive Pap test. They were given psychological tests and interviewed prior to diagnosis and none of the subjects had any gross abnormality that would lead the physician to suspect cervical cancer. On the basis of high life events scores 6 months prior to the first positive Pap smear, the authors then predicted who would ultimately be diagnosed as having cervical cancer. It was found that there was a significantly high level of accuracy in their judgements, based almost solely on life events immediately preceding the first tests.

In a later investigation of premorbid breast cancer, Greer[21] studied 160 women admitted to hospital for a breast tumor biopsy; for the purpose of the study, a breast tumor was defined as being "a tumor with or without palpable axillary nodes, with no deep attachment and no distant metastases", that is, women with either very early breast cancer, which is operable, or women with some benign breast disease. These patients were interviewed on the day prior to the biopsy and detailed information was collected on stressful life events (e.g., events that caused them severe and prolonged emotional distress). All recorded events were verified by husbands or close relatives. Psychometric data were also collected on depression, hostility, extraversion/neuroticism, and other social and psychiatric states. After the operation, 69 women were found to have breast cancer and 91 a benign breast disease. The cancer and control (benign disease) groups were matched in most respects (e.g., social class, marital state, etc.), except that the cancer patients were significantly older. No significant differences were found with respect to the occurrence of stressful life events, including loss of a loved person, or depression, or denial as the characteristic response to life stresses. Although an effort was made to design the research in a way that would minimize the effects of diagnosed cancer on personality and the recall of life events, the author admits to having "no control over what surgeons told patients before admission". He was also unable to control for the fear of having surgery that could result in the diagnosis of breast cancer and the removal of a breast. As well, the cancer group was significantly older, which could have biased the results. Most importantly, since breast cancer may take several years to develop and the stressful life events responsible may have taken place years before that, there was a strong potential "memory falsification" problem.

Subsequently, Priestman and co-workers[22] reported a study of 200 women presenting at a surgical clinic with a newly discovered breast lump or attending a radiotherapy department for treatment of stage I/II breast cancers diagnosed within the previous 3 months; 100 of the women had breast cancer and 100 had benign breast disease. These women were compared against a group of 100 healthy controls. Unfortunately, 93 of the cancer group and 66 of the benign disease group knew their diagnosis at the time of assessment. The controls were found to have experienced *more* stressful life events, but the types of events experienced were similar in all three study groups. No differences were found on the standard EPI personality scale. The cancer group was significantly older than the other two groups, and the control group was selected from a higher socioeconomic status, but neither imbalance appeared to have affected the study findings.

Cheang and Cooper[23] studied 121 women undergoing a breast lesion biopsy and a control group of 42 women selected from a well-woman clinic. Subsequently, 46 of the lesion group were diagnosed as having cancer while the remaining 75 had benign breast disease; however, all women were studied prior to histological diagnosis being completed. The three groups were well-balanced demographically, although the cancer group was slightly older on average. In this study, the cancer patients experienced significantly more events than the other two groups; the types of events reported by the cancer group were proportionally more loss-related and/or illness-related.

More recently, Edwards et al.,[24] reporting a study of 1052 women interviewed while awaiting diagnosis of a breast problem, found few significant relationships between psychosocial variables and breast cancer after controlling for age and history of the disease. The relationships that were identified were moderated by coping style, type A behavioral traits, and availability of social support. Conversely, in a study carried out over the same time period, Forsen[25] found significantly more life events, more bereavement/loss events, and more difficult life situations immediately prior to the diagnosis of a breast tumor in a group of 87 women compared with a group of 87 matched controls. A greater use of repressive defence mechanisms was also found in the cancer group.

In common with most stress-related research involving life event methodology, these studies into the role of life events as antecedents to the detection of a breast cancer have tended to use the Holmes and Rahe Social Readjustment Rating Scale (SRRS)[26] as the prime measuring tool. However, there have been other studies that have explored traumatic life events and cancer, without using the SRRS.

In one such study, Smith and Sebastian[27] examined the emotional history of 44 cancer patients and 44 patients with physical abnormalities that were noncancerous. Structured interviews were carried out to try and identify the frequency, intensity, and duration of emotional states in each person's life, which involved questions about family life, childhood, social and sexual life, career, religion, etc. Critical incidents were then recorded and rated as either high, medium, or low, and the intensity and duration of the emotional events for each person were rated on a 15-point scale. It was found that there were significantly more frequent and intense emotional events prior to diagnosis among cancer patients than in the comparison group.

Another interesting, much earlier, study along these lines was undertaken by Witzel,[28] of 150 cancer patients and 150 patients with other serious diseases. He took personal histories of past illnesses and found that noncancer patients had a significantly larger number of reported incidents of medical problems throughout their lives than cancer patients. They reported being out-patients three times more often, being in a hospital bed three times more often, having temperatures in excess of 38.5°C seven times more often, and experiencing twice as many minor illnesses and operations. The authors contend that this does not necessarily contradict the other research on adverse life events, as these critical medical incidents may signal the disease process itself. As Fox[29] has suggested "developing cancer had mobilised the immune response, which is capable of fighting many diseases, and which, because of its aroused status, could do so more successfully than that of non-cancer patients".

Problems associated with life events methodology

As previously stated, most studies on the role of life events as antecedents to the detection of a breast cancer have used the SRRS as the prime measuring tool. This scale and others that have followed it (Paykel[30]) produce scores based on weightings allocated to each of a series of listed life events. These weightings are mainly generated from either a large general population sample or from a smaller, but more representative, sample drawn from the specific population under investigation.

There are, unfortunately, methodological problems common to all instruments involving the use of generic weightings—these may inadvertently bias or distort study findings, which may go some way in explaining the apparent lack of any consistent thread to the results published in this field. There are two major areas of concern. Firstly, all of the scales present a list of items that are a mixture of critical incidents (such as marital breakdown, redundancy, etc.) and events that may be symptoms or consequences of an underlying illness. In the case of the latter category, the illness itself may serve to impede or even prevent the patient from recalling accurately the times and order of events, particularly if these are now

viewed as relatively trivial in the light of more serious events that have occurred in the interim.[31] Secondly, and much more importantly, each event
on the scale is likely to have a differential meaning for each subject, but individual perceptions are rarely taken into account; conversely, indeed, the
items are usually allocated rigid weightings (scores) for all subjects. These
weightings will also have limited validity if applied to subjects in other
centers, particularly if cultural boundaries are crossed (e.g., a scale developed in the U.S. may have little clinical value if used in Europe, and possibly no value at all if applied in a developing nation in the so-called Third
World).

In a retrospective study designed specifically to address these problems,[17] weightings based on a subsample drawn from the population to be
studied in detail were found to be frequently in conflict with individual
perceptions of such events. A 10-point Likert-type rating scale was devised
to provide a rating for each of 42 life events generated from a U.K. female
sample in terms of its degree of stressfulness or upset to the individual.[23]
A total of 18 life events were common to the SRRS and the Cheang/Cooper
inventory. Using data obtained from 53 women attending a breast screening clinic (all of whom were ultimately diagnosed as having breast cancer)
and 418 "well-women" attending for an annual medical screen, these perceptual ratings were compared with the weighted items common to the
SRRS. A number of interesting findings emerged which raise doubts about
the validity of using standardized weighted life event scales.

- The SRRS weights for many of the life events investigated were substantially different from the Cheang/Cooper perception ratings of
  both the cancer group and the well-woman control group. As the
  SRRS weights were devised in the U.S. using both males and females,
  whereas the Cheang/Cooper scale was devised in the U.K. using
  only females, these differences could reflect cultural and/or gender
  differences. Interestingly, events related to the stability of the family
  (such as family member left home or a difficult relationship within
  the family unit) were rated higher both in the U.K. sample and by
  female respondents relative to the general U.S. population studied.
- Substantial differences were found between the Cheang/Cooper
  perception ratings provided by the cancer and control groups for
  the same life event. Thus, if the proportions of individuals in the
  two groups with a given event were equal, no significant difference
  would be found using the SRRS, even though the cancer patients
  were apparently perceiving these events to be as much as twice as
  stressful as the women in the control group. (The cancer group provided higher perception ratings than the controls for 29 of the 42
  items on the Cheang/Cooper scale.)
- In extensive, in-depth interviews with 200 of the women studied, a
  number of significant life events were identified as being important

to include on an inventory but which did not appear on many of the standardized scales. In many cases, these events were discovered in between 25 to 35% of the study sample, and included events such as illness of a close family member, increased nursing responsibility for elderly parents or other family member, and (temporary) separation from a loved one.

Another, often glaring, weakness in the published literature is statistical inadequacy of the sample sizes employed. Total sample sizes rarely exceed 200 patients, with individual diagnosis group sizes often considerably less than 100. This raises the inevitable question as to how representative the samples are of the population from which they have been selected. Many studies have found loss-related and illness-related events to be closely associated with diagnosis; both types of event occur relatively infrequently in the general population. This problem is further exacerbated if the time scale over which these events are studied is relatively short (commonly the 2 to 3 years immediately preceding diagnosis). The more infrequent the event, the larger the sample that is required to obtain an acceptably precise estimate of the true population frequency and to establish statistical significance between diagnostic subgroups.

Despite these methodological concerns, the area of stressful life events and the pathogenesis of cancer remains a potentially fruitful field of future research. The published evidence, with all of its shortcomings, suggests strongly that, at the very least, adverse life events must act as an intervening, if not primary, source of illness behavior.

Coping strategies and breast cancer

The process by which a person selects coping strategies when attempting to deal with stress has been the subject of surprisingly little published research. Equally little appears to be known about the way in which the strategies chosen are then implemented. Nevertheless, a widely held recognition exists that the ability to cope with stress is an important determinant of well-being.[32-36] Several attempts have been made to advance theories to explain the coping process. All contain inherent flaws.

Building on the writings of Freud, Adler, and Jung, one theory suggests a psychoanalytic stratagem. A hierarchical structure is postulated, within which coping is defined as a form of adjustment. Realistic thoughts and actions directed towards the solution of problems are placed above (i.e., are considered to be more efficient) than less reality-oriented strategies, such as denial and avoidance. Unfortunately for this theory, there are many documented circumstances in which the denial of reality can prove to be a most effective method of coping. For example, when an individual is initially overwhelmed by an event or judges the situation as being uncontrollable, denial may actually help to reduce the stress levels produced by the event.[37-39] On this basis, avoidance coping strategies may well have short-term efficacy, although nonavoidance coping skills will invariably emerge as having long-term superiority. Furthermore, this general approach defines coping strategies solely in terms of their (successful) outcome; failure to meet the demands of a stressful event is defined, per se, as failure. By thus defining coping itself in terms of the (often short-term) outcome, any possibility of investigating the relationship between coping and well-being is effectively neutralized at the source.[33]

The traits which, when used by an individual, provide an increased predisposition to handle stressful situations have been sought by a number of researchers. Hardiness, locus of control, and type A personality are the three major characteristics that have been specifically implicated; the evidence linking these to improved well-being, however, is decidedly equivocal.[40] By definition, coping must be one-dimensional and stable, both over time and across situations, under this theory. The limited empirical evidence available suggests that the exact converse is probably true.[33,41]

A clearly defined sequence of discrete responses activated by an individual as the course of a stressful event unfolds has been postulated. Under this theory, coping becomes a sequence of stages. Kubler-Ross[42] attempted to justify this thesis using the specific example of his research on terminally ill patients; he claimed that, in his study, these patients passed through stages of denial, anger, bargaining, depression, and acceptance. Again, however, no consistent empirical evidence has emerged to support this theory. Most critically, the nature of the trigger mechanism required to provoke the transition between stages has not been identified. Indeed, the restricted amount of evidence that is available tends to support the exact antithesis (that individuals appear to employ a complex and varying cocktail of strategies rather than a fixed sequence of predictable responses when attempting to cope with stress).

The classification of coping techniques by virtue of the methods used or according to the targets (foci) of the strategies used has also been attempted by several researchers. Several classifications of this sort exist. The most widely used are those schemes which discriminate between "problem-focused coping" and "emotion-focused coping". In the former, individuals adopt strategies with the purpose of directly changing either the stress situation itself or their assessment of the situation; in the latter, conversely, individuals select strategies with the intention of moderating their emotional response to the stress event. Moos and Billings[43] have attempted to expand this basic dichotomy, categorizing coping methods into appraisal-focused, problem-focused, and emotion-focused strategies. A criticism of this classification, however, is that each of the three categories is itself defined in terms of a coping strategy. Thus, some forms of appraisal-focused coping methods are described as involving "mentally rehearsing possible actions and their consequences".

Although this theory does have some advantages, it ultimately falters due to the inherent absence of any clearly defined distinction between the methods of coping and their supposed foci. Folkman and Lazarus[33] have pointed out that, because a particular coping strategy may involve several methods or may be directed at a multiplicity of foci, there is also the problem of establishing satisfactory boundaries within the two classifications. Janis and Mann,[44] among others, have observed that inadequate attention has been directed towards the decision process involved in the selection both of coping strategies and of foci, without which a proper understanding of the determinants of stress is impossible. In addition, the mechanisms by which stress and (more importantly) well-being are influenced by coping strategies are also poorly understood.

Finally, a "process" theory of coping has been postulated by Edwards.[45] In this model, emphasis is given to "the process by which person and situation factors combine to influence coping and the mechanisms by which coping, in turn, influences stress and well-being". Stress is defined as an important, negative discrepancy between an individual's perceived and desired states. By definition, therefore, stress has a negative effect on well-being, whereas coping comprises the efforts made to reduce this negative impact by changing the determinants of the stress. The degree of importance given by individuals to the discrepancy between their perceived and desired states will directly affect both well-being and coping. The model predicts that increasing this importance will reduce well-being and subsequently increase the efforts being made to cope. As a consequence, a negative feedback loop is created. Within this loop, discrepancies between desire and perception reduce well-being; this produces efforts to resolve the discrepancies; these efforts are evaluated to determine their effectiveness. The loop is subsequently repeated in an iterative manner. Uniquely, in order to conform with the empirical evidence, the model allows the use of a multiplicity of coping strategies. These may be selected using less than rational criteria; however, there is a built-in inference that a small number of coping methods chosen in a rational fashion will have the most positive (and hence productive) impact on well-being.

The most recent empirical research strongly supports the theory that coping ability may be related to a proneness to breast cancer. In a study of 91 women awaiting a breast biopsy, Hughson et al.[46] found high levels of psychosocial morbidity, but the levels of anxiety and depression were similar to those measured in a control group of 30 women awaiting elective cholecystectomy. Hilton[47] identified a phenomenon which she described as "uncertainty" in women with breast cancer; this included not being able to foretell the future, not feeling secure and safe from danger, being in doubt, being undecided, perceptions of vagueness, and not being able to rely on someone or something.

Using the Millon Behavioral Health Inventory (MBHI), which categorizes repressive coping styles into "introversive", "cooperative", and "respectful", Goldstein and Antoni[48] compared 44 women recently diagnosed as having breast cancer with 34 healthy controls. The cancer patients reported disproportionately high levels of repressive coping styles and attained a clinically significant score on the "respectful" scale; the controls were found to prefer the use of sensitizing coping strategies. Finally, Liiceanu and co-workers[49] studied 813 women with breast cancer and 685 nonmalignant controls. They found the cancer group exhibited a greater tendency to internal rather than external locus of control, producing "a rigidity of the self expressed by resistance to change and low self-confidence".

The evidence supporting a link between coping skills and cancer is not new. Evans' seminal work postulating that some people, when experiencing grief, direct their psychic energies inwards against their own natural body defences has already been noted.[4] Tarlau and Smalheiser[50] reported negative attitudes towards sexuality, rejection of the female role, and patterns of mother dominance in a study of 22 women with tumors. Similar findings were reported by Bacon et al.[51] in a case history study of 40 women with breast cancer; one of the major behavioral characteristics of this group was an inability to discharge or deal appropriately with anger, aggressiveness, or hostility covered over by a facade of pleasantness. A similar result was observed by LeShan and Worthington[52] in their study of 152 breast cancer patients and 125 control women using a projective test developed by Worthington. The cancer group differed from the controls in that they had difficulty expressing hostile feelings, they suffered the loss of a "dear one" in the period preceding diagnosis, and they showed greater potential anxiety about the death of a parent.

Kissen[53] carried out a study among 335 patients, of whom 161 had been diagnosed as having lung cancer, while the others had some other less severe illness. He discovered that, both in their childhood and adult lives, the cancer patients had suffered from a reduced ability for "emotional discharge". In an unpublished study of 93 lung cancer patients and 82 subjects with tubercular disease, Booth[54] found similar patterns among his cancer patients. He found that they responded very differently on an inkblot test compared with the tubercular patients, emphasizing inward direction of anger, a vulnerability to emotional loss, and emotional repression. Grissom and colleagues[55] compared patients with bronchial carcinoma with a group of healthy subjects and found that the former group had lower "personal integration" scores on the Tennessee Self Concept scales, indicating an increased tendency to direct frustration, anger, and failure inward, and a vulnerability to the loss of an important relationship.

Greer and Morris[56] reported a consecutive series of 160 women attending for a breast biopsy. Of these, 69 were subsequently diagnosed histologically as having breast cancer while the remaining 91 were found to have benign breast disease. Few differences emerged between the groups, although the cancer women were (predictably) older. However, a significantly increased proportion of the cancer group manifested extreme suppression of anger and other emotions; this ability to release emotions was found to be positively correlated with age. A similar relationship with anger suppression was found by Bageley,[57] who observed a significant correlation between breast cancer and a chronic behavior pattern of abnormal emotional expression, specifically concealment of emotions and bottling up of anger, in a study including 45 women with breast cancer.

Morris and colleagues[58] evaluated 71 women awaiting a breast biopsy and found that those women diagnosed as having cancer were less likely to experience "feelings of anger" or "loss of control in anger". Similarly in a study of 56 women undergoing a breast biopsy, Wirsching et al.[59] discovered that the women found to have a malignancy showed an increased difficulty in expressing anger, tended to avoid trouble and conflict, were less accessible (i.e., were more aloof), and were less anxious about the likely diagnosis of their lump. Simultaneously, however, these women were also less realistic about the clinical outcome. The women in the cancer group also claimed to be more self-sufficient and altruistic but less aggressive than the women with benign breast disease, tending to sacrifice themselves, particularly to their family.

Jansen and Muenz[60] studied 222 women selected from out-patient clinics for study prior to their being told the diagnosis of their breast complaint. The 69 women ultimately found to have a malignancy recorded reduced levels of aggression and exhibitionism. Relative to the women in the remainder of the sample, the patients with cancer emerged as timid, nonassertive, noncompetitive, calm, easy-going, and inclined to suppress feelings of anger. These findings remained after statistical adjustment for significant group differences with respect to age, ethnic group, educational status, socioeconomic status, and marital status. Tozzi and Pantaleo[61] compared 50 women diagnosed as having breast cancer with 50 diabetic women and 50 healthy women. They found that the stresses of a major loss event (including death or separation from a loved one), depression, repressed hostility towards parents, and desperation, in combination with personality characteristics such as suppression and denial of emotions, appeared to increase the risk of breast cancer.

Bremond and co-workers[62] conducted an age-matched case-control study on 50 women with breast cancer and 105 healthy controls. The cases reported more depleting life events in the 5 years prior to diagnosis, were more committed to prevailing social norms and to the external appearance of being a nice/good person, and had an increased tendency to suppress and internalize their feelings (particularly those of anger). In a study of the psychological characteristics of 76 women awaiting a breast biopsy, Grassi and Cappellari[63] discovered trait characteristics of more emotional suppression and state characteristics of less hostility and irritability under stress among the 41 ultimately found to have a malignant growth. These results support the hypothesis that women prone to breast cancer tend to inhibit emotions, are eager to please, and manifest a calm exterior under stress.

Finally, as an interesting footnote, Kreitler and colleagues[64] compared the psychological profile of 210 women who self-referred for breast screening with 210 matched nonattending women. The attenders were found to score higher on measures of emotion repression, neuroticism, and health orientation, manifesting a profile similar in construct to that of women found to have breast cancer (i.e., to the so-called "cancer prone personality").

General criticisms

A number of general criticisms apply globally to all aspects of the research into the relationship between psychosocial factors and cancer. Those relating specifically to studies of life events have already been dealt with. Several additional problems recur commonly in studies directed at the more subjective areas of coping styles and personalities.

A common problem, particularly in studies of women with breast cancer, is the choice of control group. Many studies restrict their attention to a cancer and a benign disease group. However, the mere presence of a symptom suggestive of a carcinoma can alter some personality factors and the way in which life events are dealt with. Thus, a benign group cannot be reasonably regarded as an adequate control sample for studies into breast cancer. A group of healthy subjects with no known illness or pathology drawn from the same general population as the two disease groups should also be included. Furthermore, if the detection of a potentially malignant lump could affect measures of personality and life events, there is an even greater likelihood that the histological diagnosis will do so. Thus, it is essential that assessment of psychosocial factors is carried out prior to diagnosis, and, if at all possible, before the biopsy is carried out.

Finally, in addition to design problems, there are often considerable concerns relating to the statistical methodology used. Many researchers assume that their measures are statistically independent, with no intercorrelations present, and do so often in the face of overwhelming evidence that this is not the case. For example, the most consistent finding to emerge from studies in breast cancer is that a randomly selected group of women with this type of malignancy will tend to be older on average than groups of women with benign breast disease or normal breasts randomly selected from the same population. Age is thus a major potential confounding factor, but is rarely adjusted for. This problem increases in severity if the measures being used in the study are themselves known to be, or are found to be, age dependent. This property has been established for a number of the more commonly used personality measures; the frequency of loss-related and illness-related events is, intuitively, also likely to increase with age.

Analyzing variables univariately (i.e., in isolation from each other) is thus inadequate.

Statistical adjustment for known confounding factors using appropriate multivariate methods can provide useful insight into the complex interrelationship between psychosocial factors and disease processes. This has been shown in a series of papers[65–69] reporting a quasi-prospective study of 2145 women attending a surgical out-patients clinic or a general health screen, the majority of whom were complaining of breast symptoms; all were unaware of the diagnosis when assessed. Ultimately, 169 women were found to have breast cancer, 155 a cyst, 1107 benign breast disease, and the remaining 714 women were healthy, normal controls. Each woman completed a detailed questionnaire eliciting information on her demographic background, major life events experienced in the previous two years and their impact, strategies used for coping with stressful situations, personality, and social support available.

The four diagnosis groups differed with respect to their demographic characteristics. Most importantly, the women with cancer were 15 years older on average than the other groups; as breast cancer is a disease known to be more prevalent in old age, the emergence of age as a major confounding factor was not unexpected. The four groups also differed significantly with respect to the number and types of life events experienced, the perceived stressful impact of life events, the coping strategies used to handle stress, personality and amount/type of social support available during difficult problems. All of these factors were also correlated significantly with the age. Multivariate statistical methods were used to identify those psychosocial factors which correlated independently with diagnosis, having first adjusted out the effect of age. All four dimensions were found to be implicated in the disease process. Using relative risk estimates, life events outside the locus of control of an individual (e.g., bereavement, serious illness in the family) significantly increased the risk of developing breast cancer, as did more minor life events perceived as having a major stress impact. Women who handled stress by using "internalizing" strategies (i.e., through dependence on their inner resources), who concealed their emotions, and whose personalities made it difficult for them to mobilize support from family and friends were at highest risk of a serious breast diagnosis. Supportive partners and/or mothers mediated risk. However, as levels of social support decreased with advancing age, the mediating effect of this factor diminished, to be replaced by improved personal coping and behavioral skills.

The results obtained suggest that stress tends to break down the effectiveness of the immune system, creating an environment that can cause a tumor to be formed or, if already present, can cause its development to accelerate, but that counseling to provide individual women with "externalizing" (i.e., emotion releasing) coping skills and good interpersonal skills could potentially mediate the clinical implications of the stress.

References

1. Mettler, C. C. and Mettler, F. A., *History of Medicine*, Blackiston, Philadelphia, 1947.
2. Guy, R., *An Essay on Scirrhous Tumours and Cancers*, The Wellcome Historical Medical Library, J. and A. Churchill, London, 1759.
3. Snow, H. L., *Cancer and the Cancer Process*, J. and A. Churchill, London, 1893.
4. Evans, E., *A Psychological Study of Cancer*, Dodd Mead, London, 1926.
5. LeShan, L., Psychological states as factors in the development of malignant disease: a critical review, *J. Natl. Cancer Inst.*, 22, 1, 1959.
6. Cooper, C. L. and Payne, R., *Personality and Stress: Individual Differences in the Stress Process*, John Wiley & Sons, Chichester, 1991.
7. Jenkins, D., Recent evidence supporting psychological and social risk factors for coronary disease, *N. Engl. J. Med.*, 294, 987, 1976.
8. Haynes, S. G., Feinleib, M., Levine, S., Scotch, N., and Kannel, W. B., The relationship of psychosocial factors to coronary heart disease in the Framingham study, *Am. J. Epidemiol.*, 107, 483, 1980.
9. Cooper, C. L., Faragher, E. B., Bray, C. L., and Ramsdale, D. R., The significance of psychosocial factors in predicting coronary artery disease in patients with valvular heart disease, *Soc. Sci. Med.*, 20, 315, 1985.
10. Newton, R. W. and Hunt, L. P., Psychosocial stress in pregnancy and its relation to low birth weight, *Br. Med. J.*, 288, 1191, 1984.
11. Lehrer, S., Life change and gastric cancer, *Psychosom. Med.*, 42, 499, 1980.
12. Jacobs, T. J. and Charles, E., Life events and the occurrence of cancer in children, *Psychosom. Med.*, 42, 11, 1980.
13. Eysenck, H. J., Lung cancer and stress personality inventory, in *Psychosocial Stress and Cancer*, Cooper, C. L., Ed., John Wiley & Sons, Chichester, 1984, 49.
14. Cooper, C. L., Ed., *Psychosocial Stress and Cancer*, John Wiley & Sons, New York, 1984.
15. Cooper, C. L., *Stress and Breast Cancer*, John Wiley and Sons, Chichester, 1988.
16. Cooper, C. L. and Watson, M., *Cancer and Stress: Psychological, Biological and Coping Studies*, John Wiley & Sons, Chichester, 1991.
17. Cooper, C. L., Cooper, R., and Faragher, E. B., Psychosocial stress as a precursor to breast cancer: a review, *Curr. Psychol. Res. Rev.*, 5, 268, 1986.
18. LeShan, L., An emotional life history pattern associated with neoplastic disease, *Annu. NY Acad. Sci. J.*, 125, 780, 1966.
19. Muslin, H. L., Gyarfas, K., and Pieper, W. J., Separation experience and cancer of the breast, *Annu. NY Acad. Sci. J.*, 125, 802, 1966.
20. Schmale, A. H. and Iker, H. P., The effect of hopelessness and the development of cancer, *J. Psychosom. Med.*, 28, 714, 1966.
21. Greer, S., Psychological enquiry: a contribution to cancer research, *J. Psychol. Med.*, 9, 81, 1979.
22. Priestman, T. J., Priestman, S. G., and Bradshaw, C., Stress and breast cancer, *Br. J. Cancer*, 51, 493, 1985.
23. Cheang, A. and Cooper, C. L., Psychological stress and breast cancer, *Stress Med.*, 1, 61, 1985.
24. Edwards, J. R., Cooper, C. L., Pearl, S. G. et al., The relationship between psychosocial factors and breast cancer: some unexpected results, *Behav. Med.*, 16, 5, 1990.

25. Forsen, A., Psychosocial aspects of breast cancer, *Psychiatr. Fenn.*, 21, 189, 1990.
26. Holmes, T. H. and Rahe, R. H., The social readjustment rating scale, *J. Psychosom. Res.*, 11, 231, 1967.
27. Smith, W. R. and Sebastian, R., Emotion history and pathogenesis of cancer, *J. Clin. Psychol.*, 32, 63, 1976.
28. Witzel, L., Anamnese und Zweiterkrankungen bei Patienten mit bösartigen Neubildingen. (Anamnesis and second diseases in patients with malignant tumours), *Med. Klin.*, 65, 867, 1970.
29. Fox, B. H., Premorbid psychological factors as related to cancer incidence, *J. Behav. Med.*, 1, 45, 1978.
30. Paykel, E. S., Methodological aspects of life events research, *J. Psychosom. Res.*, 27, 341, 1983.
31. Napier, J. S., Metzner, H., and Johnson, B. C., Limitations of morbidity and mortality data obtained from family histories: a report from the Tecumseh studies, *Am. J. Public Health*, 62, 30, 1972.
32. Antonovosky, A., *Health, Stress and Coping*, Jossey-Bass, Washington, 1979.
33. Folkman, S. and Lazarus, R. S., If it changes, it must be a process: a study of emotion and coping during three stages of a college examination, *J. Personality Soc. Psychol.*, 48, 150, 1985.
34. Holroyd, K. A. and Lazarus, R. S., Stress, coping and somatic adaptation, in *Handbook of Stress: Theoretical and Clinical Aspects*, Goldberger, L. and Breznitz, S., Eds., The Free Press, New York, 1982, 21.
35. Lazarus, R. S. and Launier, R., Stress-related transactions between person and environment, in *Perspectives in Interactional Psychology*, Pervin, L. A. and Lewis, M., Eds., Plenum Press, New York, 1978.
36. Pearlin, L. I. and Schooler, C., The structure of coping, *J. Health Soc. Behav.*, 9, 2, 1978.
37. Hamburg, D. A. and Adams, J. E., A perspective on coping behaviour: seeking and utilising information in major transactions, *Arch. Gen. Psychiatry*, 17, 277, 1967.
38. Lazarus, R. S., The costs and benefits of denial, in *Denial of Stress*, Breznitz, S., Ed., International Universities Press, New York, 1983, 1.
39. Miller, S. M. and Grant, R., The blunting hypothesis: a view of predictability and human stress, in *Trends in Behaviour Therapy*, Sjoden, P. O., Bates, S., and Dockens, W. S., Eds., Academic Press, New York, 1979.
40. Cohen, S. and Edwards, J. R., Personality characteristics as moderators of the relationship between stress and disorder, in *Advances in the Investigation of Psychological Stress*, Neufeld, W. J., Ed., John Wiley & Sons, New York, 1988, 235–283.
41. McCrae, R. R., Situational determinants of coping responses: loss, threat and challenge, *J. Personality Soc. Psychol.*, 46, 919, 1984.
42. Kubler-Ross, E., *On Death and Dying*, Macmillan, New York, 1969.
43. Moos, R. H. and Billings, A. G., Conceptualising and measuring coping resources, in *Handbook of Stress: Theoretical and Clinical Aspects*, Goldberger, L. and Breznitz, S., Eds., The Free Press, New York, 1982, 212.
44. Janis, I. L. and Mann, L., *Decision Making*, The Free Press, New York, 1977.
45. Edwards, J. R., The determinants and consequences of coping with stress, in *Causes, Coping and Consequences of Stress at Work*, Cooper, C. L. and Payne, R., Eds., John Wiley & Sons, London, 1988, 233–263.

46. Hughson, A. M., Cooper, A. F., McArdle, C. S., and Smith, D. C., Psychosocial morbidity in patients awaiting breast biopsy, *J. Psychosom. Res.*, 32, 173, 1988.

47. Hilton, B. A., The phenomenon of uncertainty in women with breast cancer, *Issues Mental Health Nursing*, 9, 217, 1988.

48. Goldstein, D. A. and Antoni, M. H., The distribution of repressive coping styles among non-metastatic and metastatic breast cancer patients as compared to non-cancer patients, *Psychol. Health*, 3, 254, 1989.

49. Liiceanu, A., Toufexi, E., and Xenitidis, I., The unhappy personal events and their etiological value in breast cancer: experiencing the psychological trauma, *Rev. Psychol.*, 35, 101, 1991.

50. Tarlau, M. and Smalheiser, I., Personality patterns in patients with malignant tumours of the breast and cervix, *Psychosom. Med.*, 13, 117, 1951.

51. Bacon, C. L., Renneker, R., and Cutler, M., A psychosomatic survey of cancer of the breast, *Psychosom. Med.*, 14, 453, 1952.

52. LeShan, L. and Worthington, R. E., Some psychological correlates of neoplastic disease: preliminary report, *J. Clin. Exp. Psychopath.*, 16, 281, 1955.

53. Kissen, D., Personality characteristics in males conducive to lung cancer, *Br. J. Med. Psychol.*, 36, 27, 1963.

54. Booth, G., Cancer and culture: psychological disposition and environment, Unpublished Rorschach study, 1964.

55. Grissom, J., Weiner, B., and Weiner, E., Psychological correlates of cancer, *J. Consult. Clin. Psychol.*, 43, 113, 1975.

56. Greer, S. and Morris, T., Psychological attributes of women who develop breast cancer: a controlled study, *J. Psychosom. Res.*, 19, 147, 1975.

57. Bageley, C., Control of events, remote stress and the emergence of breast cancer, *Am. J. Clin. Psychol.*, 6, 213, 1979.

58. Morris, T., Greer, S., Pettingale, K. W., and Watson, M., Patterns of expression of anger and their psychological correlates in women with breast cancer, *J. Psychosom. Res.*, 25, 111, 1981.

59. Wirsching, M., Stierlin, H., Hoffman, F., Weber, G., and Wirsching, B., Psychological identification of breast cancer patients before biopsy, *J. Psychosom. Res.*, 26, 1, 1982.

60. Jansen, M. A. and Muenz, L. R., A retrospective study of personality variables associated with fibrocystic disease and breast cancer, *J. Psychosom. Res.*, 28, 35, 1984.

61. Tozzi, V. and Pantaleo, M. T., Psicosomatica del cancro della mammella (Psychosomatic elements in breast cancer), *Med. Psicosom.*, 30, 217, 1985.

62. Bremond, A., Kune, G. A., and Bahnson, C. B., Psychosomatic factors in breast cancer patients: results of a case-control study, *J. Psychosom. Obstet. Gynaecol.*, 5, 127, 1986.

63. Grassi, L. and Cappellari, L., State and trait psychological characteristics of breast cancer patients, *N. Trends Exp. Clin. Psychiatry*, 4, 99, 1988.

64. Kreitler, S., Chaitchik, S. and Kreitler, H., The psychological profile of women attending breast screening tests, *Soc. Sci. Med.*, 31, 1177, 1990.

65. Cooper, C. L., Cooper, R., and Faragher, E. B., A prospective study of the relationship between breast cancer, life events, coping skills, type A behaviour and social support, *Stress Med.*, 2, 271, 1986.

66. Cooper, C. L., Cooper, R., and Faragher, E. B., Incidence and perception of psychosocial stress: the relationship with breast cancer, *Psychol. Med.*, 19, 415, 1989.

67. Faragher, E. B. and Cooper, C. L., Type A stress prone behaviour and breast cancer, *Psychol. Med.*, 20, 663, 1990.
68. Cooper, C. L. and Faragher, E. B., Coping strategies and breast disorders/cancer, *Psychol. Med.*, 22, 447, 1992.
69. Cooper, C. L. and Faragher, E. B., Psychosocial stress and breast cancer: the interrelationship between stress events, coping strategies and personality, *Psychol. Med.*, 23, 653, 1993.

chapter nine

Stress and occupational exposure to HIV/AIDS

Lawrence R. Murphy, Robyn M. Gershon, and Dave DeJoy

Introduction

Health care workers are exposed to a variety of health-endangering factors at work, including physical agents, chemical agents, infectious diseases, and psychosocial stressors. One of the most recent occupational exposures for health care workers, and a very stressful one, is HIV/AIDS (human immunodeficiency virus/acquired immunodeficiency syndrome).[1] Since the early 1980s, a good deal of information has accumulated on HIV/AIDS, and its epidemiology in work and nonwork settings. In occupational settings, health care workers are exposed to HIV/AIDS primarily via needlestick injuries, and secondarily by contaminated blood/body fluid splashes to the eyes or mucus membranes.[1,2]

The research literature indicates that health care workers experience heightened stress associated with caring for HIV/AIDS patients,[3] and additional stress associated with fear of exposure to HIV/AIDS. Regarding the latter, Gerbert and colleagues,[4] reviewed research studies that explored the various reasons why HIV/AIDS generates stress among health care workers. These authors identified three primary reasons for the continuing fear among health care professionals: (1) the risk of occupational transmission of HIV is real, and the consequences are serious; (2) infection control procedures cannot prevent all occupational exposures, such as accidental needlesticks; and (3) communication barriers exist between experts and health care providers. Stress generated from fear of contracting AIDS at work has been displayed by symptoms like nightmares, anxiety, constant worry, and overall distress. Education and informational strategies have been only partially successful in alleviating the fear of AIDS.[3,4]

A primary stress prevention strategy would involve reducing or eliminating the exposure to HIV/AIDS, thereby reducing fear and associated stress among health care workers.[5] In this regard, the Centers for Disease Control and Prevention (CDC) Cooperative Needlestick Surveillance Group estimated that nearly 40% of occupational HIV/AIDS exposures were preventable via compliance with Universal Precautions (UP) recommendations.[6] Universal Precautions are a set of recommended work practices designed to provide barrier protection for health care workers against occupational exposure to bloodborne pathogens such as hepatitis B virus (HBV) and HIV. Specific precautions include proper disposal of sharp objects, never recapping used needles, and wearing disposable gloves.[7]

The value of UP for preventing occupational HIV/AIDS exposure was demonstrated in a prospective study, which found that an increase in the frequency of barrier use, from 54 to 73%, was associated with a significant decrease in exposures to blood/body fluids, from 5.07 exposures per patient care month to 2.66 exposures per patient care month.[8]

Levels of compliance with universal precautions

Despite the publication of work practice guidelines, and the enactment into law of the Occupational Safety and Health Administration (OSHA) Bloodborne Pathogens Standard,[9] compliance with UP among health care workers is not "universal". For example, Kellen et al.[10] found only 44% compliance with UP in an observational study conducted at the emergency room of the Johns Hopkins University Medical Center. Likewise, Hammond et al.[11] found that among house officers, only 16% adhered strictly to UP, and Gershon[12] found only 27% compliance with UP among hospital workers. Gershon[12] also reported a significant correlation between compliance with UP and occupation, with physicians reporting the lowest levels of compliance, and laboratory technicians the highest levels. Finally, in a national survey of over 3000 health care workers, Hersey and Martin[13] found that only 43% of patient care staff "always" wore gloves to draw blood, and 61% "always" washed their hands after removing gloves. Rates of compliance for use of outer garments, masks, and protective eyewear were even lower.

Job and organizational factors

Few studies have explored specific reasons why health care workers do not follow UP more frequently. Kellen and colleagues[10] asked workers why they did not follow UP, and the most common reasons were insufficient time (47%), interference with job duties (37%), and UP are uncomfortable (23%). However, no statistical relationships were explored among these reported reasons and actual lack of compliance with UP. Further, no studies have examined the influence of organization-level factors on compliance. Relevant organization-level factors would include management attitudes toward HIV/AIDS and UP, availability of personal protective equipment (PPE) in the work area, provision of performance feedback with respect to compliance with UP, and management commitment to safety. Indeed, prior studies in the occupational safety and health literature suggest that these types of organization-level factors are important predictors of employee work behavior, including safe work behavior.[14-16]

This chapter describes a study of compliance with UP among nurses at a large U.S. hospital. The study utilized a multidisciplinary approach to explore factors associated with lack of compliance. Principles and constructs from diverse research areas, including occupational safety, job stress/health, public health, and organizational behavior, were used to develop a questionnaire survey for high-risk workers, including nurses, physicians, laboratory technicians, and dentists. Specifically, the survey contained items and scales measuring demographics, personal attitudes, job/task characteristics, and organizational-level factors.

Method

The questionnaire measured a variety of personal, job/task, and organization-level factors, and was administered to over 3000 health care workers in hospitals at three geographic sites. This chapter presents data obtained from nurses at one geographic site (northeastern hospital). The questionnaire return rate for this hospital was 81%, and the sample contained responses from 450 nurses.

Unless otherwise noted, the response scale for all questionnaire items was a 4-point Likert scale, where 1 = strongly agree, 2 = agree, 3 = disagree, 4 = strongly disagree. Similar items were grouped together to form composite scales, and for these scales, responses were averaged over all items in the scale. Responses to some questionnaire items were reverse scored so that items in each composite scale would be scored in the same direction. For each composite scale, a measure of internal consistency (average correlation among items) was calculated (alpha coefficient).

Four sets of variables were analyzed in this study to assess their relative influence on worker compliance with UP.

Demographics

Three demographic variables were used: age, number of years in the job, and number of years in the field of nursing.

Employee personal characteristics

Two personal characteristics were measured, risk-taking tendencies, and worry about HIV/AIDS. *Risk-taking tendencies* (alpha = 0.76) were measured using six items selected from Zuckerman's[17] Sensation Seeking Scale. Examples of items in this scale are "I enjoy taking risks in life"; "I do dangerous things sometimes just for the thrill of it"; and "I prefer an exciting, unpredictable life". On the basis of reliability analyses, two items were dropped from the scale. *Worry about HIV at work* was measured using a single item which assessed the degree to which workers worried about acquiring HIV/AIDS at work ("I frequently worry about acquiring HIV/AIDS because of my work").

Job/task factors

Four scales assessed factors that dealt with the job or task. *Perceived job hindrances* (alpha = 0.71) were measured using four items that were developed for this study. The scale measured worker perceptions of the extent to which their job or job duties interfered with following UP. Examples of items were: "UP keep me from doing my job to the best of my abilities"; "My job duties interfere with my being able to comply with UP"; and "I can't always comply with UP because patients' needs come first". The *Workload* scale (alpha = 0.81) consisted of three items taken from Caplan et al.,[18] and measured quantitative workload, that is, having too much work to do. Examples of items in this scale were "How often does your job require you to work very hard"; and "How often is there a lot of work to be done". The response scale was 1 = always, 2 = often, 3 = sometimes, 4 = rarely/never.

Role ambiguity (alpha = 0.83) was measured using three items taken from Caplan et al.,[18] and measured the clarity of worker expectations on the job. Examples of *role ambiguity* items were "How often are you clear on what your job responsibilities are"; and "How often do you feel you know exactly what is expected of you at work". The response scale was 1 = always, 2 = often, 3 = sometimes, 4 = rarely/never.

Finally, *physical comfort at work* (alpha = 0.77) was measured using seven items that assessed how often workers were bothered by aspects of the physical work environment, such as temperature extremes, loud noise, dust, and poor air quality. The response scale was 1 = always, 3 = sometimes, 5 = never.

Organization-level variables

Organization-level variables refer to variables that go beyond the specific job or task, and reflect the attitudes and actions of the organization as a whole. The first organizational-level scale measured *availability of personal protective equipment* (alpha = 0.84). This scale contained five items, which were developed specifically for this study. The scale measured the extent to which personal protective equipment (PPE) were provided to workers. Examples of items in this scale were "All of the necessary equipment and devices to help me avoid contact with HIV are readily available"; "Sharps containers are readily available in my facility"; and "My facility provides me with all of the necessary equipment and devices in order to protect myself from HIV exposures".

Performance feedback (alpha = 0.75) was measured using eight items, which were developed for this study. The scale sought to measure the extent to which workers received feedback on their compliance with safe work practices, including compliance with UP from both management and co-workers. Sample items were "I am given feedback on how safely I perform my job"; "In my facility, employees' compliance with UP procedures and practices are part of their annual written evaluations,"; and "Employees are told when they do not follow UP".

The *organizational safety climate* (alpha = 0.83) scale contained seven newly developed items that assessed the general level of safety awareness and management commitment to safety and to UP. Although the provision of PPE and performance feedback scales described above could be considered components of the overall safety climate of an organization, the safety climate scale was designed to measure the general climate for safety, or the shared perceptions of workers regarding safety, without specific reference to HIV/AIDS. As defined in this study, safety climate included the general level of safety awareness, management commitment to safety, and the general level of cooperation among workers and management to reduce safety problems. Examples of items in this scale were "Where I work, employees, supervisors, and managers work together to insure the safest possible working conditions"; and "In my organization (or office, or facility), all reasonable steps are taken to minimize hazardous job tasks and procedures". One item ("Employee carelessness or disregard of safe procedures is almost always the cause of occupational exposure to contaminated materials") was deleted from the scale based on item analyses.

Criterion variable

Compliance with UP (alpha = 0.73) was measured using 12 items crafted from statements contained in the UP recommendations published by CDC, and the OSHA Bloodborne Standard.[9] The scale assessed how often nurses followed specific UP recommendations in their work (Table 1 contains the complete list of questions in this scale). The response scale for these items was, 1 = always, 2 = often, 3 = sometimes, 4 = rarely/never.

Examples of items were: "Dispose of sharp objects into a sharps container"; "Treat all patients as if they are infected with HIV"; "Follow all Universal Precautions with all patients regardless of their diagnosis"; "Wash my hands after removing my disposable gloves"; "Wear a disposable outer garment that is resistant to blood and body fluids whenever there is a chance of soiling my clothes at work"; and "Recap needles that have been contaminated with blood". Responses were reverse-scored where necessary, and then averaged to form a single, composite UP compliance scale.

Table 1   Compliance with Universal Precautions Scale (alpha = 0.73)

Please indicate how *frequently* you do the following things on your job:
(Never = 1, Rarely = 2, Sometimes = 3, Often/Always = 4)

	Mean	S.D.
Dispose of sharp objects into a sharps container	3.90	0.43
Treat all patients as if they are infected with HIV	3.42	0.85
Wash my hands after removing my disposable gloves	3.62	0.64
Wear a disposable outer garment that is resistent to blood and body fluids whenever there is a chance of soiling my clothes at work	2.56	1.09
Wear disposable gloves whenever there is a possibility of exposure to blood or other body fluids	3.74	0.53
Wear protective eye shields whenever there is a possibility of a splash or splatter to my eyes	2.72	1.16
Wear a disposable face mask whenever there is a possibility of a splash or splatter to my mouth	2.56	1.17
Dispose of all potentially contaminated materials into a red (and/or labeled) bag for disposal as biomedical waste	3.80	0.53
Promptly wipe up all potentially contaminated spills with a disinfectant	3.29	0.94
Eat or drink while working in an area where there is a possibility of becoming contaminated with blood or body fluids	3.40	0.96
Take special caution when using scalpels or other sharp objects	3.77	0.68
Recap needles that have been contaminated with blood	3.34	0.99

Data analysis procedures

Hierarchical, multiple regression analyses were performed to determine the relative influence of individual worker characteristics, job/task variables, and organizational factors on worker compliance with UP. The hierarchical procedure was designed as a progression from individual-level characteristics, through job/task variables, to organization-level factors. In the hierarchical procedure, groups of variables are entered into the regression equation simultaneously, and the total amount of variance in compliance (i.e., R^2) is calculated. In succeeding steps, other groups of variables are entered, and the increment in R^2 at each step is determined. All variables entered in earlier steps were automatically included in succeeding steps.

In the present study, demographics (age, job tenure, tenure in the nursing field) were entered as a group at Step 1, and the R^2 determined. At step 2, personal characteristics (risk-taking tendencies and worry about HIV at work) were entered as a group, and the R^2 for the model calculated. The difference in R^2 values at step 2 relative to step 1 reflects the unique variance accounted for by step 2 variables. At step 3, job/task factors (perceived job hindrances to UP, workload, role ambiguity, and physical discomfort) were entered into the regression model, and at step 4, organization-level variables (provision and availability of PPE, worker performance feedback, organizational safety climate) were entered. After step 4, backward elimination of nonsignificant variables was performed to produce a final, reduced regression model.

Results

Table 1 shows descriptive statistics for the 12 items comprising the compliance with UP scale. Compliance with certain elements of UP was very high (e.g., dispose of sharp objects into sharps container), while other precautions were less frequently followed (e.g., wear disposable outer garment, and wear disposable face mask). The overall internal consistency for the scale was 0.73.

Table 2 presents descriptive statistics for each study variable, and correlations among all variables. The average age for nurses in this study was 33.9 years (S.D. = 8.33), and 95% were female. The average tenure in the current job was 5.6 years (S.D. = 6.02), and the average tenure in nursing was 9.7 years (S.D. = 7.28).

Compliance with UP was generally good; the average for the 12 items was 3.34 on a 4-point response scale. Scores on the compliance with UP scale were not significantly correlated with age ($r = .04$), job tenure ($r = -.03$), tenure in the profession of nursing ($r = .05$), personal risk-taking tendencies ($r = -.09$), nor worry about HIV at work ($r = .04$). Compliance was significantly correlated with job hindrances ($r = .34$), availability of PPE ($r = .23$), performance feedback ($r = .27$), and organizational safety climate ($r = .28$). The three organization-level scales were moderately to highly intercorrelated ($r = .30$ to .56), while the four job/task scales (role ambiguity, workload, physical comfort, and job hindrances) were only slightly to moderately intercorrelated ($r = .02$ to .31).

Multiple regression analyses

Table 3 shows the results of the hierarchical multiple regressions. Demographic variables were entered at step 1, but did not explain significant variance in compliance with UP. The addition of employee personal characteristics at step 2 also did not explain significant variance. Only after the addition of job/task factors did the model become significant, and explain significant variance in compliance ($R^2 = 12\%$). Among the scales entered in this step, only perceived job hindrances was significant in the regression model (see Table 3). Finally, the addition of organization-level variables at step 4 further increased the model R^2 to 18%, indicating that this

Table 2   Means, Standard Deviations, and Correlations Among Study Variables (*N*= 450)

	Mean	S.D.	1	2	3	4	5	6	7	8	9	10	11	12	13
Demographic factors															
1. Age	33.87	8.33	—												
2. Years in job	5.60	6.02	.48	—											
3. Years in profession	9.69	7.28	.74	.63	—										
Personal factors															
4. Risk-taking tendencies	2.11	0.55	-.20	-.16	-.16	(.76)									
5. Low worry about HIV	2.50	0.81	.02	-.09	-.01	.09	—								
Job/Task Factors															
6. Low job hindrances	3.38	0.49	.03	-.07	.07	-.09	.18	(.71)							
7. Low workload	1.95	0.92	-.11	.02	.06	-.11	.04	.03	(.81)						
8. Role ambiguity	1.63	0.54	.09	-.18	-.10	.15	-.02	-.17	-.02	(.83)					
9. Physical environment	3.09	0.72	.09	-.02	.00	-.13	.10	.13	.31	-.18	(.77)				
Organizational Factors															
10. Availability of PPE	3.40	0.50	.10	.03	.06	.00	.15	.24	.06	-.21	.24	(.84)			
11. Performance feedback	2.96	0.44	.02	.02	.07	.02	.04	.21	-.02	-.16	.07	.30	(.75)		
12. Safety climate	3.04	0.50	.09	.00	.08	-.04	.15	.35	.10	-.22	.22	.46	.56	(.83)	
Criterion Variable															
13. Compliance with UP	3.34	0.44	.04	-.03	.05	-.09	.04	.34	.05	-.07	.04	.23	.27	.28	(.73)

Note: $r > 0.10$, $p < = .05$; $r > 0.13$, $p < = .01$; $r > = 0.16$, $p < = .001$.
Alpha coefficients are shown in parentheses on diagonal.

Table 3 Hierarchical Regression Analyses

	Variable Entered	Standardized Estimate	t	$p < =$
Demographics				
Step 1	Age	.01	.92	ns
	Years in job	−.09	−1.52	ns
	Years in profession	.10	−.78	ns

Step 1 model $F(3,450) = 1.11$, $p < = 0.34$, $R^2 = .007$

	Variable Entered	Standardized Estimate	t	$p < =$
Personal factors				
Step 2	Risk-taking	−.10	−2.13	0.03
	Low worry about HIV	.04	.90	ns

Step 2 model $F(5,448) = 1.67$, $p < = 0.14$, $R^2 = .02$

	Variable Entered	Standardized Estimate	t	$p < =$
Job task factors				
Step 3	Low job hindrances	.33	−6.91	.001
	Low workload	.02	0.43	ns
	Role ambiguity	−.01	−0.40	ns
	Physical comfort	−.03	−0.53	ns

Step 3 model $F(9,448) = 6.61$, $p < = 0.001$, $R^2 = .12$

	Variable Entered	Standardized Estimate	t	$p < =$
Organizational factors				
Step 4	Availability of PPE	.11	2.27	.02
	Performance feedback	.15	2.86	.01
	Organization safety climate	.07	1.22	ns

Step 4 model $F(12,446) = 9.91$, $p < = 0.001$, $R^2 = .18$

Table 3   (*Continued*)

Final Reduced Model (Backward Elimination)

Variable	Standardized estimate	t	$p < =$	R^2
Low job hindrances	.26	5.34	.001	.06
Availability of PPE	.11	2.45	.02	.01
Performance feedback	.18	3.94	.001	.03

Model $F(4,446) = 22.66, p < = .001, R^2 = .17$

group of variables explained 6% of the variance in compliance with UP over and above that explained by the other nine variables in the model. The scale measuring performance feedback had the largest standardized regression coefficient, followed by availability of PPE. Organizational safety climate was not significant in the model, probably owing to its high correlation with performance feedback ($r = 0.56$).

After all of the variables had been entered into the model at step 4, a final regression was performed, this time with backward elimination of nonsignificant variables. The final, reduced regression model contained four significant variables, low job hindrances, availability of PPE, and performance feedback, which together explained 17% of the variance in compliance with UP.

Additional analyses

Additional regression analyses were performed to explore which individual, job/task, and organizational factors were associated with the three best predictors of compliance with UP identified in the final, reduced model (i.e., perceived job hindrances, performance feedback, and availability of PPE). Essentially, we were trying to predict the "predictors". These analyses would identify the direct and indirect pathways through these variables to compliance with UP. Separate multiple regression analyses (with backward elimination of nonsignificant variables) were performed on perceived job hindrances, performance feedback, and PPE. The results are shown in Table 4. The best predictor of all three variables, perceived job hindrances, performance feedback, and PPE, was organizational safety climate, which explained 6, 32, and 14% of the variance, respectively. Other variables that were significant predictors of perceived job hindrances were tenure in nursing ($R^2 = 2\%$), tenure in the job ($R^2 = 1\%$), worry about HIV/AIDS ($R^2 = 1\%$), and personal risk-taking tendencies ($R^2 = 1\%$). For *PPE*, role ambiguity and comfortable work environment also were significant variables in the regression model. No variables other than safety climate were significant in the regression model of performance feedback.

Table 4   Hierarchical Regression Analyses for Criterion Variables

A. Criterion Variable: Perceived Job Hindrances

Variable entered	Standardized estimate	$p < =$	R^2
Safety climate	.27	.001	.06
Tenure in nursing	.21	.01	.02
Tenure in job	−.16	.01	.02
Low worry about HIV	.12	.01	.01
Risk-taking tendencies	−.10	.02	.01

Final reduced model $F(7,446) = 12.70$, $p < = .001$, $R^2 = .17$

B. Criterion Variable: Performance Feedback

Variable entered	Standardized estimate	$p < =$	R^2
Safety climate	.57	.001	.32

Final reduced model $F(2,446) = 105.86$, $p < = .001$, $R^2 = .32$

(check final model for last variable . . . same as prior variable!)

C. Criterion Variable: PPE

Variable entered	Standardized estimate	$p < =$	R^2
Safety climate	.40	.001	.14
Comfort	.12	.01	.01
Role ambiguity	−.10	.02	.01

Final reduced model $F(2,446) = 105.86$, $p < = .001$, $R^2 = .32$

Discussion

The results of this study indicated that compliance with UP recommendations among nurses was generally high, but not ideal. Certain precautions were almost universally followed (e.g., disposal of sharps, mean = 3.91, scale: 1 = never/rarely, 4 = always). Other precautions were less frequently followed, and these included wearing a disposable face mask when there is a possibility of a splash to mouth (mean = 2.54) and wearing a disposable outer garment that is resistant to blood/body fluids (mean = 2.56). Also, the relatively low reliability of the compliance with UP scale suggests that compliance with UP may not be a unidimensional construct. Additional research is needed to examine the dimensionality of this construct.

The hierarchical regression analyses revealed that demographic factors, and worker personal characteristics, were not good predictors of compliance with UP. On the other hand, job/task factors, notably worker perceptions of job hindrances, were the best predictors of compliance with UP. These job hindrances included perceptions that job duties interfered with practicing UP, failure to follow UP because "patients needs come first", and perceptions that UP prevented workers from doing their job to the best of their abilities. More traditional measures of job characteristics like workload and role ambiguity, however, did not predict significant variance in compliance with UP.

Significance of organization-level factors

The significance of organization-level factors in the regression models predicting compliance with UP highlights the important effects of management attitudes and actions on worker behavior. Of the organization-level factors, the performance feedback scale was the best predictor of worker compliance with UP, and was highly correlated with general safety climate. The performance feedback scale contained items assessing all types of performance feedback, including feedback from managers as well as coworkers. A second organizational-level variable, safety climate, is noteworthy in that it was significant in regression models of all three key predictors of compliance with UP, that is, performance feedback job hindrances, and availability of PPE. This suggests that safety climate influences worker compliance with UP indirectly via its effects on perceived job hindrances, performance feedback, and availability of PPE.

Relationship to prior studies

The results confirm and extend an earlier, preliminary report by Murphy and co-workers,[19] and suggest that efforts to improve worker compliance with UP should include attention to job/task factors and organizational factors, in addition to worker education and training. With respect to the former, engineering controls and the redesign of jobs/tasks can be initiated to reduce perceived hindrances to adherence. Regarding organization-level factors, management provision of PPE, in the form of sharps disposal units, disposable gloves, eye protection, etc., is a necessary, but not sufficient, condition for worker compliance with UP. In order to make substantial improvements in worker compliance, organizations should (1) evaluate jobs/tasks to identify and then reduce hindrances to compliance, (2) insure top management commitment to UP, and (3) encourage managers to provide feedback (and reinforcement) to employees on their compliance with UP. Other organization-level actions that foster a positive safety climate at work, and a high level of safety awareness, also should be implemented, since safety climate occupied a central role in the regression models.

Engineering controls and other management actions

Improving worker compliance with UP will reduce the number of occupational exposures to HIV/AIDS, but will not eliminate exposures due to accidental needlesticks and other sharps injuries. For these types of exposures, it is necessary to conduct detailed analyses of jobs to identify high-risk job activities or tasks, and ways of redesigning the job or restructuring the task to reduce sharps injuries.[20] Examples of high-risk tasks/duties include handling of sharps, placement of sharps containers, and ergonomically designed sharps containers. Use of anti-needlestick devices and needleless systems should provide additional protection for workers. As Kearns[21] pointed out, management actions and planned organizational change strategies usually meet with resistance, and this resistance needs to be examined and reduced for the change to be accepted by workers and to be effective. Ultimately, a combination of management actions to improve safe work behavior, and engineering controls to redesign hazardous job tasks, should produce substantial reductions in occupational exposure to HIV/AIDS.[13]

References

1. Henderson, D. K., Perspectives on the risk for occupational transmission of HIV-1 in the health-care workplace, in *Occupational Medicine State of the Art Reviews: Occupational HIV Infection: Risk and Risk Reduction*, Becker, C. E., Ed., Hanley and Belfus, Philadelphia, 1989, 7.
2. Gershon, R. M. and Vlahov, D., HIV infection risk to health care workers, *Am. Ind. Hyg. Assoc. J.*, 51, 801, 1991.
3. Scott, C. D. and Jaffe, D. T., Managing occupational stress associated with HIV infection: self-care and management skills, in *Occupational Medicine State of the Art Reviews: Occupational HIV Infection: Risk and Risk Reduction*, Becker, C. E., Ed., Hanley and Belfus, Philadelphia, 1989, 85.
4. Gerbert, B., Maguire, B., Badner, V., Altman, D., and Stone, G., Fear of AIDS: issues for health professional education, *AIDS Educ. Prev.*, 1, 39, 1989.
5. Akabogu-George, J. B., AIDS as a psychological factor at work, *Afr. Newsl. Occup. Health Safety*, 3, 69, 1993.
6. Marcus, R. R., Surveillance of health-care workers exposed to blood from patients infected with human immunodeficiency virus, *N. Engl. J. Med.*, 319, 1118, 1988.
7. Hughes, J. M., Universal precautions: CDC perspective, in *Occupational Medicine State of the Art Reviews: Occupational HIV Infection: Risk and Risk Reduction*, Becker, C. E., Ed., Hanley and Belfus, Philadelphia, 1989, 13.
8. Wong, E. S., Stotka, J. L., Chinchilli, V. M., Williams, D. S., Stuart, G. C., and Markowitz, S. M., Are Universal Precautions effective in reducing the number of occupational exposures among health care workers? *JAMA*, 265, 1123, 1991.
9. Occupational Safety and Health Administration (OSHA), Occupational Exposure to Bloodborne Pathogens. Title 29 of the Code of Federal Regulations (CFR) 1910.1030. Washington, D.C., U.S. Government Printing Office, 1991.

10. Kellen, G. D., DiGiovanna, T. A., Celentano, D. D., Kalainov, D., Bisson, L., Junkins, E., Stein, A., Lofy, L., Scott, C. R. J., Siverston, K. T., and Quinn, T. C., Adherence to universal (barrier) precautions during interventions on critically ill and injured emergency department patients, *J. AIDS*, 3, 987, 1990.

11. Hammond, J. S., Eckes, J. M., Gomez, G. A., and Cunningham, D. N., HIV, trauma, and infection control: Universal Precautions are universally ignored, *J. Trauma*, 30, 555, 1990.

12. Gershon, R. M., Barriers to Precaution Adoption Among Health Care Workers at Risk of Occupational Exposure to HIV-1. Dissertation Submitted to the School of Hygiene and Public Health of the Johns Hopkins University, Baltimore, Maryland, 1990.

13. Hersey, J. C. and Martin, L. S., Use of infection control guidelines by workers in healthcare facilities to prevent occupational transmission of HBV and HIV: results from a national study, *Infect. Control Hosp. Epidemiol.*, 15, 243, 1994.

14. DeJoy, D., A behavioral-diagnostic model for self-protective behavior in the workplace, *Professional Safety*, December, 26, 1986.

15. Sheey, N. P. and Chapman, A. J., Industrial accidents, in Cooper, C. L. and Robertson, I. T., Eds. *International Review of Industrial and Organizational Psychology*. John Wiley & Sons, Chichester, 1987, 201–228.

16. Zohar, D., Safety climate in industrial organizations. Theoretical and applied implications. *J. Appl. Psychol.* 65, 96, 1980.

17. Zuckerman, M., Buschbaum, M. S., and Murphy, D. L., Sensation seeking and its biological correlates, *Psychol. Bull.*, 88, 187, 1980.

18. Caplan, R. D., Cobb, S., French, J. R. P., Jr., Harrison, R. V., and Pinneau, S. R., Job Demands and Worker Health. DHHS (NIOSH) Publication No. 75–160, Washington, D.C., U.S. Government Printing Office, 1975.

19. Murphy, L. R., Sturdivant, K., and Gershon, R., Organizational and Employee Characteristics Predict Compliance With Universal Precautions. Paper Presented at the American Psychological Society Meeting, Chicago, June 25–28, 1993.

20. DeJoy, D., Murphy, L. R., and Gershon, R. M., The influence of employee, job/task, and organizational factors on adherence to universal precautions among nurses, *Int. J. Ind. Ergonomics*, in press.

21. Kearns, K. P., Universal precautions: employee resistance and strategies for planned organizational change, *Hosp. Health Services Admin.*, 33, 521, 1988.

Section 3

Personality, stress, and illness

chapter ten

Personality and cancer

Hans J. Eysenck

Introduction: personality and disease

There is a long-standing belief that certain types of persons are more likely to develop cancer than others; this notion of a "cancer-prone personality" dates back to Galen, and good historical accounts of the development of this belief over the centuries are available (Greer, 1983; Mettler and Mettler, 1947; Rosch, 1979). As Sir William Osler (1906) pointed out: "It is many times much more important to know what patient has the disease, than what kind of disease the patient has" (p. 758–759). The major characteristics of the cancer-prone person were believed to be (1) a tendency to suppress emotions like fear and anger, and present a bland surface towards other people; and (2) to make inappropriate and ineffectual reactions to stressful circumstances, leading to feelings of hopelessness, helplessness, and finally depression. Early workers in this field provided some observational evidence in favor of these views (e.g., Bahnson, 1969; Greene, et al., 1956; Le Shan, 1966). Surveys of many of these early studies are given by Scherg (1986) and Temoshok and Dreher (1992). Typical are studies like those of Le Shan, who claims to have found "loss of hope" in between 70 and 80% of his cancer patients, but in only 10% or so of his control group. Criticisms of these early studies relate to the fact that investigators knew the composition of their samples, used subjective methods of investigation, employed inappropriate control groups, or none at all, confounded possible differences between people suffering from different types of cancer, etc.

The work of David Kissen may serve as the point at which proper controls were introduced. His empirical work began in collaboration with this author (Kissen and Eysenck, 1962) and continued until his untimely death (Kissen, 1963, 1964, 1966a,b, 1967, 1968). The crucial features of his work are already apparent in the early joint study: (1) putting up a specific hypothesis to be tested, in this case the relationship between lung cancer and suppression of emotion; (2) choice of a suitable control group; (3) double-blind procedure; (4) choice of an objective measuring device; and (5) proper statistical analysis. These factors, now commonplace, were quite alien to workers in psychosomatics at the time, and Kissen is rightly regarded as

0-8493-2908-6/96/$0.00+$.50
© 1996 by CRC Press, Inc.

a pioneer in this field. Subjects in our study were 239 patients attending Kissen's chest clinic; they were tested with the Maudsley Personality Inventory, designed as a measure of neuroticism-emotionality (Eysenck, 1959). The hypothesis was that low scores would indicate suppression of emotion, and that those diagnosed later as suffering from lung cancer (n = 116) would have lower scores than those in whom cancer in any organ was excluded (n = 123). I was ignorant of the diagnosis, which was made *after* administration of the inventory, and Kissen was ignorant of the scores made by the patients when he made his diagnosis.

It was found that the control group had much higher neuroticism scores than the cancer group, significant at the $p < .01$ level. Smoking was ruled out as a likely intermediary. Kissen in his later work (Kissen and Rowe, 1969) repeated this study several times, always with similar results. Altogether, as he stated, the probability of a person having a low score on the N (anxiety) scale being diagnosed as suffering from lung cancer was six times as high as a person with a high score being so diagnosed. This estimate, based on several large samples, suggests that even a single personality factor may be quite strongly related to the occurrence of lung cancer (Eysenck, 1990a). It is interesting to note that Kissen (1964) already predicted, and found evidence for, a synergistic relationship between smoking and personality. As he said, it would appear from his studies that "*the poorer the outlet for emotional discharge the less the exposure to cigarette smoke required to induce lung cancer.*" (p. 213) (emphasis in original). This important point will be taken up again later on.

Many investigations have taken up this paradigm and replicated our findings, extending them to other forms of cancer, e.g., cancer of the breast in women (Berndt et al., 1980; Eysenck, 1981). A summary of all this work is given by Eysenck (1985); it is notable that practically all give positive results supporting the hypothesis. We may conclude that there is some acceptable evidence for the hypothesis that cancer is *correlated substantially with suppression of emotion.*

The original Kissen and Eysenck (1962) study, and those following it, suffered from one obvious fault. Low scorers on N, or anxiety, may indeed be suppressing genuine feelings of anxiety or anger, but their score may also signify true *absence* of such feelings. It is now customary to measure suppression of emotions by combining low N scores with *high* scores on the Eysenck Lie Scale; or the Crown-Marlowe Social Desirability scale (e.g., Gudjonsson, 1981; Weinberger, et al., 1979). It seems likely that the differentiation achieved in studies comparing cancer patients with controls would have been much better had this new technique been used.

Even better are experimental studies like that of Kneier and Temoshok (1984). They contrasted "type C" cancer patients to "type A" coronary heart disease (CHD) patients, whose personality is supposed to be governed by the "AHA" trio of anger, hostility, and aggression, i.e., traits opposite to the emotion-suppressive personality of the cancer-prone patient.

Also included was a healthy control group, predicted to be intermediate between the other two. Participants were shown 50 slides designed to disturb the subjects emotionally, and provoke anger, sadness, anxiety, threats to self-esteem, or threats to interpersonal needs. Psychophysiological measures of autonomic arousal were taken, and subjects were asked how "bothered" they had been by the slides. Subjects were scored as repressive, if they denied being bothered but had strong autonomic reactions; as predicted, cancer patients had the highest score on this emotional repression index. CHD patients had the lowest, with normal (healthy) subjects right in the middle. Such experimental designs lend much-needed support to such studies as the Kissen and Eysenck one, and immeasurably strengthen one's belief in the correctness of the theory in question. Note also that the choice of control group was dictated by theory, a design much better than the usual choice, being dictated by availability! (There is of course a good deal of evidence regarding the differential reactions of cancer-prone and CHD-prone people—e.g., Dixon and Dixon, 1991; Eysenck, 1985, 1991a; Grossarth-Maticek, et al., 1985.) Pettingale and co-workers (1984) may also be quoted as giving experimental support for the "suppression" theory.

How about the second trait suggested by the early workers in this field, namely a tendency to fail to cope with stress, give up, and develop feelings of hopelessness and helplessness? Here the crucial initial study is one by Schmale and Iker (1971). The population consisted of women recommended for a diagnostic cone biopsy because of repeated evidence of suspicious cervical cells; of 68 women so recommended, 28 were found to have cancer of the cervix, 40 not to have cancer. Interviews held prior to diagnosis based prediction of diagnostic outcome "on the presence or absence of reported evidence of a high hopelessness potential and/or a reaction of hopelessness six months prior to the first abnormal (suspicious) smear" (p. 96). Of the 28 women with cancer, 19 had been accurately predicted to have cancer, 9 erroneously not to have cancer, whereas of the 40 noncancerous women, 31 had been correctly predicted to be noncancerous and 9 had been erroneously predicted to have cancer. Thus, 50 out of 68 had been correctly predicted to have cancer, i.e., 74%, significant at p <.001. Other later studies have usually borne out this finding, mainly with other types of cancer (e.g., Greer and Morris, 1975; Goodkin et al., 1986; Horne and Picard, 1979; Wirsching et al., 1981).

Correlations, causality, and criticisms

These studies strongly suggest a correlation between personality and cancer, and it may be argued that they establish personality as a risk-factor for cancer. They are clearly not in a position to establish personality as a causal factor in the initiation or propagation of malignant cells. It is possible that cancer, even before diagnosis, causes feelings of hopelessness and helplessness, or has other influences on personality, thus reversing the assumed causal relationship. Or it might be that the link between cancer and personality is indirect; people with a cancer-prone personality may smoke more, drink more, and have a more unhealthy type of diet. The complexity of the situation is indicated by the well-known fact that cancer of the cervix is more often found in women who are promiscuous, and smoke, than in women who are monogomous and do not smoke. Nuns do not often have cancer of the cervix; hookers do. But what is the causal relation? Is smoking the causal agent, with promiscuity only indirectly associated with cancer through its correlation with smoking? Or is promiscuity the causal factor, with smoking only indirectly associated with cancer? Or are both involved, perhaps interacting significantly? Or is extraversion to blame, which is correlated with both smoking and promiscuity? The permutations are endless, and obviously univariate analyses are inadequate to answer the causal questions that arise. The problem of how causality can be established empirically will be dealt with later.

There are other problems. Critics of more recent studies, like Scherg (1986) and Fox (1978) often argue that there are a number of negative studies that should be taken to counterbalance the positive studies reported, and carry out what is a kind of meta-analysis of all published work. Thus, Scherg lists details of 40 separate studies; by now this number could be doubled. I have several times argued against the use of meta-analysis (e.g., Eysenck, 1992), for the simple reason that it is not reasonable to argue that a good study, properly conducted and analyzed, should be averaged with a bad study, using inappropriate methodology and statistics. Consider the following example, discussed at some length by Eysenck (1990b). It concerns the Schmale and Iker (1971) study already mentioned, in which they had found that cancer could be predicted by means of interviews concerning "hopelessness" feelings. They also used the Minnesota Multiphasic Personality Inventory (MMPI) and the Rorschach, and failed to find any correlations with cancer! This is hardly surprising—the MMPI is a multipurpose questionnaire having little relevance to the theory being tested, and the Rorschach lacks reliability and validity (Zubin et al., 1965), and is equally irrelevant. Yet any busy meta-analyst would have scored the study a "failure" if only these two tests had been used!

The problem with so many published papers is precisely this: they are not designed to test a specific theory, they use tests that are not relevant to the purpose, and often apply these to badly chosen groups. The frequent use of the MMPI or the Rorschach is a case in point: neither test is designed to test the major theories in the field, so that any failure to distinguish cancer patients or cancer-risk probands from controls is irrelevant to the theories that have held the stage for such a long time. When a proper measure is being used, as in the Schmale and Iker study, high levels of prediction can be attained. To combine good and bad studies in a meta-analysis, and conclude that there is inconsistency, is not very illuminating; no psychologist knowledgeable in the field would have expected anything else from the use of badly chosen tests.

There is another point. In the Schmale and Iker study the successful technique used a focused interviewing technique, and this has also been found significantly more successful than questionnaires in prediction studies of the type A-type B concept of coronary heart disease (Eysenck, 1990a); possibly an interviewing procedure elicits better cooperation than merely handing out questionnaires. Grossarth-Maticek et al. (1993) have put this hypothesis to the test in a large-scale prospective study, and found marked differences in predictive accuracy for the eventual occurrence of cancer and coronary heart disease, depending on the degree of interviewer participation. The use of interviewers may be more expensive and time-consuming than simply handing out questionnaires, but if theories of cancer-personality correlation are to be tested properly, this clearly is the method of choice; negative results not using optimal methods of data collection cannot be used to discredit positive results achieved by using trained interviewers.

Prospective studies: survival

Prospective studies, involving follow-up of groups studied at point T_1 and analyzed for mortality at point T_2, are the "gold standard" of mind-cancer research (Temoshok and Dreher, 1992). There are two clearly differentiated types of prospective studies. One, to be discussed in this section, studies cancer patients at T_1, measuring theoretically relevant personality and stress factors, and at T_2 determines how many have survived. Alternatively survival time might be the dependent variable, so T_2 is not fixed.

There are two problems with data of this kind. In the first place, many of the traits suggested to favor survival may be correlated with known physical risk factors. Thus, trait X, supposedly favoring survival, may be correlated with low frequency of drinking and smoking, good eating habits, etc.

A second problem is the fact that the effects of drinking (and probably smoking, too) are dependent on motivational factors (Grossarth-Maticek and Eysenck, 1991a). People drinking alcohol suffer greater mortality if they drink to drown their sorrows than if they drink to celebrate, or for fun. And finally, some types of nonalcoholic drink, i.e., coffee, have opposite effects on the probability of developing cancer and CHD, increasing the probability of CHD and lowering that of cancer (Grossarth-Maticek and Eysenck, 1990a); presumably alcohol has the opposite effect. We have tried to explain these effects as far as cancer is concerned (Grossarth-Maticek et al., 1991), but whatever the explanation clearly these effects are very complex, and taken together with the evidence later to be presented that psychological and physical factors in cancer genesis are synergistic, it must be obvious that simple presentation of single factor correlations, as is customary in the literature, is not sufficient for proper causal analyses.

Greer and co-workers (1979) found that survival 5 years after the diagnosis of breast cancer was significantly related to psychological traits assessed at 3 months. Women considered on the basis of a structured interview to show "fighting spirit" had a better prognosis than those displaying stoic acceptance or helplessness and hopelessness. Thus, cancer-prone women, using the traditional conception of that term, survived less well than those showing the opposite type of personality. Similarly, Derogatis et al. (1979) found that women with breast cancer who survived more than 1 year had higher ratings on measures of hostility or anger ("fighting spirit") than those who died within the first year. In an even earlier study, Blumberg and colleagues (1954) studied two groups of cancer patients matched for age, intelligence, and stage of cancer, administering a personality questionnaire following initial treatment. The study was more focused than many others; they found that those dying in less than 2 years, as compared with those dying after more than 6 years, had higher depression scores and lower neurotic outlet scores, as well as very low acting-out scores at the time of first assessment. Stavrakay et al. (1968) found their long-term survivors angrier, but without loss of control; they showed an underlying hostility or aggressiveness.

In the original study by Greer and co-workers (1979) the authors had categorized coping styles of their patients, in addition to the "fighting spirit" category, such as denial, stoic acceptance, and hopelessness-helplessness; 81% of "fighting spirit" patients were still alive, but only 20% of the hopeless/helpless group. Follow-up studies were done at 10 and again at 15 years from the outset of the study (Greer et al., 1985, 1990), finding that the original results held strongly. Fighters and deniers were more than twice as likely to be alive than helpless/hopeless patients. This is one of the most persuasive studies in the field. The main results were replicated in a similar study by Di Clemente and Temoshok (1985), using patients suffering from malignant melanomas. Among women, stoic acceptance made for a low or bad prognosis; among men, hopelessness/helplessness made for a relapse.

Another important set of results has been reported by Cooper and Faragher (1992, 1993), Cooper et al. (1989), and Faragher and Cooper (1990). In a quasi-prospective study they investigated women attending a breast screening out-patient clinic, as well as women attending a general out-patient clinic. Each of the 1596 women had presented to their general practitioners complaining of breast lumpiness or tenderness. Questionnaires were filled in prior to diagnosis, as in the Kissen and Eysenck (1962) study. In addition a symptom-free group of 567 women was included in the study. Comparisons were made between women with breast cancer, benign tumors, and normal breasts. The main findings were that women with cancer had more interpersonal problems rated by the individual as having high impact. "Denying the existence of the problem proved to be counter-productive, being associated with an increased risk of cancer" (Cooper and Faragher, 1993, p. 660). "The ability to express anger as a mechanism for handling the stress event again proved to be positive in the sense that it reduced the risk of a poor diagnosis (i.e. cancer)" (ibid). "Denial coping strategies" increased the risk of a woman being found to have breast cancer (p. 659). Interestingly, "women diagnosed as having benign breast disease were most likely to be cigarette smokers".

An interesting finding in this study provided evidence for Eysenck's (1983) "inoculation" theory. Based on numerous animal studies (e.g., Justice, 1985; Newberry, 1978; Sklar and Anisman, 1981) that had shown inhibitory effects of chronic stress on tumor cell proliferation, and adaptation to the effects of the stressor with repeated exposure, Eysenck (1983) had argued that adaptation to chronic stress had an "inoculation" effect on the organism. As Sklar and Anisman (1981) put it: "Acute stress results in depletion of catecholamines and increased acetylcholine (ACh), increased synthesis and secretions of hormones, and immune-suppression. Adaptation to these biological mechanisms is observed with chronic stress, such that normal levels of functioning or alteration opposite to those induced by acute stress are apparent" (p.391). In good agreement with this "inoculation" hypothesis, Cooper and Faragher (1993) found that "a high number of interpersonal problems continued to be related to a non-malignant diagnosis" (p. 660). In contrast, "women who experienced a loss-related event which they perceived as having a major impact on their lives had a significantly increased risk of being diagnosed as having a malignancy relative to all other women in the study" (p. 660). In assessing research on the effects of stress on cancer, the existence of such adaptation or inoculation factors should always be taken into account.

What is particularly interesting in these studies, to which many others could be added, e.g., Cella and Holland (1988), Pettingale et al. (1984), Temoshok (1985), and Temoshok et al. (1985), is that results are in good agreement with predictions from the other studies reviewed in preceding sections, and with the theories and observations described. It seems that the cancer-prone person is not only more likely to develop cancer, but if ill with cancer is less likely to survive. Of course there are many problems inherent in this type of study; how, for instance, can we be sure that the patients less likely to survive are equal to the longer-term survivors with respect to stage of illness? Personality factors are known to influence when in the development of cancer the sufferer seeks medical help (Berndt et al., 1980); perhaps this is another factor linking personality and survival? But it seems unlikely that these difficulties can be entirely responsible for the congruence observed. This conclusion will be strengthened when we consider the results of prospective studies of the second kind, in which healthy subjects are interviewed and/or given questionnaires, and then followed up for lengthy periods to check on mortality.

Prospective studies: mortality

These studies have been concerned with survival; those now to be considered are devoted to efforts to predict mortality from cancer (and/or
other diseases) in healthy individuals investigated at T_1, and followed up
for a period of years to a point T_2, when mortality and incidence are ascertained, i.e., who have died of cancer (or other causes), and who have
been so diagnosed, but are still alive. In the nature of things there are few
such studies, for obvious reasons. Large numbers of probands are required
at the beginning if sufficient numbers dying of a specified type of cancer
(e.g., bronchial carcinoma) are to be found at T_2. Even specifying "bronchial
carcinoma" may not be specific enough; we may have to distinguish between epidermoid and adeno-type cancers. Even more refined subclasses
may be asked for by oncologists. In one of our studies dealing with cancer
of the breast, we started with 8051 women; of these, 108 died of mammary
carcinoma after a 15-year follow-up. Clearly investigators must decide just
how specific a diagnosis to investigate. The more specific, the more likely
that the group will be homogeneous, but equally, the larger the T_1 population tested will have to be. A compromise is essential, and will inevitably
be criticized. If you look at cancer in general, you may get away with a
starting group of 1000; if you look at a specific type of cancer, you may
need 5000 to 10,000. Success in finding a connection between personality/stress at T_1 and mortality/incidence at T_2 will justify your choice; failure is ambiguous.

Another problem is the selection of the original sample. It is of course
necessary to have as random a sample as possible, but limitations are
needed as far as sex and age are concerned. If you are concerned with cancer of the breast, or the cervix, you obviously require only women. As far
as age is concerned, probands under 40 are out; with the average life expectancy between 70 and 80, it would take too long for any reasonable percentage to die in the lifetime of the investigator! But choosing the age limits of one's sample has other problems. If cancer-proneness bears a
dose-response relationship to mortality/incidence, as it probably does,
then the most prone would be expected to die relatively young; this suggests a relatively young sample. But that would require a much larger sample, because not many would die of cancer! Decisions of this kind are difficult to make, but they may determine outcome. A very old sample will
have high mortality in minimum time, but may show much less connection between cancer-proneness and personality/stress than a relatively
young sample. Such differences in selection may lead to "failures to replicate", where different age samples are being compared.

Some of the studies to be reviewed are relatively restricted in their coverage, but nevertheless relevant. Often they are unplanned outcomes of
analyses carried out because the data were available; these might be called
"convenience" studies, without a strong theoretical basis. Kaplan and

Reynolds (1988), in a 1-year follow-up study of 6848 healthy people, found an increased risk for cancer incidence and mortality among those who were "socially isolated". Shekelle et al. (1981) and Persky et al. (1987), in the Western Electric Study, discovered that those found on the original test to be depressed had twice as high a risk of death from cancer as those low on depression. At first this seems to contradict the Kissen and Eysenck results, showing a *negative* relation between neuroticism and cancer, but Temoshok and Dreher (1992, p.115) point out that the correlation was with death from cancer, not with onset. Hence, it is related negatively to the lack of fighting spirit shown in the previous section to prolong life.

More in line with expectations are the findings of Dattore and co-workers (1980), who followed up 200 disease-free veterans who had been tested upon entry into a hospital. Comparing the records of 75 who went on to contract cancer with 125 who remained healthy, or developed other diseases, the cancer patients were far *less depressed*, and significantly *more repressed*, than the control subjects. This agrees with the Kissen and Eysenck (1962) results, and, as Temoshok and Dreher put it, is "compelling evidence that Type C is a cancer-risk factor" (p.116).

One of the oldest and long-continued studies was started by C. B. Thomas (Shaffer et al., 1987) and continued to be followed for 40 years; Temoshok and Dreher (1992) give a list of references to successive reports. Thomas never suspected a correlation of personality with cancer, being concerned with coronary heart disease; thus, her findings are all the more convincing, confounding the chance of any possible prejudice dictating results. She found that those who were "loners" and suppressed their emotions "beneath a bland exterior" had the highest risk of cancer; in fact, the loners were 16 times more likely to develop cancer than those who gave vent to their emotions! The fact that this and other prospective studies support the Kissen and Eysenck (1962) result, and indeed produce even better discrimination between cancer and non-cancer patients, suggests strongly that it is not cancer that causes personality changes, but personality/stress that causes cancer.

We must finally turn to the work of Grossarth-Maticek, which is more voluminous than most (Eysenck, 1991a, has presented the major results in book form). Grossarth-Maticek has published three major follow-up studies, one from Yugoslavia (Grossarth-Maticek et al., 1982), and two from Heidelberg (Grossarth-Maticek et al., 1985, 1988). In all cases, healthy individuals were selected on a randomized basis, interviewer-applied questionnaires were used, medical tests applied, and information collected on smoking, drinking, and other lifestyle habits, by trained interviewers. Mortality and incidence were assessed after a 10-year (or longer) follow-up, with independent supervision. Two types of data were collected to assess personality/stress. The first was by means of a set of trait inventories theoretically based to predict cancer or CHD. Particularly relevant to the concept of type C are two questionnaires, namely number of traumatic life events evoking chronic helplessness, and rational-antiemotional behavior (suppression of emotion). A third questionnaire deals with anger, and is predictive of CHD, as opposed to cancer: number of traumatic life events evoking chronic excitement. A path model with cancer as the dependent variable was constructed, and these three variables had standardized partial regression coefficients of 0.43, 0.41, and –0.32, exactly as predicted from theory (Grossarth-Maticek et al., 1982, p.297). Four other questionnaires added very little, and the explained variance for the seven variables combined, in the prediction of cancer, is 0.55, with the contribution of the first three components amounting to 0.49. In other words, about half the cancer variance is due to personality/stress factors (Eysenck, 1988). Psychological predictors were found more important in the prediction of cancer and coronary heart disease than physical factors like smoking (Grossarth-Maticek et al., 1988).

An alternative method was to construct four "type" questionnaires, high scores on which described a person as type 1 (cancer-prone), type 2 (coronary heart disease-prone), type 3 (hysterical, but healthy), or type 4 (autonomous, healthy personality). Several studies, summarized by Eysenck (1991a) have shown that the type scores were highly predictive 10 years later of mortality and incidence of cancer (for type 1) and CHD (of type 2), with types 3 and 4 relatively immune.

These studies have been much criticized (see Eysenck [1991b] for a target article describing the Grossarth-Maticek studies, and Eysenck's [1991c] replies to invited critics). Some of the criticisms are well taken, but do not impair the evidential value of the final results. Running through much of the criticism seems to be a belief that the results are "too good to be true"; this is not easy to understand because the results are no better than those reported in the follow-up of the Thomas studies, in spite of the fact that her data collection was not theoretically based, had far more restricted material to work on, and covered a much larger life-span. However, at my suggestion, C. R. Reynolds funded a thorough re-analysis of existing data, and a continuation of the Heidelberg study for another 4½ years, under my supervision. (The re-analysis was supervised by C. Spielberger.) The detailed results of the extended follow-up have been published elsewhere (Eysenck, 1993) and are shown in Figure 1; they show a continued significant effect along the same lines, and caused the main critic, who had available all the accumulated data, to withdraw his criticisms, after carrying out his own analysis. These data seem to be quite definitive.

There are further studies extending the list of types to six, using a new inventory, adding two more to the original four types, and a different population (Grossarth-Maticek and Eysenck, 1990b). Results continue to be supportive of theory, but a detailed discussion would not be appropriate. Instead it may be useful to discuss quite briefly a number of independent replication studies, because nothing is more convincing than successful independent replication. Among the more interesting of these studies are those of Amelang and Schmidt-Rathjens (1992, 1993), Brengelmann (1993),

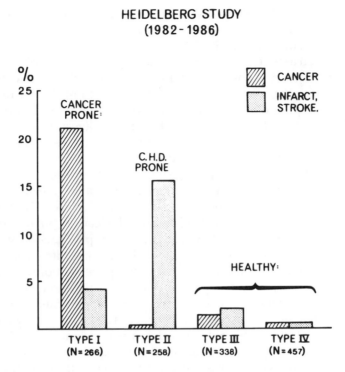

HEIDELBERG STUDY
(1982-1986)

Figure 1 Mortality of cancer-prone and coronary heart disease-prone probands, as compared with healthy types. Heidelberg follow-up continuation of the original 1972–1982 study (Eysenck, 1993).

van der Ploeg and colleagues (1989), Quander-Blaznik (1991), Ranchor et al. (1992), Sandin et al. (1993a, 1993b), Schmitz (1992), Shigehisa (1991), Shigehisa and co-workers (1989, 1991), Shigehisa and Oda (1993), Spielberger (1993). Schmitz used the 6-type questionnaire (Grossarth-Maticek and Eysenck, 1990b) and found high predictability for both cancer and CHD. He also found high correlations between the types and the three components of the Eysenck personality model (Eysenck and Eysenck, 1985). Types 1, 2, and 3 correlated positively with neuroticism, whereas type 4 correlated –.57 with N. The pattern was inverted for extraversion; psychoticism correlated positively with type 2, and negatively with type 5, as expected. Psychosomatic complaints correlated positively with types 1 and 2, but negatively with type 4.

Sandin et al. (1993a, 1993b) reported results similar to Schmitz, also very favorable to Grossarth-Maticek's theories. Spielberger (1993) reported excellent psychometric properties for some of the Grossarth-Maticek scales, as well as predictive validity. Schmitz (1992) also reported good psychometric properties of the scales, in good agreement with the original analyses by Grossarth-Maticek and Eysenck (1990b).

The theory endorsed in this chapter considers that psychosocial factors like personality reactions to stress constitute an important risk factor for cancer, whether through initiation or (more probably) propagation. It has never been asserted (as critics sometimes pretend) that this is the only risk factor, or that psychosocial factors cause cancer. There are very many risk factors (genetic, smoking, drinking, unhealthy eating habits, radon gas inhalation, air pollution, etc.), and an important question that arises concerns the *mode of interaction* of these risk factors. I have already mentioned that the results of the early Kissen-Eysenck work suggested a synergistic relationship between lung cancer and smoking, and this was borne out in the Eysenck (1988) paper comparing smokers and non-smokers with high or low scores on rationality-antiemotionality; the table given there shows that of those who never smoked only one died of cancer. Of those who smoked, but had low scores on R-E, none died of cancer. But of those who smoked *and* were high on R-E, 31 died of cancer (p.459). Clearly, it is the combination of smoking and personality that is important. This point is amplified in the Grossarth-Maticek et al. (1988) paper. A more detailed discussion of our work is given by Eysenck et al. (1991), and a more general discussion by Eysenck (1994). A good deal of evidence is cited in both studies to show that physical risk factors for cancer act synergistically with psychological risk factors. This conclusion is very important (Eysenck, 1991a); it demonstrates the extreme difficulty of using epidemiological evidence in this field. Univariate analyses are quite unequal to the demands of any rational model of risk factor interaction, yet most analyses of the effects of smoking have relied on univariate analyses, and used these to extrapolate to population estimates concerning the number of deaths "caused" by smoking. Such extrapolations are totally inadmissible in the presence of large numbers of risk factors interacting synergistically. Smoking seems to have little effect in the absence of personality/stress, or other risk factors, and cannot therefore be said to "cause" cancer or CHD. The term "cause" has a very definite meaning in science, and is clearly inappropriate here (Eysenck, 1991a).

Therapeutic intervention studies

Is it possible to interpret the studies discussed so far in a causal manner? They would seem to establish a correlational relation between the cancer-prone personality and death from cancer, but that connection could be via causally effective intermediaries (even if that is not a likely possibility). More convincing would be an intervention, perhaps along therapeutic lines, which would lead to measurable changes in personality, and a reduction in the cancer mortality of cancer-prone individuals. Alternatively, such intervention might be used to prolong life expectancy of people with inoperable cancers. I shall discuss the latter type of research first.

There are many early studies, not very rigorously controlled, that have given a positive answer. Le Shan (1977), Simonton and colleagues (1978) and Achterberg et al. (1977) are typical of this group. In the Simonton studies, for instance, 159 "incurable" cancer patients were treated by psychological methods. Two years later, 63 were alive, 22% had "no evidence of disease", and 19% had tumors that were shrinking.

Particularly impressive are some more rigorous recent studies. Grossarth-Maticek (1980) reports on 24 pairs of terminally ill cancer patients matched for type of cancer, and then allocated randomly to treatment or control, using his own autonomy-training method of psychological treatment (Grossarth-Maticek and Eysenck, 1991b). Mean survival time was 3.09 years for the control group, 5.07 years for the therapy group. Spiegel et al. (1989) reported in a study of terminally ill women that those receiving psychological treatment survived about twice as long as those who did not. Women with terminal cancer of the breast were also subjects of another study (Eysenck and Grossarth-Maticek, 1991) in which half had agreed to chemotherapy, half had refused; half of each group received autonomy training, half did not. Both chemotherapy and behavior therapy did significantly better than no therapy in prolonging life; both together did specifically better than the *sum* of their individual effects, i.e., there was a synergistic effect. These various studies definitely suggest that psychological intervention does have a significant effect on survival.

Levy and colleagues (1985) have produced evidence that psychological interventions can increase cancer patients' optimism and reduce feelings of hopelessness; in addition an increase in the number of natural killer cells was reported; these are an important part of the immune defence system against cancer (Seligman, 1991). Similarly, Fawzy et al. (1990) have reported that melanoma patients who received group treatment improved psychologically and also had higher amounts of natural killer cells. These and other studies are discussed in detail by Temoshok and Dreher (1992).

Autonomy training of healthy type 1 and type 2 probands as a prophylactic measure are perhaps even more indicative of the causal nature of psychosocial factors. Table 1 shows the effects of such prophylactic therapy for two groups, split randomly into therapy and control groups. Group 1 was made up of 100 type 1 (cancer-prone) individuals, group 2 of 92 type 2 (CHD-prone) individuals. Results show the highly significant effect of autonomy training. Similar effects have been found for group therapy (Eysenck and Grossarth-Maticek, 1991).

These studies are in urgent need of replication because it is very difficult to sort out the influence of the method of treatment, and the influence of the therapist; in these studies Grossarth-Maticek, who is a charismatic type of personality, carried out the major part of the treatment. Other successful therapists (e.g., Le Shan, Simonton, Spiegel) used rather different methods, and it is obviously important to know to what extent different methods may combine identical effective elements—a universal problem

Table 1   Mortality and Incidence of Cancer and Coronary Heart Disease

	n	Cancer		Other causes of death	Living
		Deaths	Incidence		
Control	50	16	21	15	19
		32%	42%	30%	38%
Therapy	50	0	13	5	45
		0	26%	10%	90%
Total	100	16	34	20	64
		16%	34%	20%	64%

	n	CHD		Other causes of death	Living
		Deaths	Incidence		
Control	46	16	20	13	17
		34.8%	43.5%	28.3%	36.9%
Therapy	46	3	11	6	37
		6.5%	23.9%	13%	80.4%
Total	92	19	31	19	54
		20.6%	33.7%	20.7%	58.7%

Note: Measured in both therapy and control groups treated prophylactically by individual autonomy training.

in psychotherapy (Giles, 1993). However, this question is irrelevant to the clear demonstration of psychological effectiveness on cancer prevention and prolongation of life.

The body-mind relation

The possibility that personality can influence the development of cancerous growths seems counterintuitive to many people still under the spell of Cartesian dualism. There is now sufficient evidence to demonstrate the existence of causal connections between personality and stress, on the one hand, and cancer on the other, through the intermediary of the immune system. The general theory linking the two has been discussed in some detail by Eysenck (1991a), together with a review of the evidence. We may begin with a statement of Solomon's (1987) postulates:

1. Enduring coping style and personality factors (trait characteristics) should influence the susceptibility of an individual's immune system to alteration by exogenous events, including reactions to events. (Thus, an "immunosuppression-prone" behavioral pattern is hypothesized.)
2. Emotional upset and distress (state characteristics) should alter the incidence, severity, and/or course of diseases that are immunolog-

ically resisted (infections and neoplastic) or are associated with aberrant immunologic function (allergic and autoimmune).

3. Severe emotional disturbance and mental dysfunction should be accompanied by immunologic abnormalities.
4. Experimental behavioral manipulation (e.g., stress, conditioning) should have immunologic consequences.
5. Experimental manipulation of appropriate parts of the central nervous system (CNS) should have immunologic consequences.
6. Hormones and other substances regulated or elaborated by the CNS should influence immune mechanisms.
7. Biochemical and functional similarities might be expected between the substances modulating the function and reactivity of the CNS (neuropeptides) and the substances with comparable effects on the immune system (cytokines).
8. Behavioral interventions (such as psychotherapy, relaxation techniques, imagery, biofeedback, and hypnosis) should be able to enhance or optimize immune function.
9. Altered CNS neurotransmitter receptor-site sensitivities believed to be associated with mental illnesses should be reflected in lymphocyte receptors.
10. The "functional" modes of expression of the CNS and immune system should be similar.

Research since has in large measure replicated and extended the studies reviewed by Solomon and Eysenck; there is far too much material to give anything but a very brief review of it here. The main intermediary between *stress response* and *immunodepression* has been cortisol, but other intermediaries (ACTH; endogenous opiates) should also be taken into account. Vickers (1988) showed that, for those individuals who demonstrate affective disruptions and low defensive reserve, there is a high correlation between repressive behavior, personality, and plasma cortisol secretion rate following a stressful event. It is of course well known that cortisol impairs several components of cell-mediated immunity (Cuppa and Fauci, 1982; Gorman and Kertzner, 1991). Vickers provided cumulative evidence from five studies that over 16% of the variance in cortisol level could be predicted from (often suboptimal) emotionality scores. Thus, the theory would suggest a causal pathway as follows: stress-strain (ineffectual personality response to stress)—cortisol secretion—immunodepression—cancer growth—death. Recent reviews document each of these links; good summaries are the following: O'Leary (1990), Stein (1989), Weisse (1992), Herbert and Cohen (1993), Antoni (1987), Zakowski et al. (1992), Kiecolt-Glaser and Glaser (1992), Gorman and Kertzner (1991), Locke (1986), Pletnikoff et al. (1986), and Kennedy et al. (1988). Of the more interesting recent studies not reviewed in these summaries, one may be worthy of special mention. Wiedenfeld et al. (1990) were successful in showing that the development of strong perceived self-efficacy to control phobic stressors, in an intervention design, had an immunoenhancing effect.

Human reactions are of course of main interest, but animal work (e.g., Borysenko and Borysenko, 1982; von Metzler, 1979; von Metzler and Nitsch, 1986) also supplies convincing evidence that carcinogenesis is intimately connected with events in the CNS. The demonstration by Ader and Cohen (1975) that immunosuppressors could be conditioned along Pavlovian lines points to the same conclusion. It would be difficult nowadays to deny the existence of a strong link between personality, reaction to stress, immunological reaction, and cancer, or of the possibility of psychological intervention altering the various parts of this system in the direction of increasing immunological efficacy.

This conclusion is particularly important in the context of this chapter. However compelling the studies linking personality with cancer, doubts must always remain as long as there is no evidence of a possible causal link between the two. To find that there is indeed good evidence for a strong link, susceptible to stress and also to intervention, makes the general argument much more compelling. There are of course other intermediaries, some of which are of interest in possibly mediating the opposition between cancer and CHD. Plasma cholesterol concentration is one example. There is a definite positive correlation between cholesterol and CHD, and an almost equally strong negative correlation between cholesterol and cancer (Isles et al., 1989). Unfortunately little is known about the correlation between personality and cholesterol, but this should certainly be the subject of a determined research effort, testing the obvious suggestion of a positive correlation with type A and a negative one with type C.

Summary and conclusions

The evidence surveyed suggests a number of conclusions:

1. Personality factors, concerned mainly with reaction to stress and coping mechanisms, play a powerful part in longevity (autonomous; self-regulating; hardy).
2. Specific personality traits play a part in predisposing certain people (cancer-prone, type C) to cancer.
3. Specific personality traits, differing in many ways from those characteristic of the cancer-prone personality, predispose certain people (CHD-prone; type A) to coronary heart disease.
4. Personality traits characteristic of the cancer-prone personality serve to shorten the life-span of people already suffering from cancer.
5. Prophylactic psychological therapy can cause cancer-prone people to avoid developing carcinomas, at least for a time.
6. Psychological therapy can help people suffering from inoperable cancer to live longer than controls.

7. There is much experimental support for a theory linking personality factors with immunosuppressive agents, like cortisol, and through immunosuppression with cancer.
8. It has been shown that cortisol level and the state of the immune system can be improved by means of psychological treatment.
9. Physical risk factors for cancer have been found to act synergistically, not additively.
10. Psychosocial and physical treatments have been found to act synergistically, not additively.
11. Measurements of the cancer-prone personality are only relevant if they are geared to testing the major theories developed by the leading experts in the field.
12. Measurement using personal contact (interviewing methods) is significantly more likely to give positive results than simply handing out questionnaires.

In all, the evidence supports the underlying theories of a cancer-personality link, although of course much remains to be discovered concerning the specific nature of that link. Critics have drawn attention to the fact that, in addition to articles giving positive results, there are also others that fail to show a correlation between personality and cancer. This is true, but as already pointed out, negative results are likely when certain essential conditions are not met. There has to be a specific theory to be tested, the instruments have to be appropriate, methods of data collection have to be pertinent (interviewer-assisted applications of inventories), control groups have to be apposite, and quite generally psychological considerations have to be taken into account. Too many studies fail on one or more of these points, and should not be held up as disproving the theory linking personality with cancer. As Newton pointed out, in his letter to Oldenburg, 18th August, 1676: "For it is not number of experiments, but weight to be regarded; where one will do, what need of many?"

References

Achterberg, J., Lawlis, G. F., Simonton, D. C., and Simonton, S. (1977). Psychological factors and blood chemistries as disease outcome predictors for cancer patients. *Multivariate Exp. Clin. Res.*, 3, 107–122.

Ader, R. and Cohen, N. (1975). Behaviorally conditioned immuno-suppression. *Psychosom. Med.*, 37, 333–340.

Amelang, M. and Schmidt-Rathjens, C. (1992). Personality, stress and disease: some results on the psychometric properties of the Grossarth-Maticek and Eysenck inventories. *Psychol. Rep.*, 71, 1251–1263.

Amelang, M. and Schmidt-Rathjens, C. (1993). Personalichbeit, Stress und Krankheit: Untersuchungen zu den psychometrischen Gutekriterien der Krankheitspradikatoran von Grossarth-Maticek und Eysenck. *Z. Gesundheitspsychol.*, 1, 160–182.

Antoni, M. H. (1987). Neuroendocrine influences in psychoimmunology and neoplasia: a review. *Psychol. Health*, 1, 3–24.

Bahnson, C. B. (1969). Psychophysiological complementarity in malignancies: past work and future vistas. *Ann. NY Acad. Sci.*, 164, 319–339.

Berndt, H., Gunther, H., and Rahte, G. (1980). Persoenlichkeitsstruktur nach Eysenck bei Kranken mit Brustdruesen- und Bronchial Krebs und Diagnosenverzoegerung durch die Patienten. *Arch. Geschwuestforsch.*, 40, 359–368.

Blumberg, E. M., West, P. M., and Ellis, F. W. (1954). A possible relation between psychological factors and human cancer. *Psychosom. Med.*, 16, 277–286.

Borysenko, M. and Borysenko, J. (1982). Stress, behavior, and immunity: animal models and mediating mechanisms. *Gen. Hosp. Psychiatry*, 4, 59–67.

Brengelmann, H. (1993). *Erfolg und Stress*. Hemsbach: Beltz.

Cella, P. F. and Holland, J. (1988). Methodological consideration in studying the stress-illness connection in women with breast cancer. In C. L. Cooper (Ed.), *Stress and Breast Cancer*. pp. 197–214. New York: Wiley.

Cooper, C. L. and Faragher, E. B. (1992). Coping strategies and breast disorders/cancer. *Psychol. Med.*, 22, 447–455.

Cooper, C. L. and Faragher, E. B. (1993). Psychosocial stress and breast cancer: the inter-relationshp between stress events, coping strategies and personality. *Psychol. Med.*, 23, 653–662.

Cooper, C. L., Cooper, R. D., and Faragher, E. B. (1989). Incidence and perception of psychosocial stress: the relationship with breast cancer. *Psychol. Med.*, 19, 415–422.

Cuppa, T. and Fauci, A. (1982). Corticosteroid-mediated immunoregulation in man. *Immunol. Rev.*, 65, 132–155.

Dattore, P., Shontz, R., and Coyle, L. (1980). Premorbid personality differentiation of cancer and non-cancer groups: a test of the hypothesis of cancer proneness. *J. Consult. Clin. Psychol.*, 43, 380–384.

Derogatis, L. R., Abeloff, M., and Melisaratos, N. (1979). Psychological coping mechanisms and survival time in metastatic breast cancer. *J. Am. Med. Assoc.*, 242, 1504–1508.

Di Clemente, R. J. and Temoshok, L. (1985). Psychological adjustment to having cutaneous malignant melanoma as a predictor of follow-up clinical states. *Psychosom. Med.*, 47, 87–89.

Dixon, J. P. and Dixon, J. K. (1991). Contradictory tendencies in the perception of life conflicts in persons with cardiovascular disease and persons with cancer. *Personality Individual Differences*, 12, 791–799.

Eysenck, H. J. (1959). *Manual of the Maudsley Personality Inventory*. London: University of London Press.

Eysenck, H. J. (1981). Personality and cancer: Some comments on a paper by H. Berndt. *Arch. Geschwuelstforsch.*, 51, 442–443.

Eysenck, H. J. (1983). Stress, disease and personality: the "inoculation effect". In C. L. Cooper (Ed.), *Stress Research*. pp. 121–146. New York: Wiley.

Eysenck, H. J. (1985). Personality, cancer and cardiovascular disease: a causal analysis. *Personality Individual Differences*, 6, 535–556.

Eysenck, H. J. (1988). The respective importance of personality, cigarette smoking and interaction effects for the genesis of cancer and coronary heart disease. *Personality Individual Differences*, 9, 453–464.

Eysenck, H. J. (1990a). Type of behavior and coronary heart disease. The third stage. *J. Soc. Behav. Personality*, 5, 25–44.

Eysenck, H. J. (1990b). The prediction of death from cancer by means of a personality/stress questionnaire. Too good to be true? *Perceptual Motor Skills*, 71, 216–218.

Eysenck, H. J. (1991a). *Smoking, Personality and Stress: Psychosocial Factors in the Prevention of Cancer and Coronary Heart Disease*. New York: Springer Verlag.

Eysenck, H. J. (1991b). Personality, stress and disease: an interactionist-perspective. *Psychol. Inquiry*, 2, 221–232.

Eysenck, H. J. (1991c). Reply to criticisms of the Grossarth-Maticek studies. *Psychol. Inquiry*, 2, 297–323.

Eysenck, H. J. (1992). Meta-analysis: sense or nonsense? *Pharm. Med.*, 6, 113–119.

Eysenck, H. J. (1993). Prediction of cancer and coronary heart disease mortality by means of a personality inventory: results of a 15-year follow-up study. *Psychol. Rep.*, 72, 499–516.

Eysenck, H. J. (1994). Synergistic interaction between psychosocial and physical factors in the causation of lung cancer. In C. Lewis, C. O'Sullivan, and J. Baraclough (Eds.), *The Psychoimmunology of Cancer*. pp. 163–178. Oxford: Oxford University Press.

Eysenck, H. J. and Eysenck, M. W. (1985). *Personality and Individual Differences*. New York: Plenum Press.

Eysenck, H. J. and Grossarth-Maticek, R. (1991). Creative novation behaviour therapy as a prophylactic treatment for cancer and coronary heart disease. II. Effects of treatment. *Behav. Res. Ther.*, 29, 17–31.

Eysenck, H. J., Grossarth-Maticek, R., and Everitt, B. (1991). Personality, stress, smoking, and genetic predisposition as synergistic risk factors for cancer and coronary heart disease. *Integrative Physiol. Behav. Sci.*, 26, 309–322.

Faragher, E. C. and Cooper, C. L. (1990). Type A stress prone behaviour and breast cancer. *Psychol. Med.*, 20, 663–670.

Fawzy, F. I., Kemeny, M. E., and Fawzy, N. (1990). A structural psychiatric intervention for cancer patients. II. Changes over time in immunological measures. *Arch. Gen. Psychiatry*, 47, 729–735.

Fox, B. H. (1978). Premorbid psychological factors as related to incidence of cancer. *J. Behav. Med.*, 1, 45–133.

Giles, T. R. (Ed.) (1993). *Handbook of Effective Psychotherapy*. New York: Plenum Press.

Goodkin, K., Antoni, M. H., and Blaney, P. H. (1986). Stress and hopelessness in the promotion of cervical intra-epithelial neoplasia to invasive squamous cell carcinoma of the cervix. *J. Psychosom. Res.*, 30, 67–76.

Gorman, J. and Kertzner, R. (Eds.) (1991). *Psychoimmunology Updated*. Washington, DC: American Psychiatric Press.

Greene, W., Young, I., and Swisher, S. N. (1956). Psychological factors and reticuloendothelial disease. II. Observation on group of women with lymphoma and leukemias. *Psychosom. Med.*, 18, 284–303.

Greer, S. (1983). Cancer and the mind. *Br. J. Psychiatry*, 143, 535–543.

Greer, S. and Morris, T. (1975). Psychological attributes of women who develop breast cancer: a controlled study. *J. Psychosom. Res.*, 19, 147–153.

Greer, S., Morris, T., and Pettingale, K. W. (1979). Psychological response to breast cancer: effect on outcome. *Lancet*, II, 785–787.

Greer, S., Pettingale, K., Morris, T., and Haybittle, J. (1985). Mental attitudes to cancer: an additional prospective factor. *Lancet*, 1, 750.

Greer, S., Morris, T., Pettingale, K., and Haybittle, J. (1990). Psychological responses to breast cancer: a fifteen-year outcome. *Lancet*, 1, 49–50.

Grossarth-Maticek, R. (1980). Social psychotherapy and course of the disease. *Psychother. Psychosom.*, 33, 129–138.

Grossarth-Maticek, R. and Eysenck, H. J. (1990a). Coffee-drinking and personality as factors in the genesis of cancer and coronary heart disease. *Neuropsychobiology*, 23, 153–159.

Grossarth-Maticek, R. and Eysenck, H. J. (1990b). Personality, stress and disease: description and validation of a new inventory. *Psychol. Rep.* 66, 355–373.

Grossarth-Maticek, R. and Eysenck, H. J. (1991a). Personality, stress, and motivational factors in drinking as determinants of risk for cancer and coronary heart disease. *Psychol. Rep.*, 69, 1027–1093.

Grossarth-Maticek, R. and Eysenck, H. J. (1991b). Creative novation behaviour therapy as a prophylactic treatment for cancer and coronary heart disease. I. Description of treatment. *Behav. Res. Ther.*, 29, 1–16.

Grossarth-Maticek, R., Kanazir, D., Schmidt, P., and Vetter, H. (1982). Psychosomatic factors in the process of cancerogenesis. *Psychother. Psychosom.*, 38, 284–302.

Grossarth-Maticek, R., Bastiaans, J., and Kanazir, D. T. (1985). Psychosocial factors as strong predictors of mortality from cancer, ischaemic heart disease and stroke: the Yugoslav prospective study. *J. Psychosom. Res.*, 29, 167–176.

Grossarth-Maticek, R., Eysenck, H. J., and Vetter, H. (1988). Personality type, smoking habit and their interaction as predictors of cancer and coronary heart disease. *Personality Individual Differences*, 9, 479–495.

Grossarth-Maticek, R., Eysenck, H. J., and Barrett, P. (1993). Prediction of cancer and coronary heart disease as a function of method of questionnaire administration. *Psychol. Rep.* 73, 943–959.

Grossarth-Maticek, R., Eysenck, H., and Rakic, L. (1991). Central nervous system and cancer. In O. F. Nygaard and A. C. Upton, (Eds.), *Anticarcinogenesis and Radiation Protection*. Vol. 2. pp. 429–435. New York: Plenum.

Gudjonsson, G. H. (1981). Self-reported emotional disturbance and its relation to electrodermal reactivity, defensiveness and trait anxiety. *Personality Individual Differences*, 2, 47–52.

Herbert, T. B. and Cohen, S. (1993). Depression and immunity: a meta-analytic review. *Psychol. Bull.*, 113, 472–486.

Horne, R. L. and Picard, R. S. (1979). Psychosocial risk factors for lung cancer. *Psychosom. Med.*, 41, 503–514.

Isles, C., Hole, D. J., Gillis, C. R., Hawthorne, V. M., and Lever, A. E. (1989). Plasma cholesterol, coronary heart disease, and cancer in the Renfrew and Paisley survey. *Br. Med. J.*, 298, 920–924.

Justice, A. (1985). Review of the effects of stress on cancer in laboratory animals: importance of time of stress application and type of tumour. *Psychol. Bull.*, 98, 108–138.

Kaplan, G. and Reynolds, P. (1988). Depression and cancer mortality: prospective evidence from the Alameda County study. *J. Behav. Med.*, 11, 1–13.

Kennedy, S., Kiecolt-Glaser, J., and Glaser, R. (1988). Immunological consequences of acute and chronic stressors: mediating role of interpersonal relationships. *Br. J. Med. Psychol.*, 61, 77–85.

Kiecolt-Glaser, J. and Glaser, R. (1992). Psychoimmunology: can psychological interventions modulate immunity? *J. Consult. Clin. Psychol.*, 60, 569–575.

Kissen, D. M. (1963). Aspects of personality of men with lung cancer. *Acta Psychother.*, 11, 200–210.

Kissen, D. M. (1964). Relationship between lung cancer, cigarette smoking inhalation and personality. *Br. J. Med. Psychol.*, 37, 203–16.

Kissen, D. M. (1966a). Psychosocial factors, personality and prevention of lung cancer. *Med. Officer*, 116, 135–138.

Kissen, D. M. (1966b). The significance of personality in lung cancer in men. *Ann. NY Acad. Sci.*, 125, 820–826.

Kissen, D. M. (1967). Psychosocial factors, personality and lung cancer in men aged 55–64. *Br. J. Med. Psychol.*, 40, 29–43.

Kissen, D. M. (1968). Some methodological problems in clinical psychosomatic research with special reference to chest disease. *Psychosom. Med.*, 30, 324–335.

Kissen, D. M. and Eysenck, H. J. (1962). Personality in male lung cancer patients. *J. Psychosom. Res.*, 6, 123–137.

Kissen, D. M. and Rowe, L. G. (1969). Steroid excretion patterns and personality in lung cancer. *Ann. NY Acad. Sci.*, 164, 476–482.

Kissen, D. M., Brown, R., and Kissen, M. R. (1969). A further report on the personality and psychological factors in lung cancer. *Ann. NY Acad. Sci.*, 164, 539–545.

Kneier, A. W. and Temoshok, L. (1984). Repressive coping reaction in patients with malignant melanomas as compared to cardiovascular disease patients. *J. Psychosom. Med.*, 28, 145–155.

Le Shan, L. (1966). An emotional life-history pattern associated with neoplastic disease. *Ann. NY Acad. Sci.*, 125, 780–793.

Le Shan, L. (1977). *You Can Fight for your Life: Emotional Factors in the Causation of Cancer*. New York: M. Evans.

Levy, S., Horberman, R. B., Maluish, A. M., Schlien, B., and Lippman, M. (1985). Prognostic assessment in primary breast cancer by behavioral and immunological parameters. *Health Psychol.*, 4, 99–113.

Locke, S. E. (Ed.)(1986). *Psychological and Behavioral Treatments for Disorders Associated With the Immune System: An Annotated Bibliography*. New York: Institute for the Advancement of Health.

Mettler, C. C. and Mettler, F. A. (1947). *History of Medicine*. Philadelphia: Blakiston.

Newberry, B. H. (1978). Restraint-induced inhibition of 7,12-dimenthylbenz(*a*) anthracene-induced mammary tumour: relation to stages of tumour development. *J. Natl. Cancer Inst.*, 61, 725–789.

O'Leary, A. (1990). Stress, emotion, and human immune function. *Psychol. Bull.*, 108, 363–382.

Osler, W. (1906). *Aequanimitas*. New York: McGraw-Hill.

Persky, V., Kempthorne-Rawson, J., and Shekelle, D. (1987). Personality at risk of cancer: 20-year follow-up of the Western Electric Study. *Psychosom. Med.*, 49, 435–449.

Pettingale, K. W., Watson, M., and Greer, S. (1984). The validity of emotional controls as a factor in breast cancer patients. *J. Psychosoc. Oncol.*, 2, 21–30.

Pletnikoff, N. P., Faith, E., Murgo, A. J., and Good, R. A. (Eds.) (1986). *Enkephalins and Endorphins: Stress and the Immune System*. New York: Plenum Press.

Quander-Blaznik, J. (1991). Personality as a predictor of lung cancer: a replication. *Personality Individual Differences*, 12, 125–130.

Ranchor, A., Sanderman, R., and Bouma, J. (1992). The empirical basis of the personality types of Grossarth-Maticek and Eysenck. Paper presented at the 6th European Conference of Personality. Groningen, June 15–19, 1992.

Rosch, P. J. (1979). Sress and cancer: a disease of adaptation? In J. Tache, H. Selye, and S. B. Day (Eds.), *Stress and Cancer*. pp. 187–212. New York: Plenum Press.

Sandin, B., Chorot, P., Jimenez, P., and Santed, M. (1993a). Stress behaviour types, psychosomatic complaints and disease. Paper presented at the 23rd European Congress of Behaviour and Cognitive Therapies, London, September 22–25, 1993.

Sandin, B., Chorot, P., Santed, M., and Jimenez, P. (1993b). Stress behavior types, personality, alexithymia, coping and state-trait anger expression. Paper presented at the 23rd European Congress of Behaviour and Cognitive Therapies, London, September 22–25, 1993.

Scherg, H. (1986). Zur Kausalitatsfrage in der psychosozialen Krebsforschung. *Psychother. Med. Psychol.*, 36, 98–109.

Schmale, A. H. and Iker, H. (1971). Hopelessness as a predictor of cervical cancer. *Soc. Sci. Med.*, 5, 99–100.

Schmitz, P. G. (1992). Personality, stress-reactions, and disease. *Personality Individual Differences*, 13, 683–691.

Seligman, M. (1991). *Learned Optimism*. New York: Alfred A. Knopf.

Shaffer, J., Graves, P., Swanck, R., and Pearson, T. (1987). Clustering of personality traits in youth and the subsequent development of cancer among physicians. *J. Behav. Med.*, 10, 441–447.

Shekelle, R., Raynar, W., Ostfield, A., Garron, D., Bielanskas, L., Lin, S., Maliza, C., and Paul, O. (1981). Psychological depression and 17-year risk of death from cancer. *Psychosom. Med.*, 43, 117–125.

Shigehisa, T. (1991). The role of behavioral and psychosocial factors in the etiology of cancer and cardiovascular disease. *Tokyo Kasai Gakuin Univ. J.*, 31, 227–240.

Shigahisa, T. and Oda, M. (1993). Premorbid personality, anger and behavioral health. The multifactorial approach to health and disease. *Jpn. Health Psychol.*, 2, 43–53.

Shigehisa, T., Fukui, I., and Motoakis, H. (1989). Stress coping strategy and mode of coping, in relation to proneness to cancer and cardiovascular disease. I. Analyses in males, in relation to their parents. *Jpn. J. Health Psychol.*, 2, 1–11.

Shigehisa, T., Fukui, I., and Motoakis, H. (1991). Stress coping strategy and mode of coping. II. Analyses in females and their parents, in comparison with males and their parents. *Jpn. J. Health Psychol.*, 4, 8–22.

Simonton, O. C., Mathew-Simonton, S., and Creighton, J. (1978). *Getting well again*. Los Angeles: J. P. Tarcher.

Sklar, L. S. and Anisman, H. (1981). Stress and Cancer. *Psychol. Bull.*, 89, 396–406.

Solomon, A. (1987). Psychoimmunology: interactions between central nervous systems and immune systems. *J. Neurosci. Res.*, 18, 1–9.

Spiegel, D., Bloom, J. R., Kraemer, H. C., and Gottheil, E. (1989). Effects of psychosocial treatment on survival of patients with metastatic breast cancer. *Lancet*, 2, 888–891.

Spielberger, C. (1993). Anger lifestyle, defence motivation and cancer. In F. J. McGuigan Research Lecture, APA Annual Convention, Toronto, August 20–24.

Stavrakay, N. M., Buyck, C., Lott, J., and Wancklin, J. (1968). Psychological factors in the outcome of human cancer. *J. Psychosom. Res.*, 12, 251–259.

Stein, M. (1989). Stress, depression, and the immune system. *J. Clin. Psychiatry*, 50, 35–42.

Temoshok, L. (1985). Biopsychosocial studies in cutaneous malignant melanoma: psychosocial factors associated with prognostic indicators, progression, psychophysiology and tumour-host response. *Soc. Sci. Med.*, 20, 833–840.

Temoshok, L. and Dreher, H. (1992). *Type C Behavior and Cancer*. New York: Random House.

Temoshok, L., Heller, B., Sagebiel, R., Blois, M., Sweet, D. M., Di Clemente, R., and Gold, M. (1985). The relationship of psychosocial factors to prognostic indicators in cutaneous malignant melanoma. *J. Psychosom. Med.*, 29, 139–154.

van der Ploeg, H., Kleijn, W. C., Mook, J., van Hunge, M., Pieters, A., and Leer, J.-W. (1989). Rationality and anti-emotionality as a risk factor for cancer: concept differentiation. *J. Psychosom. Res.*, 33, 217–225.

Vickers, R. P. (1988). Effectiveness of defense: a significant predictor of cortisol secretion under stress. *J. Psychosom. Res.*, 32, 21–29.

von Metzler, A. (1979). Zur antineoplastischen Wirkung zentral nervos wirksamer Pharmaka auf chemisch induzierte Tumoren der Ratte. *J. Cancer Res. Clin. Oncol.*, 95, 11–18.

von Metzler, A. and Nitsch, C. (1986). Carcinogenesis and the central nervous system. *Cancer Detect. Prev.*, 9, 259–277.

Weinberger, D. A., Schwartz, G. D., and Davidson, R. J. (1979). Low-anxious, high-anxious and repressive coping styles: psychometric patterns and behavioral and physiological response to stress. *J. Abnorm. Psychol.*, 88, 319–380.

Weisse, C. S. (1992). Depression and immunocompetence: a review of the literature. *Psychol. Bull.*, 111, 475–489.

Wiedenfeld, S., Bandura, A., Levine, S., O'Leary, A., Brown, S., and Raska, H. (1990). *J. Personality Soc. Psychol.*, 59, 1082–1094.

Wirsching, M., Shirlin, H., Weber, G., Wirsching, B., and Hoffman, F. (1981). Brustbrebs im Kontext: Ergebnisse einer Vorhersagestudie und Konsequenzen fur die Therapie. *Z. Psychosom. Med.*, 27, 239–252.

Zakowski, S., Hall, M. H., and Baum, A. (1992). Stress, stress management, and the immune system. *Appl. Prev. Psychol.*, 1, 1–13.

Zubin, J., Eron, L. D., & Schumer, F. (1965). *An Experimental Approach to Projective Techniques*. New York: Wiley.

chapter eleven

Personality, behavior patterns, and heart disease

Ray H. Rosenman

This chapter will consider a possible role of certain emotions and personality and behavioral variables in the pathogenesis of cardiovascular diseases, but will not, conversely, be concerned with the latter's effects on these variables.

As early as 200 BC, Hippocrates recognized a relationship between emotions and health when he advised "Let no one persuade you to cure the headache until he has first given you his soul to be cured. For this is the great error of our day in the treatment of the human body, that physicians separate the soul from the body." Historical interest appeared to reside particularly in relationships between emotions and functional cardiovascular symptoms. For example, Harvey is credited with stating[1,2] in 1628 that "Every affection of the mind that is attended with either pain or pleasure, hope or fear, is the cause of an agitation whose influence extends to the heart." John C. Williams emphasized the differences between nervous palpitations and organic heart disease in his classic text in 1836,[3] and many clinicians then became interested in the functional nature of cardiovascular symptoms associated with anxiety. These were well described by MacLean in 1867[4] in British soldiers in the Crimean War, independently by DaCosta in 1871[5] in U.S. Civil War soldiers, and by many others.[6] The concept of functional cardiovascular disorders was also supported by introduction of the term neurasthenia by George Beard in 1867.[7] Its widespread international use was replaced by terms such as neurocirculatory asthenia and anxiety neurosis in the First World War, and others followed.[6] It seems appropriate to first consider the role of anxiety.

Anxiety and the hypothalamic defense reaction

Ecology is concerned with interrelationships between organisms and their environment, and evolution with their ability to adapt to environmental changes. Anxiety may influence both, since maintenance of internal milieus is basic to mammalian physiology, and external threats and challenges mobilize the organism into adaptive efforts to regain equilibrium by homeostatic adjustments. Anxiety has a fundamental role in the biologically useful reaction to danger that enhances alertness and prepares the organism for fight or flight. It is an affective response that underlies the basic, physiological reaction to perceived threats and probably evolved from primitive protoplasmic irritability. Anxiety may therefore be the universal emotion that served as an evolutionary force, contributed to biological adaptation, and reinforced the processes of social bonding and communal living. The protective benefits of social networks may operate by suppressing anxiety, and covert anxiety may even underlie coronary-prone type A behaviors. Its importance may explain why no major cerebral dysfunction has ever been identified for anxiety, despite its involvement with neurotransmitters such as gamma-aminobutyric acid (GABA), norepinephrine, dopamine, and serotonin.

The well-coordinated neurohormonal changes in the hypothalamic defense reaction to external challenges are described by Folkow[8] as a highly differentiated response that overrides homeostatic brainstem mechanisms and adjusts the cardiovascular system in anticipatory fashion to prepare for vigorous physical activity. It is therefore highly suited for fight-flight,[9] easily provoked in conscious organisms in response to sudden or novel environmental stimuli, and characterized by increased heart rate and cardiac output, vasoconstriction in skin, kidney, and splanchnic areas, and vasodilatation in skeletal muscles. The increased cardiac output is thereby actively directed to the heart and skeletal muscles, and passively to the brain. The physiological changes elicited by the defense reaction are thus very similar to those during strenuous muscular exercise.

Anxiety is an emotional reaction that includes unpleasant feelings of nervousness, apprehension, worry, tension, and that activates the sympathetic nervous system (SNS). There are thus many reasons to equate psychological stress and anxiety, and what many humans term "stress" may usually be anxiety, and the same defense reaction occurs in situations that cause anxiety and in perceived stressful situations that equate with anxiety. Moreover, this also sets off other affective responses such as fear and worry, which occur infrequently without some anxiety, and with no sharp lines of demarcation. The factors that underly anxiety are different in our urbanized, industrialized world, and new and more insidious fears associated with heightened levels of anxiety have replaced older dangers. However, the same defense reaction is still operative, and it is similarly activated when the organism is slightly alerted in usual activities as during responses to major threats.[8]

The role of anxiety in functional cardiovascular symptoms and arrhythmias

Since the hypothalamic defense reaction is associated with an acute rise of heart rate, cardiac output, and systolic blood pressure, it is not surprising that anxiety can cause functional cardiovascular manifestations that include tachycardia and palpitation. The cardiovascular changes are primarily due to increased sympathoadrenal stimulation that may be a secondary reaction to oppressive precordial sensations, hyperventilation, and other symptoms associated with anxiety. These changes thus reflect the secondary physiologic expression rather than pathology of anxiety.[10] However, increased sympathoadrenal activity during psychogenic stress reactions can provoke a wide gamut of arrhythmias, even in the absence of underlying cardiac disease.

There is ample evidence that SNS neural traffic modulates development of cardiac arrhythmias. The final common pathway is via efferent vagal and SNS fibers that act on electrophysiologic properties of the heart, and autonomic interactions regulate myocardial electrical instability (MEI) in the conscious state. Autonomic nerves are driven by preganglionic sympathetic neurons in the spinal cord and are under the control of descending brain pathways. A major source of background autonomic neural activity thus depends on the integrity of neurons that drive SNS centers that are part of contiguous adrenergic neurons. Central stimuli that increase SNS traffic and suppress baroreflex activity usually produce a rise of heart rate and systolic blood pressure and increase release of epinephrine, whereas vagal nerve activity is diminished. During the post-stimulus period the blood pressure usually remains elevated, baroreflexes are no longer inhibited, and vagal excitation occurs. Ventricular arrhythmias may occur in this vulnerable period of increased vagal tone and residual SNS neural drive, for example, after exercise, and this is relevant for sudden cardiac death that is usually due to ventricular fibrillation.[11]

Its pathophysiology is not merely ischemic heart disease, but is better comprehended as an electrophysiologic MEI which provides the substrate upon which a triggering factor such as SNS activity can precipitate ventricular fibrillation.[11-13] Increased MEI is induced by overt or silent myocardial ischemia and both MEI and triggering neurogenic and catecholamine input are related to higher central nervous system (CNS) activity. Higher neural traffic can thus precipitate sudden arrhythmic death in persons with coronary artery disease. Important triggering factors often relate to neurophysiologic activity in response to psychological stress,[11-13] and coronary vasospasm and platelet aggregation may play a role. A causal relationship between psychogenic stress and sudden death has long been folklore, but the role of higher neural traffic in the genesis of lethal arrhythmias is now more firmly based on evidence that links emotionally stressful events to sudden arrhythmic death in both animals and humans.[14]

The role of anxiety in mitral valve prolapse

Symptomatic mitral valve prolapse syndrome exemplifies an interaction of physical and psychological variables. Anxiety has long been viewed in psychological terms that convey an image of overreaction to life stress, hypochondriasis, and hysteria, with labels such as hyperventilation syndrome, hypoglycemia, neurasthenia, functional cardiovascular disorders, irritable heart syndrome, soldier's heart, effort syndrome, and neurocirculatory asthenia. It is probable that many patients so diagnosed in the past would now be adjudged to have suffered from an anxiety disorder that is associated with a high prevalence of the functional mitral valve prolapse that is commonly termed MVP.[15]

MVP refers to invagination or herniation of valve leaflets into the left atrium during ventricular systole and it has multiple causes. The valve is a complex structure whose proper function depends on the integrity of many components, including the left atrium, fibrous annulus, valve leaflets, chordae tendineae, papillary muscles, and supporting structures at their base. Abnormality of any part can lead to a failure of leaflet coaptation. Under the burden of left ventricular contraction, prolapsed valve cusps stretch, become concave toward the left atrium, and can develop a pleated or scalloped appearance. An increased tugging effect can lead to chordal elongation and thinning and an enlarged mitral annulus, consequences that can cause valve regurgitation and occasionally eventuate in a floppy or ballooning valve.

The motion of the anterior valve leaflet is restricted, as it abuts the interventricular septum during diastole, and normal leaflets are displaced posteriorly into the left atrium. Prolapse can occur when the left ventricle cavity size is disproportionately small and unable to accommodate normal leaflet motion. A disturbance of normal balance between ventricle and mitral valve sizes may cause a failure of leaflet coaptation and anatomical prolapse even in the absence of initial pathological changes in the valve apparatus, and this may occur particularly when diminished ventricle cavity size prevents maintenance of normal leaflet position and contour during ventricular systole.

A disproportion between mitral valve apparatus and ventricle cavity size can occur as the result of hemodynamic factors concerned with systolic volume and/or contractility, and subjects with MVP often exhibit both subnormal blood volume and increased contractility induced by beta-adrenergic stimulation. The predisposition for MVP in young females may partly be due to their relatively smaller left ventricle cavity size.

Functional MVP often occurs in chronic anxiety disorders, although there is no common genetic basis.[15] They coexist merely because of increased beta-adrenergic stimulation, without need to hypothesize a common genetic factor that resides in an inherited dysautonomia. The majority of healthy persons with nonejection clicks in mid-systole are asymptomatic and merely have anatomic variants of normal mitral valves or minor leaflet overlap or prolapse due to hemodynamic factors that reduce ventricular preload filling and that cause a smaller ventricle cavity size relative to the mitral orifice. Specific hemodynamic factors that can be causally related to a failure of normal leaflet coaptation include a self-sustaining cycle of hypovolemia, orthostatic intolerance, and chronic hyperadrenergic stimulation, which variously induce increased myocardial contractility, veno- and vasoconstriction, and tachycardia. Chronic anxiety stimulates adrenergic activity, hypovolemia, tachycardia, and left ventricular contractility, and these combine to cause the high prevalence of functional MVP in anxiety disorders. The factors that regulate blood volume thus appear to be of primary importance both for anatomic MVP and for the cardiovascular dysregulation that is manifested by subjects with MVP syndrome.[15]

The possible role of emotions and behaviors in essential hypertension

The central nervous system integrates information from both the organism and environment in order to provide critical neurohormonal adjustments for homeostatic regulation that is essential for maintenance of the blood pressure. Arterial blood pressure can be increased by activating central neural sites with neuroanatomic connections to the SNS, and these sites connect with higher centers that are involved in perception of the environment. External stressors are thus capable of elevating blood pressure via neurohormonal mechanisms.[16]

It is popularly hypothesized that psychosocial stressors stimulate SNS overactivity and can thereby eventuate in sustained hypertension.[17] Although animal studies find that various stressors can raise blood pressure,[18] when the stressor is removed, sustained hypertension is the exception, with lack of evidence that stress alone can induce sustained hypertension in otherwise healthy animals.[19] Evidence for an ability of emotions and other stress to induce sustained blood pressure elevation in humans is even less significant. As in animals, stress and certain emotions transiently elevate blood pressure in humans, but this is not sustained. Changing cultural norms from more primitive to more complex may be associated with a rise of blood pressure, but this involves interactions between predisposing genetic factors and dietary, alcohol, weight, renal, and other relevant variables.[20] Such combinations appear necessary for the reliable expression of emotion- and stress-induced hypertension in both animals and humans.[19]

The widespread belief that anxiety is casually related to hypertension is not supported by valid evidence that higher levels of anxiety occur in hypertensives, compared to normotensives. The diagnosis often creates anxiety; hypertension itself can affect behavior at anatomic, physiologic, and emotional levels and antihypertensive drugs can affect behavioral responses. Hypertensives may thus have alterations of physiologic function that interact with behavioral factors to further cloud causal relationships of anxiety.[21] Despite common belief to the contrary, critical analysis of the relevant studies indicates that a relationship of anxiety to sustained hypertension remains an unproven hypothesis.[22] Moreover, patients with chronic anxiety do not exhibit increased reactivity to laboratory stressors,[23] and they commonly exhibit low normal blood pressures and unusually low prevalence of hypertension.[15,24] Indeed, negative correlations found in undiagnosed hypertensives indicate that they may even have lower levels of anxiety.[25]

Evidence of a causal relationship of emotions and stress to hypertension is largely based on studies of acute responses that occur in some offspring of parents with hypertension.[26] Young borderline hypertensives and offspring of hypertensive parents are at risk to develop sustained hypertension, and some exhibit heightened cardiovascular reactivity in laboratory stress tests. This underlies the concept of psychophysiologists that exaggerated pressor responses to environmental stimuli can play a pathogenetic role in the development of essential hypertension. The theory variously postulates that individuals with heightened cardiovascular responses to behavioral challenges are predisposed to develop hypertension, and that the repetitive and summated occurrence of such responses in natural environments can eventuate in sustained hypertension.[17] The hyperkinetic state of many younger subjects with borderline hypertension is neurogenically mediated, and catecholamine levels tend to be higher in many established hypertensives.[27] Since essential hypertension has a multifactorial etiology, one contributing factor may be SNS overactivity that can be induced by various emotions and, conversely, alter emotions and behaviors, particularly in younger borderline hypertensives.[27,28]

However, the magnitude of higher cardiovascular responses is generally small, and the higher prevalence of essential hypertension in black, compared to white subjects, is not associated with consistent racial differences in reactivity. Moreover, even when present, heightened reactivity only occurs in response to cognitive stressors, and not during such other stimuli as isometric and dynamic exercise, cold pressor testing, and orthostatic stress.[29] Heightened reactivity also may occur in response to dynamic exercise in established hypertensives, compared to normotensives, but they have normal responses to static exercise, tilt, and blood volume expansion.[30]

The pattern of heightened reactivity in borderline hypertensives is thus limited to behavioral tasks. Even their response to mental stressors varies widely from high to low, and they do not exhibit any generalized autonomic dysregulation.[30,31] Moreover, neither cold pressor testing nor cognitive stressors predict blood pressure responses to antihypertensive therapy. Subjects with established hypertension may exhibit increased response to tasks that require active coping, but differences between normo- and hypertensive subjects are specific for the cardiovascular system, quantitative rather than qualitative, and there is no generalized activation of the SNS.[30,31] Furthermore, enhanced reactivity shows different patterns for systolic and diastolic blood pressure, depending on whether subjects have borderline or established hypertension.

There is some evidence of an increased risk for sustained hypertension in younger subjects with borderline hypertension who have heightened cardiovascular reactivity. However, the risk is not very great, and the substantial majority do not progress to sustained hypertension. Also, there are no population-based studies that find that hyperreactors are more likely to develop sustained hypertension with the passage of time. Furthermore, a substantial number of subjects with mild to moderately elevated blood pressure during screening examinations will subsequently be found to be normotensive,[32] exemplifying the transient effect of "white coat hypertension". It is also significant that, although repeated measurements, per se, lower blood pressure, anxiolytics do not cause a sustained fall in patients with hypertension-associated anxiety. Moreover, subjects with pressure elevated in the clinic but normal at home, do not differ in anxiety levels compared to those elevated in both settings. Regression toward the mean can account for some of the findings in borderline hypertensives, and higher cardiovascular responses to mental stressors in some offspring of hypertensives may partly be due to salt loading. It is also significant that, with few exceptions, neither cold pressor testing nor response to exercise predicts development of sustained hypertension.

The findings in subjects with type A behavior pattern (TABP) also mitigate against considering that cardiovascular reactivity plays a causal role in development of hypertension. The finding of higher SNS responses in type A than type B males to competitive, cognitive challenges in both the laboratory setting and their daily environments[33] stimulated a vast array of studies of cardiovascular reactivity. Type A–B differences in SNS and blood pressure responses have generally been found during exposure to a wide array of stressors in the laboratory setting.[34] The largest differences tend to occur during tasks associated with more rapid pace of activity, greater task difficulty, and when subjects are challenged to perform more difficult tasks in a competitive manner under time pressure.[34,35] However, the pattern of these differences and lack of consistency strongly suggest that types A and B individuals do not have intrinsic reactivity differences, but only that heightened type A perception of relevant challenging stressors stimulates a more active coping style associated with increased SNS responses. Despite the tendency of type A subjects to exhibit heightened responses to perceived relevant challenges in both the laboratory setting and natural environment, neither type A subjects in general nor those with exaggerated cardiovascular reactivity exhibit either higher levels of resting blood pressure or increased prevalence of essential hypertension.[35,36] This is particularly significant, considering that type A subjects tend to exhibit higher anger and hostility dimensions, which are variously believed to be related to higher levels of blood pressure, heightened cardiovascular reactivity, and increased blood pressure variability during ambulatory monitoring in natural environments.

The test-retest reliability for laboratory and ambulatory measures of reactivity tends to be low for many commonly used stressors.[37] Responses in children seem to generalize across laboratory test procedures that require qualitatively different behavioral responses.[38] However, this suggests that individual response patterns are more genetically determined than related to differences of cognitive perception of the tasks.

It is generally assumed that the pattern of responses that occur in the laboratory generalizes to the natural environment, with an increased variability of the ambulatory blood pressure. However, ambulatory monitoring during usual daily activities has generally failed to document hypothesized findings. There are spontaneous blood pressure fluctuations of considerable magnitude during ambulatory monitoring of all individuals in their natural environments, but blood pressure variability is not greater in those with hypertension. Thus, variability during ambulatory monitoring in the daily milieu is not increased in young borderline hypertensives.[29] Nor does it differ in subjects whose blood pressures are normal, compared to those with mild or marked elevations.[39] Although average ambulatory blood pressures obtained on different occasions in these studies tend to be reproducible, the measures of daily variability are not. Variability in the natural environment may show some correlations with resting levels, and even be greater in some subjects with higher systolic responses in the laboratory setting. However, those with heightened laboratory stress responses show only small increases of systolic pressure in natural environments. Moreover, those with heightened responses in the laboratory setting do not exhibit increased ambulatory variability in everyday life activities, and the increase in variability that is accounted for by pressor responses in laboratory stress tests is very small. Finally, although ambulatory blood pressure variability is related to resting blood pressure level, it is not related to SNS activity. Thus, cardiovascular reactivity measured in laboratory stress testing does not predict blood pressure variability in the natural environment or the blood pressure changes from one to another daily activity.

Basal and reactive blood pressures appear to be under a dual system of regulation that has different anatomic centers and pathways that are almost independently controlled.[40] It is therefore not surprising that antihypertensive therapy with a wide variety of drugs affects central regulation involved in the maintenance of basal blood pressure levels, but not that of blood pressure variability or pressor reactions to environmental stressors. Thus, there is no obvious reason why cardiovascular reactivity should be a causal determinant of sustained hypertension. The largely independent regulation of basal blood pressure and its variability[41] also underlies the fact that stressful sensory stimuli have an important effect on variability of mean blood pressure, but not on the mean blood pressure itself. The principal determinant of blood pressure variability in hypertensives may be a decline in baroreceptor reflex sensitivity, but this is regulated independently of mean blood pressure. It also should be emphasized that blood pressure regulation in hypertension is normal.[30,31]

The results of these studies lead to the conclusion that cardiovascular reactivity cannot explain the development of hypertension.[22,23,30,42] Thus, there is little evidence to indicate that transient, emotion- or stress-induced blood pressure elevations are causal precursors or otherwise contribute to sustained hypertension. Stress-induced cardiovascular responses may sometimes be a correlate or marker for the risk of developing hypertension, but not its cause.[42,43] It also is apparent that behavioral differences of cognitive perception of stressors do not explain individual differences of cardiovascular reactivity, that laboratory reactivity neither predicts hypertension nor accounts for differences of blood pressure variability in the natural environment, that hypertensive persons do not have increased blood pressure variability, and that responses to stress and emotions do not play a causal role in the development of essential hypertension. Indeed, it has been emphasized that the specificity of exaggerated cardiovascular responses in borderline hypertensives to mental as opposed to physical stressors is improperly interpreted to mean that behaviorally induced blood pressure reactivity is the mechanism by which hypertension develops.[30] It is often not realized that physiological responses result from selective neuronal activation rather than from a generalized SNS response.[30,31]

Critical reviews continue to find little evidence of a causal role in sustained hypertension for either anxiety[45] or cardiovascular reactivity.[50] However, there is stronger evidence for a greater association of blood pressure with dimensions of hostility and anger. The literature on psychosocial factors in hypertension has consistently pointed to problems of anger management and expression.[16,44–48] Borderline hypertensives have sometimes been found to exhibit suppressed anger and submissiveness that may be related to more sustained elevations of blood pressure. During ambulatory monitoring in the daily milieu, blood pressure variability also may be correlated with the level of hostility. In the laboratory setting, exaggerated and more prolonged pressor responses to a variety of stressful cognitive stimuli may occur in hypertensive persons who exhibit unexpressed hostility and anger.[48] Moreover, offspring of hypertensive parents who progress to sustained hypertension are somewhat more often those who show exaggerated pressor responses to stressors that are designed to elicit anger and, among them, an enhanced risk for sustained hypertension may be found in those who have the greatest difficulty in expressing such induced anger.[49] However, there are many difficulties for the hypothesis. Although there have been repeated attempts to differentiate SNS and cardiovascular responses to different emotional states,[46] ambulatory monitoring finds no qualitative differences in blood pressure changes that occur in response to various emotions.[51] For example, the average rise of blood pressure is the same during anger and anxiety, although both are quantitatively higher than occurs during happiness.[50] It is also pointed out that the "submissive hypertensive personality" may be a result of selection procedures for patients under investigation, and is commonly found in persons without hypertension.[45] An extensive review fails to find valid evidence for causal relationships of personality traits and hypertension, including suppressed hostility.[45]

Type A behavior pattern, hostility, and ischemic heart disease

The role of type A behavior pattern (TABP) in ischemic heart disease (IHD) represents a different relationship of personality to heart disease. Although Osler[52] and a number of other early observers[53] linked IHD to aggressive and competitive behaviors, the concept of TABP emerged only after it became apparent that conventional risk factors did not explain historical changes of IHD rates, a wide variance in geographic distribution of IHD at similar risk factor levels, or an individual specificity of risk. A significant increased incidence of IHD occurred after World War I, but primarily in middle-aged males who resided in highly urbanized and densely populated, industrialized areas, indicating a role of both psychosocial and biological variables in an interaction that was considered in the TABP concept.[53] It was also apparent that widely varying rates in different European countries could not be ascribed to differences of diet, physical activity, or usual risk factors. Moreover, neither the earlier 20th century increase or more recent decline of IHD mortality in the U.S. and other western countries can be well explained by changes of diet or classical risk factors.[54]

The historical changes and geographic differences in IHD incidence that are not explained by classical risk factors promoted a broad search for additional pathogenetic influences, resulting in a separate category of risk factors that are generally related to stress concepts and different individual perceptions of the environmental milieu.[55] Such considerations, along with direct observation of the behavior of IHD patients led to conceptualization of the TABP in the 1950s.[53] Several reviews[55] found that reliable associations do exist between certain psychological variables and IHD, and quantitative meta-analysis of relevant studies found the strongest association for the TABP.[56]

TABP is a constellation of behaviors that are used to cope with the human experience, and was conceived as an action-emotion complex which individuals use to confront milieu challenges, and which involves behavioral dispositions such as competitiveness, aggressiveness, and impatience; specific behaviors such as alertness, muscle tenseness, rapid and emphatic vocal stylistics, and accelerated pace of activities; and emotional responses such as irritation, covert hostility, and increased potential for anger.[53] A large number of studies have provided strong construct validation for the TABP, with consistent findings that type A subjects are more alert, aggressive, competitive, time-conscious, impatient and fast-paced,

self-confident, orderly, self-controlled, well-organized, deeply involved
with vocation and not distracted from task performance, less able to relax
away from work, prefer to work alone when challenged, strive to control
their environments, and have a greater potential for hostility, particularly
when compared to type B persons.[53,56]

Although TABP does not equate with anxiety, as usually considered,
it is possible that there is an underlying covert anxiety associated with a
threat of failure that, in turn, leads to type A competitiveness, aggressiveness, and accelerated pace of activities.[57] The IHD incidence is associated
with urbanization, population density, and industrialization, and an associated need for competitiveness may particularly engender TABP in susceptible individuals.[57] This is not an evolutionary development and may
therefore be regarded as inappropriately directed. Montagu emphasized[58]
that the drive for preservation of species and self leads to a type of competitiveness and aggression that is biologically adaptive, life-serving, phy-
logenetically programmed, and common both to animals and humans.
Other forms of aggression that arise solely out of the human experience
and are exclusively found in humans may be biologically maladaptive.
Indeed, Montagu finds the principal factor operating in animal evolution
to be cooperation, rather than the divisiveness and inappropriate aggression, competitiveness, and conflict that characterize much human experience and the coronary-prone facets of TABP.

TABP was independently associated with a significant incidence of
IHD in prospective studies in the U.S., Europe, and elsewhere.[57] Meta-
analysis of the literature on psychosocial variables found the strongest association for TABP,[56] particularly in cross-sectional population studies,
rather than in intervention studies,[59] an important difference, since intervention studies are often flawed by selection bias and other problems.

Early studies found a relationship between the competitive-hostility
component of TABP and IHD,[53,57,60] and this relationship has received considerable popular if not valid scientific support.

Megargee[61] noted that those who attempt to relate dimensions of anger,
hostility, or aggression to cardiovascular disease may operationally define
different constructs by using a confusing array of dissimilar techniques in
their studies, often interchangeably and without proper differentiation,
and with considerable ambiguity and inconsistency in how these constructs are defined, separated, overlap, and are measured. Impetus was
given to an hostility-IHD relationship by long-term, follow-up results in
two cohorts who had much earlier completed the Minnesota Multiphasic
Personality Inventory (MMPI) Cook and Medley "HO" scale. However,
the purported relationships are spurious since the correlation was with all
cause mortality, rather than having specificity for prediction of IHD. The
problems with hostility-anger constructs are particularly relevant for this
scale, since it is a measure of neuroticism and general psychopathology
but not of hostility or overtly aggressive behavior, and is even negatively

correlated with other psychometric measures of hostility and paranoia.[61,62] Since the "HO" scale is a measure of neurotic anxiety, which is not causally related to IHD, it is not surprising that it lacks specificity for prediction of IHD and was not predictively related either to severity of coronary artery disease or to the incidence of primary or recurring IHD events in almost all studies in which the measure was used.[60]

Space precludes inclusion of references for all of this discussion, and the reader is referred to cited literature for this purpose.

References

1. Burchell, H. B., Letter to editor, *N. Engl. J. Med.*, 311, 1520, 1985.

2. Harvey, W., Exercitatio de motu cordis et sanguinis. Cited in Hackett, T. P. and Rosenbaum, J. F., Emotion, psychiatric disorders and the heart, Braunwald, E., Ed., *Heart Disease*, Saunders, Philadelphia, 1984, 1826–1946.

3. Williams, J. C., *Practical Observations on Nervous and Sympathetic-Palpitation of the Heart*, Lingman, Rees, Orme, and Browne, London, 1836.

4. MacLean, W. C., Diseases of the heart in the British Army: the cause and the remedy, *Br. Med. J.*, 1, 161, 1867.

5. DaCosta, J. M., On irritable heart: a clinical study of functional cardiac disorder and its consequences, *Am. J. Med. Sci.*, 61, 17, 1871.

6. Rosenman, R. H., Pathogenesis of the relationship of anxiety to mitral valve prolapse, in *Anxiety and the Heart*, Byrne, D. G. and Rosenman, R. H., Eds., Hemisphere, Washington, D.C., 1990, 295–346.

7. Beard, G., Neurasthenia or nervous exhaustion, *Boston Med. Surg. J.*, 53, 217, 1867.

8. Folkow, B., Physiology of behavior and blood pressure regulation in animals, in *Behavioral Factors in Hypertension, Handbook of Hypertension*, Vol. 9, Julius, S. and Bassett, D. R., Eds., Elsevier, Amsterdam, 1987, 1–18.

9. Brod, J., Fencl, V., Hejl, Z., and Jirka, J., Circulatory changes underlying blood pressure elevation during acute emotional stress (mental arithmetic) in normotensive and hypertensive subjects, *Clin. Sci.*, 18, 269, 1959.

10. Klein, D. F., Zitrin, C. M., and Woerner, M., Antidepressants, anxiety, panic and phobias, in *Psychopharmacology: A Generation of Progress*, Lipton, M. A., DiMascio, A., and Killam, K. F., Eds., Raven Press, New York, 1978, 1401–1410.

11. Skinner, J. E., Psychosocial stress and sudden cardiac death: brain mechanisms, in *Stress and Heart Disease*, Beamish, R. E., Singal, P. K., and Dhalla, N. A., Eds., Martinus Nijhoff, Boston, 1985, 44–59.

12. Lown, B., Sudden cardiac death: the major challenge confronting contemporary cardiology, *Am. J. Cardiol.*, 43, 313, 1979.

13. Schwartz, P. J., Stress and sudden cardiac death: the role of the autonomic nervous system, *J. Clin. Psychol. Monog.*, 2, 7, 1984.

14. Reich, P., De Silva, R. A., Lown, B., and Murawski, J., Acute psychological disturbances preceding life-threatening ventricular arrhythmias, *JAMA*, 246, 233, 1981.

15. Rosenman, R. H., Pathogenesis of the relationship of anxiety to mitral valve prolapse, in *Anxiety and the Heart*, Byrne, D. G. and Rosenman, R. H., Eds., Hemisphere, Washington, D.C., 1990, 295–346.

16. Diamond, E. L., The role of anger and hostility in essential hypertension and coronary heart disease, *Psychol. Bull.*, 92, 410, 1982.
17. Chesney, M. A., Hypertension: biobehavioral influences and their implications for treatment, in *Biological and Psychological Factors in Cardiovascular Disease*, Schmidt, T. H., Dembroski, T. M., and Blumchen, G., Eds., Springer-Verlag, Heidelberg, 1986, 568–583.
18. Henry, J. P. and Stephens, P. M., *Stress, Health and Social Environment*, Springer-Verlag, New York, 1977, 1–282.
19. Brody, M. J., Natelson, B. H., Anderson, E., Folkow, B., Levy, M. N., Obrist, P. A., Reis, D. F., Rosenman, R. H., and Williams, R. B., Behavioral mechanisms in hypertension. Report of Task Force No. 3, American Heart Association Conference on Behavioral Medicine and Cardiovascular Disease, Sea Island, February 3–7, 1985, *Circulation*, Part II, 76, I-84, 1987.
20. Salmond, C. E., Prior, A. M., and Wessen, A. F., Blood pressure patterns and migration: a 14-year cohort study of adult Tokelauans, *Am. J. Epidemiol.*, 130, 37, 1986.
21. Elias, M. F. and Streeten, D. H. P., *Hypertension and Cognitive Processes*, Beach-Hill, Mount Desert, ME, 1980.
22. Rosenman, R. H. and Hjemdahl, P., Is there a causal relationship of anxiety, stress, or cardiovascular reactivity to hypertension? *Stress Med.*, 7, 152, 1991.
23. Ward, M. W., Anxiety and cardiovascular reactivity, in *Anxiety and the Heart*, Byrne, D. G. and Rosenman, R. H., Eds., Hemisphere, Washington, D.C., 1990, 347–365.
24. Devereux, R. B., Brown, W. T., Lutas, E. M., Kramer-Fox, R., and Laragh, J. H., Association of mitral valve prolapse with low body-weight and low blood pressure, *Lancet*, 2, 792, 1982.
25. Winkleby, M. A., Ragland, D. R., and Syme, S. L., Self-reported stressors and hypertension: evidence of an inverse association, *Am. J. Epidemiol.*, 127, 124, 1988.
26. Falkner, B., Onesti, G., Angelakos, E. T., Fernandez, M., and Langman, C., Cardiovascular response to mental stress in normal adolescents with hypertensive parents, *Hypertension*, 1, 23, 1979.
27. Cottier, C., Shapiro, K., and Julius, S., Treatment of mild hypertension with progressive muscle relaxation: predictive value of indexes of sympathetic tone, *Arch. Intern. Med.*, 144, 1954, 1984.
28. Esler, M., Julius, S., Zweifler, A., Randall, O., Harburg, E., Gardiner, H., and DeQuattro, V., Mild high-renin hypertension; neurogenic human hypertension? *N. Engl. J. Med.*, 196, 405, 1977.
29. Conway, J., Hemodynamic aspects of essential hypertension in humans, *Physiol. Rev.*, 63, 617, 1983.
30. Julius, S., The blood pressure seeking properties of the central nervous system (Editorial review), *J. Hypertens.*, 6, 177, 1988.
31. Hjemdahl, P., Physiology of the autonomic nervous system as related to cardiovascular function: implications for stress research, in *Anxiety and the Heart*, Byrne, D. G. and Rosenman, R. H., Eds., Hemisphere, Washington, D.C., 1990, 95–158.
32. Australian therapeutic trial in mild hypertension, *Lancet*, 1, 1261, 1980.
33. Rosenman, R. H. and Friedman, M., Neurogenic factors in pathogenesis of coronary heart disease, *Med. Clin. North Am.*, 58, 269, 1974.

34. Krantz, D. S. and Manuck, S., Acute psychophysiologic reactivity and risk of cardiovascular disease: a review and methodologic critique, *Psychol. Bull.*, 96, 435, 1984.
35. Rosenman, R. H., Type A behavior pattern and cardiovascular reactivity: is there a relationship with hypertension? in *Personality, Elevated Blood Pressure, and Essential Hypertension*, Johnson, E., Gentry, W., and Julius, S., Eds., Hemisphere, Washington, D.C., 1991, 87–111.
36. Rosenman, R. H., Type A behavior and hypertension, in *Handbook of Hypertension, Vol. 9, Behavioral Factors in Hypertension*, Julius, S. and Bassett, D. R., Eds., Elsevier, Amsterdam, 1987, 141–149.
37. Van Egeren, L. F. and Sparrow, A. W., Laboratory stress testing to assess real-life cardiovascular reactivity, *Psychosom. Med.*, 51, 1, 1989.
38. Matthews, K. A., Rakaczky, C. J., Stoney, C. M., and Manuck, S. B., Are cardiovascular responses to behavioral stressors a stable individual difference variable in childhood? *Psychophysiology*, 24, 464, 1987.
39. Pickering, T. G., Harshfield, G. A., Kleinert, H. D., Blank, S. B., and Laragh, J. H., Blood pressure during daily activities, sleep, and exercise: comparison of values in normal and hypertensive subjects, *JAMA*, 247, 992, 1982.
40. Reis, D. J. and LeDoux, J. E., Some central neural mechanims governing resting and behaviorally coupled control of blood pressure, *Circulation Suppl.*, 76, S1, 1987.
41. Reis, D. J., Ruggiero, D. A., and Morrison, S. F., The C1 area of the rostral ventrolateral medulla oblongata: a critical brainstem region for control of resting and reflex integration of arterial pressure, *Am. J. Hypertens.*, 2 (Part 2), 363S, 1989.
42. Pickering, T. G. and Gerin, W., Cardiovascular reactivity in the laboratory and the role of behavioral factors in hypertension: a critical review, *Ann. Behav. Med.*, 12, 3, 1990.
43. Rosenman, R. H. and Ward, M. W., The changing concept of cardiovascular reactivity, *Stress Med.*, 4, 241, 1988.
44. Rosenman, R. H., Health consequences of anger and implications for treatment, in *Anger and Hostility in Cardiovascular and Behavioral Disorders*, Chesney, M. A. and Rosenman, R. H., Eds., Hemisphere, New York, 1985, 103–126.
45. Cottier, C., Perini, Ch., and Rauchfleisch, U., Personality traits and hypertension: an overview, in *Handbook of Hypertension, Vol. 9, Behavioral Factors in Hypertension*, Julius, S. and Bassett, D. R., Eds., Elsevier, Amsterdam, 1987, 123–140.
46. Schwartz, G. E., Weinberger, D. A., and Singer, J. A., Cardiovascular differentiation of happiness, sadness, anger, and fear following imagery, *Psychosom. Med.*, 43, 343, 1981.
47. Schneider, R. H., Egan, B. M., Johnson, E. H., Drobny, H., and Julius, S., Anger and anxiety in borderline hypertension, *Psychosom. Med.*, 48, 242, 1986.
48. Baer, P. E., Collins, F. H., Bourenoff, G. C., and Ketchel, M. F., Assessing personality factors in essential hypertension with a brief self-report instrument, *Psychsom. Med.*, 16, 721, 1979.
49. Falkner, B., Onesti, G., and Hamstra, B., Stress response characteristics of adolescents with high genetic risk for essential hypertension: a five-year follow-up, *Clin. Exp. Hypertens.*, 3, 583, 1981.

50. Pickering, T. G. and Gerin, W., Does cardiovascular reactivity have patho-
    genetic significance in hypertensive patients? in *Personality, Elevated Blood
    Pressure, and Hypertension,* Johnson, E. H., Gentry, W. D., and Julius, S., Eds.,
    Hemisphere, Washington, D.C., 1991, 151–173.
51. James, G. D., Yee, L. S., Harshfield, H. A., Blank, S. G., and Pickering, T. G.,
    The influence of happiness, anger and anxiety on the blood pressure of bor-
    derline hypertensives, *Psychosom. Med.,* 48, 502, 1986.
52. Osler, W., The Lumleian lectures on angina pectoris, *Lancet,* 1, 829, 1892.
53. Rosenman, R. H., Current and past history of type A behavior pattern, in
    Biological and Psychological Factors in Cardiovascular Disease, Schmidt, T. H.,
    Dembroski, T. M., and Blumchen, G., Eds., Springer-Verlag, Heidelberg,
    1986, 15–40.
54. Rosenman, R. H., The questionable roles of the diet and serum cholesterol
    in the incidence of ischemic heart disease and its 20th century changes,
    Homeostasis Health Dis. (Prague), 34, 1, 1993.
55. Jenkins, C. D., Epidemiology of cardiovascular diseases, *J. Consult. Clin.
    Psychol.,* 56, 324, 1988.
56. Booth-Kewley, S. and Friedman, H. S., Psychological predictors of heart dis-
    ease: a quantitative review, *Psychol. Bull.,* 101, 343, 1987.
57. Rosenman, R. H., Type A behavior pattern: a personal overview, in *Type A
    Behavior,* Strube, M., Ed., (Special Issue) *J. Soc. Behav. Personality,* 5, 1, 1990.
58. Montagu, A., *The Nature of Human Aggression,* Oxford University Press,
    Oxford, 1976.
59. Matthews, K. A., Coronary heart disease and type A behaviors: update on
    and alternative to the Booth-Kewley and Friedman (1987) quantitative re-
    view, *Psychol. Bull.,* 104, 373, 1988.
60. Rosenman, R. H., Type A behavior pattern and coronary heart disease: the
    hostility factor, *Stress Med.,* 7, 245, 1991.
61. Megargee, E. I., The dynamics of aggression and their application to car-
    diovascular disorders, in *Anger and Hostility in Cardiovascular and Behavioral
    Disorders,* Chesney, M. A. and Rosenman, R. H., Eds., Hemisphere,
    Washington, D.C., 1985, 31–38.
62. Swan, G., Carmelli, D., and Rosenman, R. H., Cook and Medley hostility
    and the type A behavior pattern: psychological correlates of two coronary-
    prone behaviors, *J. Soc. Behav. Personality,* 5, 89, 1990.

chapter twelve

Personality, stress, and chronic fatigue syndrome

Suzan Lewis

Introduction

Chronic fatigue syndrome (CFS) is an interesting case study for stress medicine. The disabling symptoms of this condition are, as yet, unexplainable by diagnosable physical disease and debates about the nature of the illness have focused on whether it should be considered in either physical or psychological terms. The role of psychosocial factors in the development and course of the illness has received less attention. Evidence is now beginning to accumulate, however, that stressful lifestyles may render certain types of people vulnerable to CFS.

CFS is also known as post-viral fatigue syndrome (PVFS) and myalgic encephalomyelitis (ME). The term CFS is usually preferred because it makes no assumptions about etiology and does not imply a unitary phenomenon. It is characterized by a principal symptom of persistent or intermittent, disabling and unexplained fatigue, together with a range of muscular, cognitive, autonomic, and neurological symptoms, which vary from person to person,[1] and which can persist for months or years. Despite some agreement about diagnostic criteria, at least for research purposes, the etiology, symptomology, and prognosis of CFS continue to be a source of controversy.

Mind and body dualism in research on CFS

Debates about CFS have been characterized by dualistic thinking, seeking to explain the illness in either physical or psychological terms, assuming the two to be mutually exclusive rather than interdependent. One line of research has been to examine the psychiatric status of sufferers in order to establish that CFS is a psychiatric disorder. There is considerable evidence of high rates of psychiatric disturbance, especially depression, associated with CFS.[2-7] However, the nature and phenomenology of depressive symptoms in CFS appear to differ from that of patients diagnosed as clinically de-

0-8493-2908-6/96/$0.00+$.50

pressed.[8,9] The possible etiological significance of findings of psychiatric disturbance is also open to different interpretations.[10,11] Emotional disturbance may be a predisposing factor or reaction to illness, or CFS and depression may share some overlap of symptoms and neurochemical reactions. There is some evidence of a relatively high incidence of prior psychiatric episodes[2] but this may be due to individual vulnerability to psychiatric disorders and/or to ongoing demands and stress. Furthermore, not all sufferers have a history of psychiatric illness, nor do all display depressive or other psychiatric symptoms in their current illness.[2,6]

Other research has examined various physical explanations of CFS and findings are often presented as an argument for an organic basis to the illness, refuting the notion of a psychological or psychiatric basis.[12] Persistent infection with viruses such as Coxsackie A and B, herpes, and Epstein-Barr viruses are thought to be involved.[13-15] However, there is no evidence of a single virus present in all sufferers and not in the general population, and as not all sufferers report an acute viral infection prior to the onset of illness the direction of causality is unclear. There is considerable evidence of immune dysfunction in CFS,[16-19] but, again, the clinical importance of these findings is not always evident.[20,21]

Clearly, neither psychological nor physical explanations alone can encompass the complexities of this condition or set of conditions. More recently the value of a multifactorial model, based on a complex interaction of physical, psychological, and social factors, has been proposed.[10,22,23]

Themes emerging from recent literature on CFS

Although the debate about the relative significance of psychological and physical factors continues, certain themes and areas of consensus are emerging from the recent literature. One is that CFS is not a unitary condition but a set of conditions and that etiologies and prognoses are also likely to be heterogeneous. This complicates the picture, as each conflicting model of CFS may fit one subset of CFS sufferers. A second theme is that etiological and perpetuating or maintaining factors may differ. For example, regardless of whether the causes and symptoms are psychological or physical, psychological factors such as illness attributions and coping strategies may perpetuate illness.[8,24,25] There is also growing awareness of the significance of social context in this, as in other illnesses. Finally, several authors have pointed to the need to move away from an emphasis on psychiatric disorders and pathological factors to examine the significance of psychological processes in CFS.[26,27] In particular there is an emerging view that stress plays a role in the etiology of CFS and that psychosocial factors may increase vulnerability to the condition.

There are many reasons to suspect that CFS is stress related, not least that CFS sufferers themselves frequently attribute the onset of the illness or the occurrence of relapses to stress.[7,28,29] The symptoms of CFS are readily recognizable as stress related. Chronic fatigue is a form of exhaustion, which mirrors the third stage in Selye's model of the stress process, following alarm and resistance to long-term, ongoing stressors.[30] The widely reported personality and lifestyle factors associated with CFS and discussed below, including hard driving, achievement-oriented behavior,[23,25,27,31] suggests possible similarities with burnout, which has also been associated with the relentless pursuit of success.[32]

The stress model is particularly appropriate for understanding CFS, as it incorporates the dynamic interaction between psychological, physical, and social factors and has the potential to explain its psychological, immunological, and viral symptoms. Stress can cause emotional upset and distress which, in turn, impacts on the immune system and increases vulnerability to infectious and other diseases.[33] Similarly, emotional distress resulting from acute or chronic stress can influence the course and prognosis of an illness via effects on the immune system.[33] In addition, individual difference factors may determine the experience of and reaction to stressful events and these will have consequences for the immune system and psychological well-being.

This chapter examines the evidence for a relationship between stress, psychosocial factors, and CFS. No assumptions are made about the relative contributions of psychological or organic factors, as there is growing consensus that both are involved in any illness, and mind body dualistic thinking can obscure the more complex interaction of processes contributing to ill health. It is argued that stress may play a role at all levels, in interaction with physical and social factors. Neither is it assumed that CFS sufferers are a homogeneous group or that one explanation can fit all cases. The possible ways in which stress may be implicated in the etiology and in the maintenance of CFS are examined and implications for treatment, prevention, and further research are explored.

Stress, individual differences, and the development of CFS

Life events and ongoing stress as precursors to CFS

Stressful life events and ongoing situations appraised as stressful may contribute to illness via changes in the immune system[34,35] and/or through the effects on mental health.[36] Sufferers' attributions of their illness to stress[23] and the association of CFS with high achievement and a highly demanding and potentially stressful lifestyle[23,37] suggests that occupational stress may be implicated. Research has not directly examined this possibility, although the potential impact of stressful events has been explored.

Not all sufferers make the link between stress and the onset of illness, often because of a focus on other triggers, particularly viral infections, which may themselves be a consequence of acute or chronic stress and subsequent lowered resistance to pathogens. Surawy et al.[25] report that most of the more than 100 CFS patients they have observed and interviewed reported that the onset of illness occurred in association with a viral illness, but that on further questioning, patients typically revealed major psychosocial stressors preceding the onset of illness. These included chronic relationship or work problems, difficulty in adapting to life changes, and bereavement. Stressful life events have been identified as potential contributors to the development of CFS in a number of other studies,[23,27,38,39] but the evidence is not entirely consistent and is weakened by methodological flaws. Stressful life events prior to their illness were reported by a large proportion of sufferers studied by Ware[23,25] and by Wood et al.,[38] but no comparison was made with a control group. Striklen et al.[39] found CFS sufferers to have experienced more loss-related life events in the 12 months prior to the onset of illness than healthy controls, and loss-related events were also reported in other studies.[23,25] However, Lewis et al.[27] reported no significant differences between CFS sufferers and irritable bowel syndrom (IBS) patients in the overall number and severity of life events recalled in the 2 years prior to the onset of illness or those reported by healthy controls in the past two years. Of 42 events, only 2, both of which related to moving house, were reported more frequently by the CFS group. Interestingly, many of the life events reported in the past 6 months in the Wood et al.[38] study also involved changes in residence.

There is some indication, therefore, that life events involving loss, change in residence, and relationship difficulties may be implicated in the onset of CFS. However, studies are, by their very nature, retrospective and recall can obviously be affected by illness. Patients with an illness such as CFS for which there is no available acceptable explanation may also be particularly likely to search for explanations in the form of life events. The research has used the Holmes and Rahe scale or modifications of this[27,39] or simply asked one question to avoid expanding already long interviews.[25] The limitations of these approaches are well documented.[36] Research is needed using more sophisticated instruments, such as the Life Events and Difficulties Scale,[36] which helps interviewees to place events in context and attach meaning to them, and which would provide more insight into the quality and quantity of life events preceding CFS and the ways in which they are experienced. It is important also to examine the ways in which meanings attached to stressful life events and difficulties vary with individual differences. For example, difficulties with relationships or at work will be particularly stressful for those who set themselves high standards and expectations in these areas.

Personality, coping, and the onset of CFS

There are three major strands of research on personality factors and CFS. These are studies of psychological vulnerability or personality factors predisposing individuals to develop psychiatric illness, research into behavioral styles and stress-prone lifestyles associated with CFS, and studies of coping styles and strategies.

Psychological vulnerability. There is a long tradition of considering illnesses that cannot yet be explained by medical science to be psychologically determined,[40] particularly when women are overrepresented among sufferers, as in the case of CFS, and of attributing this to aspects of personality. Some researchers argue CFS may be the result of organic illness in psychologically vulnerable individuals.[6] However, the legacy of the mind/body debate has been that the vulnerability factors investigated have been mainly clinical and pathological factors and comparisons made with other physical or psychological conditions rather than with healthy controls.

The theory that CFS sufferers have psychologically vulnerable or emotionally unstable premorbid personalities has developed from a body of earlier studies indicating a relationship between personality factors such as depressive vulnerability and the development of fatigue and of prolonged recovery from what are normally minor illnesses.[41,42] No studies have been carried out prospectively on healthy populations to test this theory in relation to CFS. Rather, research has focused on current CFS sufferers, although there is evidence suggesting that the illness itself may change personality and behavioral style.[27] It is therefore difficult to disentangle personality factors that may have contributed to the development of the condition from emotional reactions that are consequences of the debilitating symptoms and the mixed responses of others to the illness.

Several studies have examined levels of personality disorders or traits increasing vulnerability to psychiatric illness among current CFS sufferers, but results are mixed and inconclusive. Some small studies with or without control groups indicated that CFS patients have severe personality pathology.[5,6] Others using various comparison groups reveal that despite high levels of depression or other psychiatric symptoms in CFS this is not easily explained by personality factors because of heterogeneity among CFS sufferers[43] or lack of significant differences between personality profiles of CFS patients and those suffering from conditions of known organic basis.[9,38] It is possible that CFS patients' resistance to a psychiatric diagnosis may cause them to categorically deny any symptoms of psychiatric disorder and hence distort responses on self-report measures, although Pepper et al., while acknowledging that this may be true of an occasional patient, report that such adamant denial was not a characteristic of the CFS patients in their study.[9] Evidence concerning the role of personality factors predisposing patients to mental illness as a basis for CFS is therefore mixed and difficult to interpret, although it is possible that this is true in some cases.

Behavioral styles. There is accumulating anecdotal, clinical, and empirical evidence that many CFS sufferers, or at least those who seek medical help, are hard-driving, perfectionist, high occupational achievers, for whom success is an important part of self image and who may be particularly distressed by any symptoms that prevent them from achieving the high standards that they set for themselves or the high expectations of others.[23,25–27,31,44]

Much of this evidence emerges from qualitative research. For example, Ware[23] and Ware and Kleinman[44] carried out in-depth semistructured interviews with 50 CFS patients to elicit data on life history and illness experience. The interview questions were open ended and therefore the data emerging were not limited by the type of *a priori* assumptions about personality categories that underpin research using standardized questionnaires. Interviewees described their lives prior to the onset of illness as characterized by intense activities, involvement, and busyness, including excessively long hours at work. Many of the interviewees attributed their illness to their hectic lifestyle, which they consistently labeled as stressful and to their apparent need to operate in this way:

> I was a driven person kind of thing. I had been working really hard for years. There was one period where I worked for three months and had one day off. Then I went to graduate school and worked at the same time, and I was just exhausted all the time (p. 64).[23]

> I was working probably 60 hours a week . . . I thought "I'm superman. I'm the guy that can get it all done. Nobody else can do it; they're all such a bunch of lazy idiots . . . I'll show them all" (p. 64).[23]

CFS sufferers in other studies also talked of high achievement orientation, perfectionism, high standards of work performance with persistent striving to meet the needs and expectations of others, often at the expense of neglecting their own personal needs.[25,31]

These findings have led to speculation that the type A behavior pattern may be related to CFS.[27,45] Several interviewees in Ware's study spontaneously referred to themselves as being type A.[23] A study by Lewis et al.[27] compared 47 CFS patients with 47 IBS patients and 30 healthy controls using the Bortner scale,[46] and also asked the two illness groups to rate their behavior prior to the onset of illness. No significant differences emerged on the global type A scale but an interesting pattern of differences emerged when subscales were compared. CFS sufferers rated themselves as better listeners (a type B characteristic) both pre- and post-illness, more hard-driving prior to illness, and reported more outside interests than healthy controls prior to illness, although not more than IBS sufferers, as has been reported in previous research.[47] Although CFS sufferers rated themselves as being somewhat less hard driving post-illness than they had been previously, they still rated themselves as higher on the good listener scale than the other groups, which suggests high self-imposed standards in interpersonal relations, which is supported by Ware's findings[23] that CFS patients tend to be highly involved in doing things for others in addition to other pressurized activities. Of course these are self-reported and not objectively observed characteristics and may result from a need to present well. However, it can be argued that the findings do at least indicate a self image of hard-driving yet interpersonally concerned individuals, or those who feel they ought to be so, which may be real in its consequences.

Ways of coping

Studies of the ways in which CFS sufferers cope with stress prior to the onset of illness are all retrospective, but consistently point to hard-driving, highly demanding strategies. Themes elicited from interview data, for example, suggest that pre-illness coping strategies included bottling up feelings, putting on a brave face, and role expansions or working especially hard to meet all demands.[23,25] Other research also suggests the use of coping strategies that may be hard on the individual. Lewis et al.[27] used an adapted version of the Ways of Coping checklist to examine the ways in which CFS sufferers reported coping with a stressful life event prior to the onset of illness and found they were significantly more likely than IBS patients and healthy controls to report using problem-focused coping, especially planful problem solving and seeking social support. The CFS sufferers in this study also reported using problem-oriented strategies in coping with their illness (although to a lesser extent than previously), suggesting a degree of consistency which may be inappropriate.

It would be useful to replicate these findings in studies that do not rely on retrospective reporting. The effectiveness of problem-focused strategies is often dependent on the extent to which the individual has some control.[48] Problem-focused strategies require individuals to dwell on problems, in contrast to more emotion-focused strategies, which can reduce stress and arousal by directing attention elsewhere. There is evidence from prospective research that the continual use of problem-focused coping can predict frequency of illness.[49] If problem-focused strategies are used consistently, the effort involved and the associated appraisals of stressful situations as problems to be solved, together with general hard-driving perfectionist behavior may thus have harmful consequences in terms of sustained arousal, distress, and associated physiological processes.

Other support for the role of hard-driving coping strategies comes from Surawy et al.,[25] who elicited thoughts and cognitions of CFS patients in treatment sessions and via patients' weekly diaries. Thoughts centered on the comparison of current performance with previous high standards and on the importance of the opinions of others and were underpinned by assumptions that imply that self-respect and the respect of others is dependent on the achievement of high standards in most spheres of life. Surawy et al. argue that, although these assumptions may have been associated with high achievements prior to illness, they make people vulnerable to illness when personal sources are depleted and/or excessive and prolonged demands threaten the achievement of these standards. The initial response to illness, they argue, appears to be a continuation of the hard-driving behavior manifested pre-illness, with sufferers intensifying efforts to cope. This can create chronic frustration, exhaustion, and distress, with associated physical and psychological symptoms. When this happens a minor illness may be a last straw precipitating failure to cope and the onset of illness.

Social support prior to the onset of illness

The nature and potential effects of social support prior to the onset of CFS has received little research attention. However, in the Lewis et al. study[27] CFS sufferers reported significantly lower levels of perceived social support than the comparison groups both pre- and post-illness. As the CFS group also reported seeking social support as a strategy for coping with a stressful life event, it appears that support was desired but not experienced as forthcoming. This may be because of life contexts or due to a lack of skill in eliciting support from others, but may increase the negative effects of potentially stressful life events. If replicated, particularly in prospective research, the association between CFS onset and low social support for stressful lifestyles may contribute to an explanation of the depression and immunological changes in this condition. It has been argued that the emotional states associated with low levels of perceived support may be linked with specific disease-producing physiological responses through emotionally induced effects on neuroendocrine or immune system functioning.[50] For example, Levy et al.[51] found that natural killer cell activity in breast cancer patients was associated with perceived quality of emotional support, even after controlling for estrogen receptor status, age, functional status, and surgical status. This evidence of a link between social support and the immune systems, together with evidence of immunological changes in CFS,[17] suggest the hypothesis that low perceived social support may increase vulnerability to this condition or underlying pathogens, either directly or indirectly by exacerbating stress. Another possibility suggested by the lack of support for highly demanding lifestyles and hard-driving behaviors is that illness may develop as a cry for help[27] or as a strategy for opting out of a culture of achievement and busyness.[23] The dynamics involved in such a process would of course require clarification.

Social context and the development of CFS

CFS has variously been called a disease of our time, a new disease, a postmodern illness.[31] The importance of locating illness within the broad social context is widely recognized.[23,26,31,45,52,53] It is important to examine the context in which the personality and behaviors associated with CFS flourish and in which the illness develops and is perpetuated.

It can be argued that the behavioral styles reported by many CFS sufferers flourish in societies that are preoccupied with achievement.[26] The overrepresentation of individuals in professional and managerial occupations and particularly career women[37] point to the increasing personal demands made in these fields and suggests that transitions in gender expectations may also be relevant. Growing numbers of women pursue demanding careers while often retaining the major responsibility for family work, while employers continue to expect committed workers to conform to the male model of continuous full-time work, making no concessions for family.[54,55] This creates overload and role conflict as women strive to fulfill the expectations of different sectors of society.[56] Often their response is to attempt to excel in traditional caring roles and in their chosen, male-dominated occupations. The need to achieve, drive oneself hard, and not admit to difficulties in coping and the irrational cognitions linking achievement and coping with self-esteem typical of many CFS sufferers is exacerbated in this context. The social expectation that women will care for others and be sensitive to others' feelings, often denying their own neediness, described by psychodynamic writers[57] combined with newer expectations of achievement may also explain why many sufferers perceive themselves as supportive to others but neglect to elicit support for themselves.[25,27,44]

Psychosocial factors in the perpetuation of illness

Social context and support

There are several aspects of the social context in which CFS is experienced that may contribute to ongoing stress and hence impact on duration of illness. The media stereotype of "yuppie flu" and the plethora of articles in the popular and medical press debating the organic or psychological nature of the illness has had the effect of trivializing CFS, perpetuating the counterproductive mind body dichotomous thinking, and promoting the construct of CFS as not being a socially acceptable illness.[26] For some sufferers, the experience of a debilitating illness which is repeatedly dismissed as being "all in the mind" exacerbates the stressfulness of the symptoms. It may also strengthen sufferers' resolve to prove that it is a physical disorder and contribute to the resistance to a psychological explanation.

To the extent that the media instill disbelief about CFS in sufferers' family members and social networks, this can also serve to reduce available social support. A sense of loss or lack of support from colleagues, friends, family, and others is vividly described in Ware's[23] interviews with sufferers and is reflected in the lower perceived support reported by current CFS than IBS sufferers.[27]

In the context of low perceived support as well as uncertainty and the need for information on their condition, it is not surprising that many sufferers participate in support groups. Groups such as the ME group in the U.K. often propound diagnoses, explanations, or treatments that may conflict with those offered by the medical establishment. Participation in support groups has been associated with ongoing disability after 2 years.[28] This may be because the more seriously ill join these groups or because support groups provide advice that perpetuates disability. It is also possible that both participation and ongoing illness may be predicted by a third factor, such as low social support. Certainly the appeal of support groups is apparent in this context.

One source of support that is very variable is that forthcoming from physicians. Some sufferers report that their doctors are highly supportive, but for others the doctor-patient relationship becomes a battleground.[31] Many physicians hold stereotypical views of, and dislike treating, CFS patients.[58] From the physician's perspective, the confusing reports available and lack of treatment possibilities can be very frustrating. They face dilemmas about whether to admit that there is no treatment, thus provoking feelings of helplessness, or to offer possible treatments and risk raising false hopes.[26] Although physicians may be accustomed to such dilemmas in cases of terminal illness, the ambiguity surrounding this condition makes it more problematic. Some physicians are also uncomfortable when their expertise is challenged by patients who have sought their own understandings.[31] Many patients, in turn, feel that doctors are dismissive of their symptoms, which may explain why they suffer greater depression than those with other debilitating yet diagnosable diseases, such as multiple sclerosis.[9] The role of the doctor-patient relationship in exacerbating stress should therefore be investigated in more comprehensive examinations of stress and the perpetuation of CFS.

Coping and the perpetuation/maintenance of illness

Much recent research has focused on the ways in which CFS sufferers cope with the illness and its unpredictability and in some cases ways of coping have been linked with possible impact on illness duration and prognosis. The hard-driving behavior and coping styles manifested prior to illness appear to continue to some extent in the ways in which sufferers cope with the experience of illness,[25,27] although there is, perhaps inevitably, some slowing down in the demands they make on themselves. For example, Lewis et al.[27] note that sufferers use more emotional focuses coping post-illness than previously, although they continue to use more problem-focused strategies than IBS sufferers in coping with their illness.

A limitation of much of the research examining coping strategies is that different measures of coping are used, assessing coping constructs that are not entirely overlapping and it is difficult to generalize or find consistency across studies. A recently developed coping scale developed specifically for use with CFS patients[53] identifies four types of coping used by sufferers: maintaining activity, accommodating to the illness, information seeking, and focusing on symptoms.

Maintaining activity includes attempts to ignore symptoms and carry on even though unwell and reflects the continuation of hard-driving preillness behavior. Accommodating to the illness, on the other hand, involves organizing and planning one's life to avoid exertion and to avoid stress, a pattern of coping that is widely reported in the CFS literature.[23,25,28] CFS sufferers frequently alternate between the two forms of coping, avoiding activity in an attempt to control symptoms, with occasional bursts of activity in attempts to overcome the self-perceived failure to live up to previous standards.[25] Several authors have argued that although avoidance of activity can reduce symptoms in the short term, the long-term consequence is the perpetuation of intolerance of physical and mental activity, thus prolonging illness.[24,25]

Information seeking as a way of coping with CFS is also widely reported[27,31,53] and may be regarded as an active strategy for reducing helplessness in the face of an illness for which no readily available explanation and advice are forthcoming. This type of coping includes a readiness to try alternative remedies.[53] However, there is evidence from the academic literature as well as from correspondence from physicians in the medical and the popular press implying that some physicians are unhappy with this patient strategy.[31] Where this happens it has the potential to increase the stressfulness of doctor-patient relationships and of the experience of illness.

The final dimension of coping identified by Ray et al.[53] is focusing on symptoms. This is described as a preoccupation with symptoms linked to an appraisal of helplessness and of one's life as dominated by these symptoms. Much of the research on this approach to coping centers on whether symptoms are attributed to physical or psychological causes. From a cognitive behavioral perspective it is argued that, regardless of the relative contribution of physical and psychological factors to the disease, a focus on the physical aspects of illness typical of the majority of CFS sufferers leads to feelings of helplessness and a focus on the need to avoid activity.[24] Most CFS sufferers reject a psychological explanation for their illness.[7] There are a number of explanations for this, including the experience of very real physical symptoms, a lack of awareness that most illnesses have both physical and psychological dimensions, and the social stigma associated with psychiatric diagnoses, especially for individuals whose self-esteem is dependent upon achievement and coping. It has been suggested that physical illness is considered a legitimate reason for not achieving high standards by CFS sufferers, whereas psychological illness is perceived as evidence of personal weakness.[25] Some evidence that illness attributions can affect outcome is provided by prospective studies[28,59] in which attribution of symptoms to viral infection or other physical cause is associated with a more delayed recovery. However, the significance of these findings is unclear, as beliefs about the cause of illness may be a consequence of more severe or different physical experiences of illness. Nevertheless, it is possible that a focus on symptoms, especially physical ones, may prevent sufferers from addressing the psychosocial stressors in their lives which may have triggered the initial illness in some cases, and may also serve to perpetuate the stress and hence immunological and psychological consequences. The life events and ongoing stressors that may have contributed to the onset of illness are not always resolved by the illness.[25] Indeed, illness may exacerbate problems associated with, for example, chronic relationship or work difficulties. The focus on symptoms may serve to draw attention away from such problems, as a way of coping, but it may also prevent people from working out solutions or modifying stress-producing situations.

A neglect of the complexity and multidimensional nature of the coping process has been a limitation of much of the research on coping and the maintenance of CFS. People cope in different ways with different aspects of their illness and different strategies may be adaptive at different times. CFS sufferers may deal in different ways with symptoms, the uncertainty of the illness, interaction with physicians, and with nonmedical areas of their lives, such as the impact of illness on relationships or work, and there may be different explanations of the strategies adopted in different areas. More sophisticated research is now needed to address the significance for recovery of different ways of coping with the many dimensions of the illness. A related limitation has been the tendency to treat ways of coping as a trait variable with a degree of consistency. The recognition that ways of coping, like other behaviors, are determined by an interaction between the person and their environment should underpin future research in this area.

Implications for treatment and future research

We have seen that there is much preliminary evidence of mind and body linkages in CFS. It appears that psychosocial factors are associated with the onset of illness and perhaps also with its perpetuation, via effects on the immune system. It follows that psychological interventions should be capable of changing psychological and immunological functioning.[33] A number of promising cognitive behavioral approaches to treatment have been reported,[24,25,60] although outcome studies are very preliminary at this stage. These approaches attempt to change ongoing cognitions which are thought to maintain illness behavior and perpetuate symptoms. This usually involves attempts to change attributions of symptoms to physical disease and to encourage sufferers to gradually increase activity.[24,60] However, the assumptions on which this is based, and hence the treatment itself, is unacceptable to many patients and therefore the treatment refusal rate is high.[60] This limits its applicability and confounds outcome studies.

Another approach is to build on patients' initial model of illness, by separating etiological from perpetuating factors and introducing the possible role of cognitive and behavioral factors in the latter process.[25] The cognitive behavioral techniques associated with this approach are based on an understanding of patient cognitions and personality and include negotiating realistic treatment targets and activity recording and discussion which places as much emphasis on reducing striving as it does on increasing activity.

The focus on current cognitions and behaviors may be effective in reducing the duration of illness, although long-term evidence is not yet available. This approach, however, deliberately does not address the etiology of the condition in any depth. Failure to address premorbid and ongoing psychosocial stressors may result in relapse. Cognitive behavioral approaches to treatment could be extended to include a more detailed examination of sources of stress prior to illness and stress management techniques. A number of stress management techniques may be useful, including, for example, training in the identification of contexts in which different coping styles are appropriate, encouragement of more effective techniques for eliciting social support, encouragement of self-valuing and looking after oneself, a questioning of social expectations attached to particular roles, and recognition that it is unrealistic to expect to fulfill all of these. The clarification of factors increasing vulnerability to CFS and the processes involved would also raise the possibility of using cognitive behavioral and stress management techniques as preventative measures for appropriate "at risk" populations.

Future research on CFS should incorporate as many as possible of the various psychosocial variables identified here in order to contribute towards a comprehensive model of CFS. The roles of life stress, personality, and social context need to be better understood. Multiple assessments of psychosocial factors, using more sophisticated measures than those used in much of the CFS research, would strengthen the findings as different measures can produce varying results,[62,63] which may explain some of the inconsistencies in the literature. The use of both psychosocial and physiological measures would also be useful in clarifying the processes involved.

Prospective studies are necessary to clarify directions of causality that are difficult to determine at this stage. As the experience of CFS can change behavioral as well as physiological processes, it is important to begin research at the earliest stage possible. One possibility might be to follow up consecutive patients presenting with postviral fatigue to general practitioners, so as to compare those who go on to develop CFS with those who recover. This would overcome some problems of patient selection bias, such as those associated with the use of patients from primary or secondary care, but would not eliminate bias as not all people suffering postviral fatigue will consult a doctor and CFS does not always begin with a viral illness. A long-term prospective study of a heathy population would be an ideal starting point. However, it must be recognized that, as CFS is not a life-threatening illness, it is unlikely to attract the necessary resources for such an undertaking. One solution might be for collaboration between those studying different illnesses, so that large prospective studies examining the etiology of other illnesses would include the psychosocial variable discussed in this chapter (whose range of applicability extend well beyond CFS) and to chart incidence of CFS in this population.

In conclusion, the evidence concerning psychosocial factors and CFS is less well developed than that relating to other illnesses. Nevertheless, there is sufficient preliminary evidence to suggest that personality factors may play a role in the etiology and possibly the perpetuation of CFS, via the stress process. The challenge for further research is to clarify the processes involved and the implications for treatment and prevention.

References

1. Sharpe, M., Archard, L. C., Banatvals, J. et al., Chronic fatigue syndrome: guidelines for research, *J. R. Soc. Med.*, 84, 118, 1991.
2. Katon, W. J., Buchwald, D., Simon, G. E., Russon, J. E., and Mease, P. J., Psychiatric illness in patients with chronic fatigue and rheumatoid arthritis, *Am. J. Med.*, 6, 227–285, 1991.
3. Manu, P., Matthews, D. A., and Lane, T. J., The mental health of patients with a chief complaint of chronic fatigue; a prospective evaluation and follow up, *Arch. Int. Med.*, 148, 2213–2217, 1988.
4. Manu, P., Lane, T. J., and Matthews, D. A., The pathophysiology of chronic fatigue syndrome: confirmation, contradiction and conjecture, *Int. J. Psychiatry*, 22 (4), 397–408, 1992.
5. Millon, C., Salvato, F., Blaney, N., Morgan, S., Martero-Atienza, E., Klimas, N., and Fletcher, M. A., A psychological assessment of chronic fatigue syndrome/chronic Epstein Barr virus patients, *Psychol. Health*, 3, 131–141, 1989.
6. Taerk, G. S., Toner, B. B., Salit, I. E., Garfinkel, P. E., and Ozersky, S., Depression in patients with neuromyasthenia (benign myalgic encephalomyelitis), *Int. J. Psychiatry Med.*, 17, 49–56, 1987.
7. Wessely, S. and Powell, R., Fatigue syndrome: a comparison of postviral fatigue with neuromuscular affective disorder, *J. Neurol. Neurosurg. Psychiatry*, 52, 940–948, 1989.
8. Powell, R., Dolan, R., and Wessely, S., Attributions of self esteem in depression and chronic fatigue syndrome, *J. Psychosom. Res.*, 34, 665–673. 1990.
9. Pepper, C. M., Kupp, L. B., Friedberg, F., Dorscher, C., and Coyle, C. K., A comparison of neuropsychiatric characteristics in chronic fatigue syndrome, multiple sclerosis and major depression, *J. Neuropsychiatry*, 5 (2), 200–205, 1993.
10. Ray, C., Interpreting the role of depression in chronic fatigue syndrome, in *Postviral Fatigue Syndrome*, Jenkins, R. and Mowbray, J., Eds., Wiley, London, 1991.

11. Ray, C., Chronic fatigue syndrome and depression. Conceptual and methodological ambiguities. *Psych. Med.*, 21, 1–9.
12. Behan, P. O. and Bakheit, A. M., Clinical spectrum of postviral fatigue syndrome, *Br. Med. Bull.*, 47(4), 793–808, 1991.
13. Bell, E. J., McCartney, R. A., and Riding, C., Coxsackie B virus and myalgic encephalomyelitis, *J. R. Soc. Med.*, 81, 329–331, 1988.
14. Cunningham, L., Bowles, N. E., and Archard, L. C., Persistent post viral infection of muscle and post viral fatigue syndrome, *Br. Med. Bull.*, 47(4), 852–871, 1991.
15. Gow, J., Behan, W., Clements, G., Woodall, C., Riding, M., and Behan, P., Entroviral RNA sequences detected by polymerase chain reaction in muscle of patients with postviral fatigue syndrome, *Br. Med. J.*, 302, 692–696, 1991.
16. Buchwald, D. and Komaroff, A., Review of laboratory findings for patients with chronic fatigue syndrome, *Rev. Infect. Dis.*, 13 (Suppl. 1), 12–18, 1991.
17. Lloyd, A. R., Immunological and psychological dysfunction in patients receiving immunotherapy for chronic fatigue syndrome, *Aust. NZ J. Psychiatry*, 26 (2), 249–256, 1992.
18. Lloyd, A. R., Wakefield, D., Boughton, C. R., and Dwyer, J. M., Immunological abnormalities in the chronic fatigue syndrome, *Med. J. Aust.*, 151 (3), 122–124, 1989.
19. Straus, S. E., Intravenous immunoglobin treatment for the chronic fatigue syndrome, *Am. J. Med.*, 77, 31–34, 1990.
20. Buchwald, D., Laboratory abnormalities in chronic fatigue syndrome, in *Postviral Fatigue Syndrome*, Jenkins, R. and Mowbray, J., Eds., Wiley, Chichester, 1989, 117–136.
21. Chase, J., Psychological factors that may lower immunity, in *Postviral Fatigue Syndrome*, Jenkins, R. and Mowbray, J., Eds., Wiley, Chichester, 1989, 365–384.
22. David, A. S., Wessely, S., and Pelosi, A. J., Postviral fatigue syndrome: time for a new approach, *Br. Med. J.*, 296, 696–699, 1988.
23. Ware, N. C., Society, mind and body in chronic fatigue syndrome: an anthropological view, in *Chronic Fatigue Syndrome*, Wiley, Chichester, 1993, 62–82.
24. Wessely, S., Butler, S., Chadler, T., and David, A., The cognitive behaviourial management of post-viral fatigue syndrome, in *Postviral Fatigue Syndrome*, Jenkins, R. and Mowbray, J., Eds., Wiley, Chichester, 1989, 305–334.
25. Surawy, S., Hackman, A., Hawton, K., and Sharpe, M., Chronic fatigue syndrome: a cognitive approach. Paper presented at the British Psychological Society Annual Conference, London, 1994.
26. Abbey, S. E., Somatization, illness attribution and the sociocultural psychiatry of chronic fatigue syndrome in *Chronic Fatigue Syndrome*, Kleinman, A. and Straus, S. E., Eds., London, Ciba Foundation, 1993, 238–261.
27. Lewis, S., Cooper, C. L., and Bennett, D., Psychosocial factors in chronic fatigue syndrome, *Psychol. Med.*, 24, 661–671, 1994.

28. Sharpe, M., Hawton, K., Seagroatt, V., and Pasvol, G., Follow up of patients presenting with fatigue to an infectious diseases clinic, *Br. Med. J.*, 305, 147–152, 1992.
29. Ray, C., Illness perception and symptom components in chronic fatigue syndrome, *J. Psychosom. Res.*, 36, 243–256, 1992.
30. Selye, H., *The Stress of Life*, Mcgraw-Hill, New York, 1956.
31. Wheeler, B. B., Feminist and psychological implications of chronic fatigue syndrome, *Feminism Psychol.*, 2, 197–204, 1992.
32. Freudenberger, H. J. and Richelson, G., *Burn-Out: The High Cost of Achievement*, Anchor Press, New York, 1980.
33. Solomon, A., Psychoimmunological interactions between central nervous systems and immune systems, *J Neurosci. Res.* 18, 1–7, 1987.
34. Kennedy, S., Kiecolt-Glaser, J. K., and Glaser, R., Immunological consequences of acute and chronic stresses: mediating role of interpersonal relationships, *Br. J. Med. Psychol.*, 61, 77–85, 1988.
35. Dorian, B. J., Garfinkel, P. E., Brown, G., Shore, A., Gladman, D., Keystone, E., and Darby, P., Stress, immunity and illness, *Psychosom. Med.*, 48, 324–328, 1986.
36. Brown, G. W. and Harris, T. O., *Life Events and Illness*, Unwin Hyman, London, 1989.
37. Shafran, S. D., The chronic fatigue syndrome, *Am. J. Med.*, 90, 730–739, 1991.
38. Wood, G. G., Bentall, R. P., Gopfert, M., and Edwards, R. H. T., *Psychol. Med.*, 21, 619–627, 1991.
39. Stricklen, A., Sewell, M., and Austad, C., Objective measurement of personality variables in epidemic neuromyasthenia patients, *S. Afr. Med. J.*, 77, 31–34, 1990.
40. Sontag, S., *Illness as Metaphor*, Farrar, Straus and Giroux, New York, 1978.
41. Imboden, J. B., Canter, A., and Cluff, L. E., Convalescence from influenza: a study of psychological and clinical determinants, *Arch. Intern. Med.*, 108, 115–121, 1961.
42. Montgomery, G. K., Uncommon tiredness among college undergraduates, *J. Consult. Clin. Psychol.*, 51, 517–525, 1983.
43. Blakey, A. A., Howard, R. C., and Soosich, R. M., Psychiatric symptoms, personality and ways of coping with chronic fatigue syndrome, *Psychol. Med.*, 21, 347–362, 1991.
44. Ware, N. C. and Kleinman, A. Culture and somatic experience: the social course of illness in neurasthenia and chronic fatigue syndrome, *Psychosom. Med.*, 54, 546–560, 1992.
45. Woods, T. O. and Goldberg, D. P., Psychiatric perspectives: an overview, *Br. Med. Bull.*, 47, 908–918, 1991.
46. Bortner, R. W., A short rating scale as a potential measure of pattern A behaviour, *J. Chronic Dis.*, 22, 87–91, 1969.
47. Riley, M. S., O'Brien, C. J., McCluskey, D. R., Bell, N. P., and Nicholls, D. P., Aerobic work capacity in patients with chronic fatigue syndrome, *Br. Med. J.*, 301, 953–956, 1990.
48. Roth, S. and Cohen, L., Approach avoidance and coping with stress, *Am. Psychol.*, 41, 813–819, 1986.
49. Nowack, K. M., Psychosocial predictors of health status, *Work Stress*, 5, 117–132, 1991.

50. Jemmott, J. B. and Locke, S. E., Psychosocial factors, immunological mediation and human susceptibility to infectious diseases: how much do we know?, *Psychol. Bull.*, 95, 78–108, 1984.

51. Levy, S. M., Ghaberman, R. B., Whiteside, T., Sanzo, K., Lee, J., and Kirkwood, J., Perceived social support and tumour oestrogen/progesterone receptor status as predictors of natural killer cell activity in breast cancer patients, *Psychosom. Med.*, 52, 73–85, 1990.

52. Kleinman, A., *The Illness Narrative: Suffering, Healing and the Human Condition*, Basic Books, New York, 1988.

53. Ray, C., Weir, W., David, S., and Miller, P., Ways of coping with chronic fatigue syndrome: development of an illness management questionnaire, *Soc. Sci. Med.*, 37, 385–391, 1993.

54. Cook, A., Can work requirements change to accommodate the needs of dual-earner families?, in *Dual-Earner Families. International Perspectives*, Lewis, S., Izraeli D., and Hootsmans, H., Eds., Sage, Beverly Hills, 1992, 204–220.

55. Cooper, C. L., *The Workplace Revolution: Managing Today's Dual Career Families*, Kogan Page, London, 1993.

56. Lewis, S. and Cooper, C. L., Stress in dual earner families, in *Women and Work. An Annual Review*, Vol. 3, Gutek, B. A., Stromberg, A. H., and Larwood, L., Eds., Sage, Beverly Hills, 1988.

57. Eichenbaum, L. and Orbach, S., *Understanding Women*, Penguin, Harmondsworth, 1983.

58. Wessely, S., Discussion in *Chronic Fatigue Syndrome*, Kleinman, A. and Straus, S. E., Eds., 258. Ciba Foundation, London, 1993.

59. Wilson, A., Hickie, I., Lloyd, A., Hadzi-Pavlovic, D., Boughton, C., and Dwyer, J., *Br. Med. J.*, 308, 756–759, 1994.

60. Butler, S., Chalder, T., Ron, M., and Wessely, S., Cognitive behaviour therapy in chronic fatigue syndrome, *J. Neurol. Neurosurg. Psychiatry*, 54, 153–154, 1991.

61. Edwards, J., Bagglioni, A., and Cooper, C. L., Examining the relationships among measures of type A behaviour: the effects of multidimensionality, measurement error and differences in underlying constructs, *J. Appl. Psychol.*, 48, 150–170, 1990.

Social support, stress, and illness

chapter thirteen

Social support and heart disease

John G. Bruhn

Social support: its relationship to health

That social bonding should be a positive influence on health, and social isolation a pathogenic factor in disease, is not surprising.[1] Each of us has had personal experiences that make the correlation between social support and health real. Yet, because social support is difficult to measure and quantify and its mechanisms are elusive, social support remains an enigma and is "unreal" to the scientific community.

Social support is thought to be a "carrier" of physical and mental health.[2] Therefore, some researchers have attempted to manipulate social support to affect a particular outcome, such as patient compliance with a medical regimen, or to assist people undergoing a medical crisis in their recovery. Because many of their studies of social support lacked designs that specified the mediating processes, our understanding of how social support works still is incomplete.[3] It has been suggested that we pay closer attention to the context and meaning of social support and how it is perceived by individuals at particular points in time. Bloom[4] has suggested that whether a life event is viewed as a source of stress may be due to the individual's style of coping. Social support may affect how the individual defines the situation.

The general relationship between social support and health is most clear when it is linked to physical health outcomes. A common thread that runs through nearly all published studies is that a broad array of diseases and causes of death are associated with social support.[5] Yet, these studies have their limitations. Most researchers have studied only white men or homogeneous populations, or have not sorted out covariates of social support to determine whether social support is the consequence or cause of illness. Despite these limitations and variations, there is a remarkable consistency in the overall finding that social relationships predict mortality for men and women in a wide range of populations, even after adjustments for biomedical risk factors for mortality.[6] Other prospective studies have shown that social relationships are predictive of all types of cardiovascular mortality in the elderly or in people who have serious illnesses.

0-8493-2908-6/96/$0.00+$.50

Social support and heart disease

A lack, or disruption, of social support appears to better predict *some* break-down in health than a specific condition or illness.[7] Yet, some animal, laboratory, and clinical evidence suggests that the link between social support and heart disease is a direct sympathetic physiologic pathway.[8] In fact, a large prospective clinical trial identified a unique set of psychosocial predictors for sudden cardiac death, while nonsudden cardiac death and nonfatal recurrences were predicted by biologic factors.[9] One of the common findings that emerge from studies of social support and heart disease is that the function, content, and quality of social ties is more important than the mere presence or quantity of social ties.[10]

Social support and the life cycle

Social support is now widely regarded as a personal experience, rather than a set of objective experiences, or even a set of interactional processes.[11] Coyne and DeLongis point out that we need to learn more about how people find, build, maintain, and end relationships; how they are constrained by personal characteristics and circumstances; and the benefits and costs they incur.[12] These authors note the distinctiveness of marriage, which can be a source of both stress and support. Indeed, Storr points out that interpersonal relationships are assumed to be the chief source of human happiness.[13] Yet, many of the world's greatest thinkers and creative poets, novelists, composers, painters, and sculptors have lived alone or not formed close personal ties.[13]

Social affiliation is a basic need, but like other needs, how it is met is highly individualistic. An individual's need for, and experience with, social support changes as he/she moves through the life cycle, grows and develops, changes social roles, and experiences life events.[14] Little is known about social support through the life course, particularly in a longitudinal sense. Kahn and Antonucci's[15] convoy model, which builds upon the work of John Bowlby and other attachment theorists, notes the importance of interpersonal relationships over a lifetime. Through its attachment relationships with parents and others, the infant begins to learn about interpersonal relationships. The process of learning and experience throughout later life stages influences how the individual perceives and utilizes the convoy network. Schulz and Rau[16] view the development of social support as analogous to a string quartet where several participants work together to produce a whole. A good support system consists of a number of different players who together cover a range of needs. Different players play different roles at different times, and the works they perform vary with time and place.[16] Social support, its meaning and usefulness, is part of the process of growing and developing throughout life. It is culture-specific and idiosyncratic. Therefore, it is reasonable to expect social support to be difficult to measure and quantify and, possibly, subtle enough that it is not observable to an outsider. Interventions or inoculations that propose to inject or enhance social support into an individual or group's life may be artificial, meaningless, and therefore, ineffective, if they are not culturally appropriate and part of the life experience of the individual or group.[17]

Definition and measurement of social support

Heitzmann and Kaplan, in reviewing the psychometric properties of 23 methods for measuring social support, concluded that the problem of accurately measuring social support is due in part, to the lack of a common definition.[18] Each researcher's definition of social support appears to be as unique as the subjects being studied. Winemiller and colleagues recently reviewed 262 empirically based articles about social support published between 1980 and 1987.[19] They found that many social support researchers utilized standardized instruments, but failed to consider the complex, multidimensional nature of social support. Most instruments were objective and assessed support received from close, nuclear relationships, such as those with family, spouse, and friends. This means that our perspective of social support generally excludes an individual's support network, focuses on the social support received rather than on its interactive nature, excludes consideration of cultural and environmental sources of support, and tends to look at an individual's perceptions of available support without concomitant consideration of the support the individual has used and is likely to use in certain circumstances.

As Heitzmann and Kaplan noted,[18] we do not need 23 separate measures of social support, especially if we are serious about extending our knowledge about the relationship between social support and heart disease. Others have come to the same conclusion.[20,21] The present author suggests that the National Institutes of Health assemble an expert panel composed of researchers of social support to reach consensus on acceptable measures of social support, much as has been done for hypertension and arteriosclerosis by the American Heart Association and National Heart Institute. This would ensure some uniformity in definitions and measurement techniques which, in turn, would facilitate the comparability of results and the ability to link specific conditions or aspects of social support and physiologic mechanisms.

Mechanisms of social support

Social support and cardiovascular reactivity

Several studies have tested whether social support can reduce cardiovascular reactivity. Kamarck and colleagues had college-age women complete mental arithmetic and concept formation tasks alone and in the presence of a female friend. During the latter support situation, the friend touched the subject's wrist throughout testing, but also wore a headset and completed questionnaires to avoid distracting or arousing apprehension in the subject.[22] This study clearly demonstrated that the presence of a supportive partner reduces the magnitude of cardiovascular response (heart rate). Gerin and co-workers also studied the possibility that social support operates as a moderator of cardiovascular reactivity.[23] An experiment was performed in which each of 40 subjects was verbally attacked during the discussion of a controversial issue. One subject and three confederates participated in each session: two of the confederates argued with the subject. In half of the groups, a third confederate defended the subject's position; in the other half, the third confederate sat quietly. Subjects' blood pressure and heart rate were continuously monitored. Subjects who received social support showed significantly smaller increases in cardiovascular measures than subjects who did not.

Edens et al.[24] tested the relative contribution of three elements of social support—the presence, in the laboratory, of another person, the presence of a person considered to be a friend, and physical touch to cardiovascular reactions to stress. Undergraduate females were assigned to one of five groups: alone, friend present–touch, friend present–no touch, stranger present–touch, stranger present–no touch. Heart rate and blood pressure measures were obtained at baseline and during the presentation of mental arithmetic and a mirror tracing. The findings suggest that the presence of a friend, rather than touch, was the important factor in reducing reactivity. Lepore and colleagues extended previous research in sampling both men and women in a study of the effect of social support on cardiovascular reactivity.[25] College students gave a speech in one of three conditions: alone, in the presence of a supportive confederate, or in the presence of a nonsupportive confederate. Supported and solitary subjects showed smaller increases in blood pressure while anticipating and delivering their speech than did nonsupported subjects. Gender did not moderate the effects of social support on cardiovascular activity.

In yet another study, in Sweden, Unden and colleagues examined the cardiovascular effects of psychosocial characteristics in the work environment in men and women representing seven different occupational groups.[26] Standardized measures of work demand, work control, and social support, and ambulatory 24-hour monitoring of electrocardiograms at home and work were performed. Subjects also underwent physical examinations and blood pressure monitoring. Mean heart rates were found to be significantly higher in persons reporting low social support at work. Systolic blood pressure was found to be higher in persons reporting low social support. Controlling for age, sex, and physical strain at work strengthened the association of low social support with elevated heart rates.

These studies affirm a connection between social support and heart rate. During recent years, a number of reports have indicated the long-term harmful effects of elevated heart rates. Beere et al. have found that lower heart rates prevent or slow the development of arteriosclerotic plaques in the coronary arteries of primates.[27]

Several psychologists have proposed models to guide future investigations of the role of social support and the etiology of physical disease.[28] McEwen and Stellar propose a new formulation of the relationship between stress and the processes leading to disease.[29] This formulation emphasizes the cascading relationships, beginning early in life, between environmental factors and genetic predispositions that lead to large individual differences in susceptibility to stress and to disease. Both physiologic and behavioral assessments require long-term time frames in order to gauge health consequences. This entails measures of cumulative effect and steady-state differences in physiologic and behavioral reactivity.

Social support and the etiology of heart disease

Social support, cultural and social variations

Among industrialized countries, Japan is remarkable for its low rate of heart disease. The low rate is unlikely to be the result of some genetically determined protection, as Japanese migrants to the U.S. lose this apparent protection. Japanese in Hawaii have higher rates of heart disease than Japanese in Japan,[30] and Japanese in California have higher rates than those in Hawaii. One hypothesis suggested is that Japanese culture is characterized by a high degree of social support. Potentially stressful situations are defused by the emotional support provided by closely knit social groups. Many observers of Japanese employment practices have noted that individual competitiveness is discouraged in favor of loyalty to the organization. To test the hypothesis that traditional Japanese cultures may protect against heart disease, Marmot[31] classified Japanese in California according to a number of indices of acculturation. Culture and social assimilation identified men with markedly different prevalence rates of heart disease. Men who were brought up in traditional Japanese fashion were found to have a lower prevalence of heart disease than men with a more Westernized upbringing. The higher prevalence among the acculturated men could not be explained by differences in smoking, plasma cholesterol, blood pressure, relative weight, blood sugar, or dietary pattern.

A 25-year study of Roseto, an Italian-American community in Pennsylvania, indicated that acculturation and changes in social institutions, especially the loosening of social ties to the family and the church, were accompanied by an increase in heart disease.[32]

Social networks and heart disease

Berkman and Syme's[8] study, in Alameda County, California, provides impressive evidence of the importance of social networks. They looked at the general availability of social support in terms of network involvement or social ties and found that the more people were "connected", as measured by marital status, contact with friends and relatives, membership in a religious group, and membership in other organizations, the lower the all-cause mortality rate over 9 years of follow-up. This association was independent of smoking, alcohol consumption, obesity, physical activity, and self-reported health status at the time of the original survey.

Orth-Gomer and colleagues found, in a study of a random sample of 736 50-year-old men in Sweden, that a lack of social support was associated with an increased risk of an acute heart attack and death from heart disease.[33] Men and women who had sparse social networks had significantly increased mortality rates from all causes and from heart disease.

Blumenthal and associates[34] studied 214 patients undergoing diagnostic coronary angiography and concluded that individuals with type A personalities who had low levels of social support had more severe coronary artery disease than did individuals with type A personalities who had high levels of social support. This relationship was not present for individuals with type B personalities.[34] Seeman and Syme found that it is the supportive function of a social network, rather than its size, or type, that most influences the development of coronary arteriosclerosis.[35]

Personality factors as predictors of heart disease

There are differences of opinion about the strength of the evidence establishing the type A behavior pattern as a precursor to heart disease. Jenkins[36] states that many published reports in different nations have demonstrated a relationship between the type A pattern and heart disease in cross-sectional and prospective studies. Matthews and Haynes[37] reach different conclusions. They note that type A behavior meets some, but not all of the epidemiologic criteria for causation, and state that there is no clear linear relationship between the type A behavior pattern and coronary heart disease. They also point out the absence of data regarding the association of type A behavior and coronary heart disease in women, blacks, Hispanics, and young adults. Margolis and co-workers suggest that, instead of singularly concentrating on personality components at the level of the individual, it is important to view type A behavior from an ecological perspective, with attention directed at the interpersonal, institutional, and cultural environments of individuals.[38] An ecological framework would help to elucidate the mechanisms of this complex disease and, thus, strategies for prevention.

Attention has also focused on the role of anger and hostility as predictors of heart attacks. In a 25-year follow-up of medical students who completed the Minnesota Multiphasic Personality Inventory while in medical school, Barefoot et al.[39] found that high levels of hostility were associated with increased levels of arteriographically documented coronary atherosclerosis. In addition, hostility scores predicted mortality from all causes. They speculate that social support could mediate hostility, which is an attitude that tends to make a person distrustful of, and isolated from, others.

Siegman recently reviewed studies that implicate the negative cardiovascular consequences of the experience and repression of anger.[40] The review suggests that it is not so much the experience of anger, or its suppression, but rather the chronic full-blown expression of anger that is a significant risk factor for heart disease. Moreover, this risk can be attenuated by learning to control one's expressive vocal behavior.

Some prospective evidence suggests that prolonged, unresolved emotional tension may result in physical and mental exhaustion ("emotional drain") which, in turn, may be a contributing factor in provoking a heart attack.[41] Appels, in a large prospective study in the Netherlands, found "vital exhaustion" present in the year prior to a heart attack.[42] Appels found the prevalence of myocardial infarction, defined as unstable angina pectoris plus electrocardiographic signs of ischemia, to be more than four times higher among exhausted and depressed persons than among persons who were not so affected.

Social support, survival, and rehabilitation from heart disease

Social support and mortality

Orth-Gomer et al.[43] studied the possible interactive or additive effects of social influences and clinical factors on total and heart disease-related mortality in 150 middle-aged men over a period of 10 years. The sample consisted of men with clinically manifest heart disease, men with elevated risk factor levels, and men in good health. The three most important predictors of total and heart disease-specific mortality were ventricular dysrhythmia, low social activity levels, and a poor perceived health status. Furthermore, the 10-year mortality experience of socially isolated type A men was 69% and that of socially integrated type A men 17%.[44] Ruberman and colleagues, in a study of 2320 male survivors of acute myocardial infarction, found that men with high life stress and high levels of social isolation had more than four times the risk of death over a period of 3 years than men with low levels of both stress and isolation.[45] Strong relationships between social network participation and mortality among males has also been documented by Kaplan et al.,[46] House et al.,[47] and Schoenbach et al.[48]

Chandra and colleagues examined the influence of marital status on the in-hospital and long-term survival rate of 1401 men and women who had experienced myocardial infarctions.[49] Married men and women who experienced myocardial infarction showed a significantly better survival rate than unmarried, independent of other factors. Case et al. found that living alone is an independent risk factor for the recurrence of a major cardiac event.[50] Williams and coworkers found that unmarried patients without a confidant had a more than threefold increase in the risk of death within 5 years of their heart attack than patients who were either married or had a confidant.[51]

Almost half of the people who die each year from coronary heart disease are women, but there has only been one study of psychosocial predictors of recurrent coronary events in women.[52] Recently, Powell and colleagues reported results from an exploratory investigation of psychosocial risk factors for mortality among 83 women with premature acute myocardial infarction.[53] Divorce and being employed without a college degree independently predicted mortality. The authors hypothesize that being divorced or employed without a college degree are markers for low socioeconomic status, low status on the job, and poor role fit. They note that these factors are likely to be interrelated. In men, post-myocardial infarction, for example, mortality was explained by a pattern of psychosocial factors including low education, high stress, and social isolation.[45]

Effects of social support on recovery

Social support appears to be a salient factor for patients with heart disease in maintaining compliance with their rehabilitation programs. Patients who receive support from family and friends are more likely than others to comply with risk factor modification and postcoronary rehabilitation programs. Interpersonal relationships may facilitate such appropriate health behaviors as complying with medical regimens. Friis and Taff[54] note that the most promising social support or social network variables isolated from a literature review appear to be the number and intimacy of social ties, satisfaction with social activities, work and financial status, perceived opportunities to discuss problems, and the level of social interaction.

Helgeson interviewed 90 post-myocardial infarction patients before their hospital discharge, to assess masculinity/feminity and social support.[55] Follow-up interviews were conducted at 3-, 6-, and 12-month intervals following discharge. After controlling for traditional risk factors, severity of myocardial infarction, and psychological distress, the amount of disclosure to one's spouse was the greatest single predictor of recovery. Married patients who were less able to disclose to their spouse were more likely to be hospitalized than unmarried patients or married patients who were more able to disclose to their spouse. Both masculinity and spouse disclosure significantly added to the prediction of post-MI chest pain. More severe post-MI chest pain was predicted by higher scores on masculinity and less spouse disclosure.

Vogt and associates found that social networks may be more effective in supporting recovery from heart disease, cancer, strokes, and hypertension than in preventing disease.[10] These authors suggest that a critical issue in surviving illness may be the degree to which different resources are available. An appropriate resource for solving a problem, regardless of the nature of that problem, is critical to recovery from illness.

Social support and the prevention of heart disease

Ruberman points out that the prevention of every public health problem is not preceded by a complete understanding of its mechanism.[56] Cigarette smoking and hypertension are examples of two risk factors for heart disease that operate through unknown mechanisms. Yet, applying what we know about risk factors or factors that are thought to inhibit risk, such as social support, may be effective even though we cannot explain why or how.

Cwikel and Israel reviewed 17 intervention studies that involved some type of social support or social network approach in the area of physical health problems.[57] They concluded that:

- Social support and social network interventions exhibit greater effects for those people who have recently experienced life crises
- Studies that used a combination of different types of social support in the intervention were more effective
- The provision of social support by peers, significant others, and professionals can affect the level of adherence to medical regimens
- Studies that incorporated both affective and appraisal support had positive results
- Stronger effects were noted when interventions provided more emotional than informational support
- Some of the more successful interventions used lay counselors or peers to deliver the intervention
- The presence of a spouse may inhibit successful interaction about emotionally laden issues

Community interventions

Major community-based cardiovascular disease prevention programs have been conducted in North Karelia, Finland; Minnesota; Pawtucket, Rhode Island; and in three communities and, more recently, five cities near Stanford, California.[58] These programs have sought to reduce cardiovascular disease by reducing risk factors in whole communities. One of the key ingredients in these intervention programs was the mobilization of support networks in a variety of ways, such as the involvement of community organizations and leaders; the delivery of interventions by peer volunteers; the monitoring, feedback, and management of educational activities; face-to-face counseling; and programs with educational contacts with community groups. Interventions mobilized existing community social support networks and created new networks.

Findings reported thus far strongly support the concept that community intervention programs can affect the levels and prevalence of major cardiovascular risk factors.[59] Cardiovascular disease mortality data from North Karelia strongly support a program effect acting through reduction in risk factors to reduce heart disease mortality. Shea and Basch[59] point out that the most important lesson from these studies is that change occurs at multiple social levels, including the individual, group, organization, and the community as a whole, for multiple risk factors; and at multiple stages in the change process, including awareness, motivation, initiation, maintenance, and support of change. Evaluation of the effectiveness of community intervention programs requires complex, multidimensional, and longitudinal tracking.

Family interventions

Family-based interventions present an opportunity for long-term changes in the family social environment that will enhance maintenance of changes in behaviors and risk factors for cardiovascular disease, yet very few family-based interventions are reported.[60]

Nader and colleagues describe the observed and reported behavioral and measured physiologic outcomes 3 years following a year-long family-based cardiovascular risk reduction intervention directed at volunteer Mexican-American and Anglo fifth and sixth grade children and their parents.[60] The intervention was based on social learning theory and principles of self-management. It was designed to assist families in making long-term changes in their physical activity and dietary habits. One of the major reasons for studying family-based interventions was that, by increasing family support of health-promoting behavior, maintenance of gains would be enhanced. There was substantial evidence to indicate that dietary gains were maintained a year after intervention. Intervention effects were found among both Anglo and Mexican-American families. This study demonstrated that with interventions that are culturally appropriate, and using group facilitators who are culturally sensitive, health behavior change can be effective even in a population disadvantaged by income and education.

Lifestyle and individual health behavior change

Health behaviors are a part of lifestyle, which is a broader concept encompassing not only behaviors and attitudes, but an outlook or philosophy of life. Lifestyle is learned and modeled and has many components that are acquired and changed as one moves through the life cyle. Lifestyle and health behavior are closely interrelated, so changes in one affect the other. Many factors, such as environment, culture, family, group, and personality, affect lifestyle. In addition, an individual's perceptions can influence the development of health behavior. Perceptions of vulnerability, susceptibility, benefits, costs, and competing needs all influence health actions or inactions.[61]

Lifestyle is modifiable, but barriers exist which need to be overcome. Often, the individual needs to choose among values and decide which, if any, trade-offs will be necessary to make one's lifestyle more risk free.

Everyone has "times" in their lives when they are more receptive to behavior change. Unfortunately, these "times" usually occur after a heart attack when a physician clearly sets out the path to recovery or early death.

Feuerstein and associates have discussed the challenge of modifying type A behavior.[62] Not all characteristics of type A are predictive of heart disease, and there is no assurance that totally altering type A behavior would benefit the productivity of an individual. An alternative to modifying the type A behavior pattern would be to alter the mechanisms that lead to increased risk, such as anger. Modification could be directed to anger management. Another approach might be to address an individual's response to challenge and develop a multifaceted training program in problem skills, communication skills, and relaxation techniques to help the individual cope with irritating stimuli.

Suinn has developed a program known as cardiac stress management training (CSMT).[63] It is Suinn's view that type A behavior is cultural in origin, and type A values have been learned and internalized. Therefore, the only way to alter type A risk is through anxiety management and vasomotor behavior rehearsal. Significant reductions in state and trait anxiety, and on the Speed, Impatience, and Hard-Driving subscales of the Jenkins Activity Scale have been reported following intervention.

Increasing attention has been paid to physical fitness programs as a beneficial preventive approach. Many large-scale epidemiological studies have associated habitual physical activity with a reduced incidence of heart disease. Type A individuals have been shown to reduce their physiological risk factors in addition to modifying their behavior traits.

Cardiological and behavioral counseling in groups, over a period of years, has also been shown to be effective among post-myocardial infarction patients. This intervention emphasizes the importance of group process. Marked reductions have been achieved in type A behavior, angina pectoris, and serum cholesterol.

Obviously, the goal is to reduce the risk of heart attacks before they occur. Often, individuals who have experienced a heart attack try and fail at behavior change, others dismiss the risks; it is only when faced with death that many heart attack victims become motivated to change their behavior patterns. The role of the health professional becomes crucial in encouraging patients (well and sick) to *consider* risk-reducing behavior change, to *attempt* behavior change, and to *support* changes they do make in their behavior.[64] Health professionals are not expected to be behavioral change experts, but they should be familiar with practitioners and programs to which they can refer patients. Ideally, one would hope that health practitioners would model healthy behaviors themselves so that their advice is not a contradiction of their own lifestyle. Of course, any change in lifestyle or behavior is the responsibility of the individual and evidence of an individual's commitment to *maintaining* a health-enhancing way of life. Certainly public laws regarding tobacco use, use of seat belts, and other behaviors help to sensitize the public to risks, and stress individual and social responsibility to protect one's health and that of others. As Norman Cousins has said, "we need to learn that survival is an option".[65]

Summary

Despite the fact that there is no commonly agreed upon definition of social support or its measurement, an impressive amount of evidence from diverse epidemiological and clinical studies, prospective and retrospective, suggests that social support and social networks do impact the course of health and illness. The pathophysiological links between behavioral factors and cardiovascular diseases appear to involve sympathoadrenomedullary activity.[66] Many pathophysiological processes are known to cause hypertension, myocardial infarction, and sudden death. The basic disease processes do not cause signs or symptoms by themselves. Clinical manifestations occur only when complications are added to the basic disease processes. Behavioral factors may influence both the basic disease processes and the clinical manifestations. The precise mechanism or mechanisms by which social support and social networks work remain a source of speculation and require continued study.

Current evidence about the positive effects of social networks could be used by clinicians in educating patients (well and sick) about the risks of heart disease and sudden death by pointing out the importance of social ties. We do not have to wait until further data are available to effectively apply what we know about the links between social support and heart disease. Indeed, we may gain greater insights into how social support works through trial and error.

References

1. Eisenberg, L., A friend, not an apple, a day will help keep the doctor away, *Am. J. Med.*, 66, 551, 1979.
2. Kaplan, R. M., Social support and social health: is it time to rethink the WHO definition of health, in *Social Support: Theory, Research and Applications*, Sarason, I. G. and Sarason, B. R., Eds., Martinus Nijhoff, Dordrecht, 1985, chap. 6.
3. Ganster, D. C. and Victor, B., The impact of social support on mental and physical health, *Br. J. Med. Psychol.*, 61, 17, 1988.
4. Bloom, J. R., The relationship of social support to health, *Soc. Sci. Med.*, 30, 635, 1990.

5. Berkman, L. F., Social networks, support, and health: taking the next step forward, *Am. J. Epidemiol.*, 123, 559, 1986.
6. House, J. S., Landis, K. R., and Umberson, D., Social relationships and health, *Science*, 241, 540, 1988.
7. Pilisuk, M. and Parks, S. H., *The Healing Web: Social Networks and Human Survival*, The University Press of New England, Hanover, 1986.
8. Berkman, L. F., The relationship of social networks and social support to morbidity and mortality, in *Social Support and Health*, Cohen, S. and Syme, S. L., Eds., Academic Press, New York, 1985, chap. 12.
9. Brackett, C. D. and Powell, L. H., Psychosocial and physiological predictors of sudden cardiac death after healing of acute myocardial infarction, *Am. J. Cardiol.*, 61, 979, 1988.
10. Vogt, T. M., Mullooly, J. P., Ernst, D., Pope, C. R., and Hollis, J. F., Social networks as predictors of ischemic heart disease, cancer, stroke and hypertension: incidence, survival and mortality, *J. Clin. Epidemiol.*, 45, 659, 1992.
11. Turner, R. J., Frankel, B. G., and Levin, D. M., Social support: conceptualization, measurement, and implications for mental health, in *Research in Community and Mental Health*, Vol. 3, Greeley, J., Ed., JAI Press, Greenwich, 1983, 67.
12. Coyne, J. C. and DeLongis, A., Going beyond social support: the role of social relationships in adaptation, *J. Consult. Clin. Psychol.*, 54, 454, 1986.
13. Storr, A., *Solitude: A Return to the Self*, Ballantine Books, New York, 1989, 9.
14. Bruhn, J. G. and Philips, B. U., A developmental basis for social support, *J. Behav. Med.*, 10, 213, 1987.
15. Kahn, R. L. and Antonucci, T. C., Convoys of social support: a life-course approach, in *Aging: Social Change*, Kiesler, S. B., Morgan, J. N., and Oppenheimer, V. K., Eds., Academic Press, New York, 1981, chap. 14.
16. Schulz, R. and Rau, M. T., Social support through the life course, in *Social Support and Health*, Cohen, S. and Syme, S. L., Eds., Academic Press, New York, 1985, chap. 7.
17. Heller, L., Price, R. H., and Hogg, J. R., The role of social support in community and clinical interventions, in *Social Support: An Interactional View*, Sarason, B. R., Sarason, I. G., and Pierce, G. R., Eds., Wiley, New York, 1990, chap. 18.
18. Heitzmann, C. A. and Kaplan, R. M., Assessment of methods for measuring social support, *Health Psychol.*, 7, 75, 1988.
19. Winemiller, D. R., Mitchell, M. E., Sutliff, J., and Cline, D. J., Measurement strategies in social support: a descriptive review of the literature, *J. Clin. Psychol.*, 49, 638, 1993.
20. Barrera, M., Distinctions between social support concepts, measures, and models, *Am. J. Comm. Psychol.*, 14, 413, 1986.
21. Bruhn, J. G. and Philips, B. U., Measuring social support: a synthesis of current approaches, *J. Behav. Med.*, 7, 151, 1984.
22. Kamarck, T. W., Manuck, S. B., and Jennings, J. R., Social support reduces cardiovascular reactivity to psychological challenge: a laboratory model, *Psychosom. Med.*, 52, 42, 1990.
23. Gerin, W., Pieper, C., Levy, R., and Pickering, T. G., Social support in social interaction: a moderator of cardiovascular reactivity, *Psychosom. Med.*, 54, 324, 1992.

24. Edens, J. L., Larkin, K. T., and Abel, J. L., The effect of social support and physical touch on cardiovascular reactions to mental stress, *J. Psychosom. Res.*, 36, 371, 1992.

25. Lepore, S. J., Mata Allen, K. A., and Evans, G. W., Social support lowers cardiovascular reactivity to an acute stressor, *Psychosom. Med.*, 55, 518, 1993.

26. Unden, A., Orth-Gomer, K., and Elofsson, S., Cardiovascular effects of social support in the work place: twenty-four hour ECG monitoring of men and women, *Psychosom. Med.*, 53, 50, 1991.

27. Beere, P., Glagov, S., and Zarins, C., Retarding effect of lowered heart rate on coronary arteriosclerosis, *Science*, 226, 180, 1984.

28. Cohen, S., Psychosocial models of the role of social support in the etiology of physical disease, *Health Psychol.*, 7, 269, 1988.

29. McEwen, B. S. and Stellar, E., Stress and the individual: mechanisms leading to disease, *Arch. Intern. Med.*, 153, 2093, 1993.

30. Reed, D., McGee, D., Yano, K., and Feinlab, M., Social networks and coronary heart disease among Japanese men in Hawaii, *Am. J. Epidemiol.*, 117, 384, 1983.

31. Marmot, M. G., Stress, social and cultural variations in heart disease, *J. Psychosom. Res.*, 27, 377, 1983.

32. Wolf, S. and Bruhn, J. G., *The Power of Clan*, New Brunswick, Transaction Publishers, 1993.

33. Orth-Gomer, L., Rosengren, A., and Wilhelmsen, L., Lack of social support and incidence of coronary heart disease in middle-aged Swedish men, *Psychosom. Med.*, 55, 37, 1993.

34. Blumenthal, J. A., Burg, M. M., Barefoot, J., Williams, R. B., Haney, T., and Zimet, G., Social support, type A behavior, and coronary artery disease, *Psychosom. Med.*, 49, 331, 1987.

35. Seeman, T. E. and Syme, S. L., Social networks and coronary heart disease: a comparison of the structure and function of social relations as predictors of disease, *Psychosom. Med.*, 49, 341, 1987.

36. Jenkins, C. D., Behavioral factors in the etiology and pathogenesis of cardiovascular diseases: sudden death, hypertension, and myocardial infarction, in *Perspectives on Behavioral Medicine*, Weiss, S. M., Herd, J. A., and Fox, B. H., Eds., Academic Press, New York, 1981, 41.

37. Matthews, K. A. and Haynes, S. G., Type A behavior pattern and coronary disease risk: update and critical evaluation, *Am. J. Epidemiol.*, 123, 923, 1986.

38. Margolis, L. H., McLeroy, L. R., Runyan, C. W., and Kaplan, B. H., Type A behavior: an ecological approach, *J. Behav. Med.*, 6, 245, 1983.

39. Barefoot, J. C., Dahlstrom, G., and Williams, R. B., Hostility, CHD incidence, and total mortality: a 25-year follow-up study of 255 physicians, *Psychosom. Med.*, 45, 59, 1983.

40. Siegman, A. W., Cardiovascular consequences of expressing, experiencing, and repressing anger, *J. Behav. Med.* 16, 539, 1993.

41. Bruhn, J. G., McCrady, K. E., and du Plessis, A., Evidence of "emotional drain" preceding death from myocardial infarction, *Psychiatr. Digest*, 29, 34, 1968.

42. Appels, A., The year before myocardial infarction, in *Biobehavioral Bases of Coronary Heart Disease*, Dembroski, T. M., Schmidt, T. H., and Blumchen, G., Eds., Karger, Basel, 1983, chap 2.

43. Orth-Gomer, K., Unden, A., and Edwards, M., Social isolation and mortality in ischemic heart disease, *Acta Med. Scand.*, 224, 205, 1988.
44. Orth-Gomer, K. and Unden, A., Type A behavior, social support, and coronary risk: interaction and significance for mortality in cardiac patients, *Psychosom. Med.*, 52, 59, 1990.
45. Ruberman, W., Weinblatt, E., Goldberg, J. D., and Chaudhary, B. S., Psychosocial influences on mortality after myocardial infarction, *N. Engl. J. Med.*, 311, 552, 1984.
46. Kaplan, G. A., Salonen, J. T., Cohen, R. D., Brand, R. J., Syme, S. L., and Puska, P., Social connections and mortality from all causes and from cardiovascular disease: prospective evidence from Eastern Finland, *Am. J. Epidemiol.*, 128, 370, 1988.
47. House, J. S., Robbins, C., and Metzner, H. L., The association of social relationships and activities with mortality: prospective evidence from the Tecumseh community health study, *Am. J. Epidemiol.*, 116, 123, 1982.
48. Schoenbach, V. J., Kaplan, B. H., Fredman, L., and Kleinbaum, D. G., Social ties and mortality in Evans County, Georgia, *Am. J. Epidemiol.*, 123, 577, 1986.
49. Chandra, V., Szklo, M., Goldberg, R., and Tonascia, J., The impact of marital status on survival after an acute myocardial infarction: a population-based study, *Am. J. Epidemiol.*, 117, 320, 1983.
50. Case, R. B., Moss, A. J., Case, N., McDermott, M., and Eberly, S., Living alone after myocardial infarction, *JAMA*, 267, 515, 1992.
51. Williams, R. B., Barefoot, J. C., Califf, R. M., Haney, T. L., Saunders, W. B., Pryor, D. B., Htlatky, M. A., Siegler, I. C., and Mark, D. B., Prognostic importance of social and economic resources among medically treated patients with angiographically documented coronary heart disease, *JAMA*, 267, 520, 1992.
52. Shekelle, R. B., Gale, M., and Norusis, M., for the Aspirin Myocardial Infarction Study Research Group, Type A score and risk of recurrent coronary heart disease in the Aspirin Myocardial Infarction Study, *Am. J. Cardiol.*, 56, 221, 1985.
53. Powell, L. H., Shaker, L. A., Jones, B. A., Vaccarino, L. V., Thoresen, C. E., and Pattillo, J. R., Psychosocial predictors of mortality in 83 women with premature acute myocardial infarction, *Psychosom. Med.*, 55, 426, 1993.
54. Friis, R. and Taff, G. A., Social support and social networks, and coronary heart disease rehabilitation, *J. Cardiopulmonary Rehabil.*, 6, 132, 1986.
55. Helgeson, V. S., The effects of masculinity and social support on recovery from myocardial infarction, *Psychosom. Med.*, 53, 621, 1991.
56. Ruberman, W., Psychosocial influences on mortality of patients with coronary heart disease, *JAMA*, 267, 559, 1992.
57. Cwikel, J. M. and Israel, B. A., Examining mechanisms of social support and social networks: a review of health-related intervention studies, *Public Health Rev.*, 15, 159, 1987.
58. Shea, S. and Basch, C. E., A review of five major community-based cardiovascular disease prevention programs. I. Rationale, design, and theoretical framework, *Am. J. Health Prom.*, 4, 203, 1990.
59. Shea, S. and Basch, C. E., A review of five major community-based cardiovascular disease prevention programs. II. Intervention strategies, evaluation methods, and results, *Am. J. Health. Prom.*, 4, 279, 1990.

60. Nader, P. R., Sallis, J. F., Abramson, I. S., Broyles, S. L., Patterson, T. L., Senn, K., Rupp, J. W., and Nelson, J. A., Family-based cardiovascular risk reduction education among Mexican and Anglo-Americans, *Fam. Community Health*, 15, 57, 1992.

61. Bruhn, J. G., Life-style and health behavior, in *Health Behavior*, Gochman, D. S., Ed., Plenum, New York, 1988, chap. 4.

62. Feuerstein, M., Labbe, E. E., and Kuczmierczyk, A. R., *Health Psychology: A Psychobiological Perspective*, Plenum, New York, 1986, chap. 10.

63. Suinn, R. M., The cardiac stress management program for type A patients, *Cardiac Rehabil.*, 5, 13, 1975.

64. Greenlick, M. R., Helping patients achieve risk-reducing behavior change, in *Advances in Disease Prevention*, Vol. 1, Arnold, C. B., Ed., Springer, New York, chap. 2.

65. Cousins, N., *Human Options*, Norton, New York, 1981.

66. Herd, J. A., Behavioral factors in the physiological mechanisms of cardiovascular disease, in *Perspectives on Behavioral Medicine*, Weiss, S. M., Herd, J. A., and Fox, B. H., Eds., Academic Press, New York, 1981, chap. 4.

chapter fourteen

Social support, secure attachments, and health

Jonathan D. Quick, Debra L. Nelson, Patricia A. C. Matuszek,
James L. Whittington, and James Campbell Quick

Over the last two decades of work in the field, theorists and researchers
have put forward a wide variety of largely complementary definitions of
social support. Social support has been conceptualized in perceptual, developmental, dynamic, structural, and functional terms. We define social
support as the provision of positive psychological, emotional, and material resources to a person through interpersonal relationships.

The absence of social support is social isolation. House and co-workers[1] argue that social isolation is a significant health risk factor for morbidity and mortality problems. Therefore, the conventional line of argument is that people need social support, secure attachments, and
community to immunize them against the health risks associated with
social isolation. The reasoning goes that social support helps prevent ill
health and serves as a therapeutic agent in healing distress and illness. In
addition, attachment behavior in humans helps the young and needy survive in times of danger.[2]

This chapter has five major sections. The first section reviews common
definitions and functions of social support, including consideration of measures of social support. The second section reviews the research on social
support and health, calling into question some of the conventional thinking about the purely positive role of social relationships in health. The third
section presents a three-level developmental framework for secure attachments, which are level I (Receiving), level II (Exchanging), and level
III (Transcending). Faith, belief, and relevant research are also discussed
in this section. The fourth section discusses ways to develop social support to prevent distress. The concluding section examines future directions
for research.

Though there is a growing body of research evidence demonstrating
a strong relationship between social support and better mental and physical health, the causal nature of this relationship can best be confirmed
through further research aimed particularly at (1) elucidating the mecha-

0-8493-2908-6/96/$0.00+$.50

nisms through which social support affects health and (2) critically assessing the impact on health of individual and organizational interventions aimed at fostering higher levels of social support.

Social support: definition and functions

Definitions of social support

Social support is a concept that is generally understood in an intuitive sense. Yet, as House[3] notes, early work on social support sometimes lacked any explicit definition of the concept. Over the last two decades of work in the field, however, theorists and researchers have put forward a wide variety of complementary definitions and concepts of social support. These concepts can be described as perceptual, developmental, dynamic, structural, and functional.

In one of the earliest major reviews on social support, Cobb[4] takes a perceptual approach, defining social support as the individual belief that one is *cared for and loved, esteemed and valued,* and *belongs to a network of communication and mutual obligation.* By contrast to the perceptual approach, a developmental approach to social support is reflected in Bowlby's[5,6] work on attachment theory. Attachment theory, considered in greater detail later in this chapter, suggests that secure attachments in childhood are rooted in instinctive human behavior. These attachments become a basis for an adult's ability to form effective social support relationships.

Social support has also been described in dynamic terms. House[3] summarizes earlier work in the field which defined social support in terms of interpersonal transactions. Later, Shumaker and Brownell[7] defined social support as, *an exchange of resources between at least two individuals perceived by the provider or recipient to be intended to enhance the well-being of the recipient.*

Several authors describe social support in structural terms. That is, what are the types and sources of social support? In an oft-cited construct of social support, House[3] described four main categories of social support:

1. Emotional support, which generally comes from family and close friends, is the most commonly recognized form of social support. It includes empathy, concern, caring, love, and trust.
2. Appraisal support involves transmission of information (as opposed to affect) in the form of affirmation, feedback, or social comparison. This information is often evaluative and can come from family, friends, co-workers, or community sources.
3. Informational support includes advice, suggestion, or directives which assist the person to respond to personal or situational demands.

4. Instrumental support is the most concrete direct form of social support, encompassing help in the form of money, time, in-kind assistance, and other explicit interventions on a person's behalf.

These four classes or types of social support actually combine elements of perceptual, dynamic, and functional definitions of social support.

Finally, several authors have taken a functional approach to social support. Quick and colleagues[8] describe the five functions of social support for executives as protective, informational, evaluative, modeling, and emotional. Using role theory, Zey[9] describes 12 supporting-cast roles representing functional ways in which individuals may support a person: advisor, catalyst, celebrator, cheerleader, constructive critic, contact, esteem-builder, financier, public-relations specialist, role model, sponsor, and technical supporter.

Measurement of social support

As there are many definitions, descriptions, and functions ascribed to the concept of social support, there are also a variety of ways in which social support is operationalized and measured. This leads to problems, as noted by writers who find a lack of any consistent method for measuring social support.[10,11] One of the earliest measures of social support in the workplace was a brief questionnaire developed by House and Wells,[12] whose three central questions were:

1. How much can each of the following people be relied on when things get tough at work? Immediate supervisor or boss; other people at work; spouse; friends; relatives.
2. How much is each of these same people willing to listen to your work-related problems?
3. How much is each of these same people helpful to you in getting your job done?

The majority of subsequent research on social support has used this genre of self-report questionnaire aimed at identifying supportive relationships and assessing the degree of support from, type of support in, and/or quality of each relationship. There are three exceptions to this general measurement approach. First, Fleury[13] used interviews to explore the role of social networks in motivating health behavior change. Second, Kulik and Mahler[14] used the number of hospital visitations as an archival measure of marital support for hospitalized patients. Third, Gerin et al.[15] used an experimental manipulation in a laboratory study in which one confederate attacked the subject as a negative social relationship and one confederate was support neutral.

Social support and health: the need for relationship?

Social support has been presented as a social-psychological agent that facilitates interpersonal immunization against life's demands. This suggests that it operates as one form of prevention against distress. This section of the chapter reviews literature from the last 7 years dealing with the links between social support, social relationship, and health. Therefore, in addition to examining the healthy consequences of social support, the review examines the negative impact of some social relationships, and the differential circumstances for social support.

Healthy consequences of social support

House et al.[1] begin by pointing out that more socially isolated or less socially integrated individuals are psychologically and physically less healthy and more likely to die. Their meta-analysis supports the notion that positive health outcomes, especially longer life span, are associated with social support. They contend that there is sufficient evidence to suggest social isolation is a risk factor of mortality and morbidity. This view is supported for chronic[16,17] as well as acute illness.[18] Horman[19] broadens this perspective, taking a life cycle view of the relationship between social support and health. He concludes that social support at all phases of the life cycle has important implications for health outcomes, and that health educators should encourage good quality relationships.

The most obvious of the positive effects of social support are the measurable differences in physiological responses to challenging or stressful situations. Several researchers have documented specific physiological responses associated with the presence, or absence, of social support. Gerin et al.[15] found that there was greater cardiovascular reactivity among people who had no social support and who faced a challenge, especially compared to people who were supported by another individual. The people with no social support actually had higher blood pressure and faster heart rate. Kulik and Mahler[14] found that coronary bypass patients who were visited by spouses while in the hospital did not require as much pain medication nor remain in intensive care nor hospital as long as patients who had relatively little spousal support during their hospital stay. Similarly, Hibbard and Pope[20] found that women who received social support at work had a lower mortality rate than nonemployed women. They further found that nonemployed women had an 80% greater risk of death than women who enjoyed even low levels of social support at work. Their findings also suggested that social support may be one aspect of employment that is protective of health. Falk and colleagues[21] also found that job strain was buffered by a positive social network and social support. In another recent study,[18] evidence was found to reinforce the effect of social support as a buffer against the physiological effects of stress. Cancer patients were found to have poorer medical outcomes when confronted with a lack of social support.

Another well-documented domain is the relationship between stress and social support. Greller et al.[22] note that the most widely identified stress buffer is social support. They also point out that social support may affect stress in one of two ways—first, by acting as a compensation for strain, and second, by changing the experience of strain. Callaghan and Morrissey's[11] review concludes that social support may play an important role in maintaining health while mitigating against the adverse effects of environmental and social stress. Kobasa and co-workers[21] suggest that social support explains relatively little about resistance to illness, but instead combines with hardiness and exercise during stressful times to decrease the likelihood of disease. A similar view is held by Cohen and Edwards,[24] who found that social support and other psychosocial assets buffered stress only after stress appraisal. There was no indication that disease was prevented because of the presence of any psychosocial assets. The Kobasa[23] study also considers social support to be only one resource for lowering illness risk and contends people with multiple resources are less likely to become ill.

Table 1 presents data previously reported by graphing age-adjusted mortality rate and level of social integration for males and females in five prospective studies.[1] The relative risk ratio of mortality at lowest versus highest level of social integration shows in each study the increased risk

Table 1   Relative Risk Ratio of Mortality versus Social Integration

Study population	Relative risk ratio of mortality[a]		Source
	Males	Females	
Alameda County, CA	2.44	2.81	Berkman and Syme[b]
Eastern Finland	2.63	1.92	Kaplan et al.[c]
Evans County, GA			
Blacks	1.08	1.59	Schoenback et al.[d]
Whites	1.83	1.07	
Gothenburg, Sweden	4.00	1.92	Welin et al.[e]
Tecumseh, Michigan	3.87	1.97	House et al.[f]

[a] Based on age-adjusted mortality in each of five prospective studies.
[b] Berkman, L. F. and Syme, S. L., Social networks, host resistance, and mortality: a nine-year follow-up study of Alameda County residents, *Am. J. Epidemiol.*, 109, 186, 1979.
[c] Kaplan, G. A., Jukka, T., Saleonen, R. D., Cohen, R. D., Brand, R. J., Syme, F. L., and Peska, P., Social connections and mortality from all causes and cardiovascular disease: prospective evidence from Eastern Finland, *Am. J. Epidemiol.*, 128 (2), 370–380, 1988.
[d] Schoenback, V. J., Kaplan, B. H., Fredman, L., and Kleinbaum, D. G., Social ties and mortality in Evans County, Georgia, *Am. J. Epidemiol.*, 213, 577–591, 1986.
[e] Welin, L., Svardsudd, K., Ander-Peciva, S., Tibblin, G., Tibblin, B., Larsson, B., and Wilhelmsen, L., Prospective study of social influences on mortality: the study of men born in 1913 and 1923, *Lancet*, 1, 915–918, 1985.
[f] House, J. S., Robbins, C., and Mertzner, H. M., The association of social relationships and activities with mortality: prospective evidence from the Tecumseh Community Health Study, *Am. J. Epidemiol.*, 116, 123–140, 1982.

of mortality, for both sexes, associated with lower levels of social integration. This suggests that social isolation is lethal and social support is healthy.

Negative impacts of social relationships

There is an implicit assumption that social relationships and networks provide positive influence for health maintenance. However, there is evidence to suggest that social relationships and networks may actually have a negative impact on the health of an individual in some cases.

A distinction between social support and social relationships is necessary at this point. By definition, social support is a positive influence in an individual's life. Conversely, social relationships are not necessarily positive. They may be negative or nonexistent, and, as a result, may have very different impacts on health outcomes. Greller et al.[22] contend that family and co-workers do not fundamentally change the effects of stressors, but may add or subtract from the experienced strain. If, for example, an individual is faced with a job that has numerous time limits, the stress experience would be exacerbated by a home life that also includes time limits. This would not allow sufficient winding down time.[25] Vinokur and van Ryn[26] conceptualize social undermining as a set of behaviors that negatively impact a target person, and empirically found changes in mental health are much more highly associated with undermining than with social support. The effects of undermining are described as volatile and extreme while the effects of support are described as weaker but stable. Auslander and Litwin[27] concluded that not all social networks were supportive, and some may be sources of stress. Further, Shumaker and Hill[28] found social networks sources of social support for women as well as sources of added demands that could deplete their resources.

Romano et al.[29] found that urban African Americans living in communities with large African American populations seemed to be at especially high risk for illness associated with smoking. In this instance, the peer pressure of the men's social group was hypothesized to outweigh the positive effects of the network that would reduce smoking; that is, the network actually increased the likelihood of a negative health behavior. Other evidence suggests that social networks may impair motivation to continue health-related activities. Fleury[13] concluded that negative communication and conflicting values discouraged patients from changing or made them question their ability to manage the necessary changes to maintain healthy lifestyles. Evans and co-workers[30] found greater psychological distress and lower social support associated with increased residential density.

In spite of possible negative impacts of social relationships, Fleury[13] notes that the most effective social support results in positive self-evaluation, improved self-esteem, control or environmental mastery, and feelings of self-worth. This is supported by Cohen and Wills,[31] who state that the best social support buffers are those that provide esteem and information support.

Circumstantial differences in the effects of social support

There is also some evidence that social support may be more (less) effective under some circumstances than others. Reifman et al.[32] concluded that benefits of social support were different at different levels of stress. While social support had a beneficial effect at low stress levels, the effects at high stress levels included increased symptoms. Timing of support may also be critical. Wilcox et al.[33] determined that people with little need for emotional support may be less distressed by a crisis and manage better until adjustment to the crisis has taken place, at which time instrumental, not social, support may be more important. This suggests that people with a high need for emotional support will be more distressed by a crisis and benefit less from practical support. Social support may also be particularly important to the elderly, who tend to suffer social isolation for a variety of reasons. Revicki and Mitchell[34] found social contact reduced psychological distress for the elderly. Marriage has been shown to be positively related to social support.[35] This is especially important when one considers the impact of spousal support (nonsupport) for health benefits.[14,17,28] Spiegel[18] notes that marital disruption can suppress immune function, thereby making it more difficult for the body to fight disease. Cummins[36] found differences in coping abilities based on the individual's locus of control. Specifically, work support was a stress buffer for individuals with internal locus of control.

There are also gender differences in the effects of social networks that should be considered as one studies the implications for health. As men age they experience a shrinking social network, because they tend to rely on a single confidant (typically a mate) as a liaison for social interaction. When comparing mortality rates among unmarried men and women, Shumaker and Hill[28] came to the conclusion that men's higher death risk was the result of fewer social resources. A study by Linden and colleagues[37] also found gender differences. Specifically, low ambulatory systolic blood pressure was associated with high social support in women but not in men and men with elevated hostility scores reported lower social support.

Conclusion

This review represents the plethora of research concerning the relationship between health and social support. The literature does not uniformly support the notion that social relationships lead to positive health outcomes. Rather, it suggests that social support may be an integral part of an ongoing process that includes a variety of factors to determine an individual's health status. Other factors that may help determine the impact of social

support on one's health include a variety of demographic and psychosocial elements. Most of the studies reviewed here may not warrant causal
inferences about the social support-health relationship, the prospective
studies in Table 1 excepted. Therefore, it is virtually impossible to determine whether social support causes improved health outcomes, or whether
improved health outcomes are responsible for a positive social network.
Nonetheless, there is substantial evidence to support the belief that the perception of positive support is healthy for most people.

A developmental framework for secure attachments

House and colleagues[1] were puzzled about the mechanism whereby social
relationships affect health. Further, they are silent on the question of the
mechanism whereby people develop social supports. Attachment theory,
proposed as an ethological approach to personality, may have explanatory
power with regard to the latter question.[2,6] This theoretical framework suggests (1) the young reach out for supportive, secure attachments in times
of danger and (2) secure attachments contribute to the healthy development of the individual.

New research on self-reliance suggests it is a healthy characteristic that
extends into adulthood,[38] resulting in self-reliant adults who are able to
form and maintain the secure attachments (i.e., social supports) essential
to their health.[8] One early study suggests that self-reliance is a personality
construct which may be measured in adults.[39] However, self-reliance is a
paradoxical pattern of behavior which leads individuals to function au-
tonomously or interdependently, as is situationally appropriate.[6,8] A central notion in attachment theory is that the person believes he or she has
access to the attachment figure in time of need and a key consequence of
secure attachments is a person's experience of felt security.

Three levels of attachment

We propose that there are in fact three levels of attachment which lead to
the experience of felt security and which form a developmental continuum, though not a hierarchy. We label them levels I, II, and III, as shown
in Table 2. The table describes the usual settings and characteristics of these
attachments.

Level I attachment: receiving

Secure attachments in childhood are rooted in instinctual human behavior, according to Bowlby's[5] original theory. Again according to Bowlby,[5] attachment behavior is a potential behavior that is normally activated in the
young by threatening and dangerous circumstances. Attachment behavior enables the young to receive essential social support from secure attachment figures and to utilize secure attachments to develop their own
strength and competence for managing the various stresses of life. The re-

Table 2 A Developmental Framework for Secure Attachments

Attachment level	Usual setting	Characteristics of relationship
I. Receiving	Childhood Incapacitating illness Requires attachment figures	Instinctive Passive One-way Perceived availability
II. Exchanging	Adulthood Support through human relationships Availability depends on others	Active Two-way Facilitates buffering effects Based on experienced interactions
III. Transcending	Adult religious belief Support through higher relationships Faith support groups	Instinctive Active or passive Facilitates transformational coping Based on faith and belief Perceived as always available

cipient of secure level I attachments is dependent on the secure attachment figure to responsibly provide for the needs, health, and well-being of the young. The emphasis in this developmental theory is on the quality (secure versus insecure) of the relationship between the attachment figure and the young. It does not explicitly address in detail any predisposition in the young to be able to be more or less receptive to the resources provided in a secure attachment. Secure level I attachments are a category of supportive relationship that contributes to health and well-being. Understanding level I attachments is particularly important for parents and caregivers who have the responsibility to provide the resources the young require. This may be particularly challenging in the case of the distressed vulnerable child who is temperamentally not predisposed to be a receiver.[40] Valliant[41] suggests that attachment, internalization, and later rediscovery are important platforms for healthy adulthood development.

Level II attachment: exchanging

The new research on adulthood attachments suggests that attachment behavior carries over into the adulthood years.[8,38] While the quality of secure level II attachments is similar to secure level I attachments, the distinguishing feature of level II attachments is their exchanging nature. Specifically, secure level II attachments may be labeled self-reliant and interdependent. They are characterized by mutual, reciprocal exchanges of various social and/or interpersonal resources in the work and home environments. As is situationally and circumstantially appropriate, secure level II attachments may vary in the amount and nature of the social exchanges that occur within them. Secure level II attachments characterize healthy adulthood behavior, being inherently flexible and responsive by nature. While the child in secure level I attachments is clearly the receiver, adults in secure level II attachments must act as secure bases for others in need as well as receiving from others in their own time of need. Level II attachments are the basis of socially supportive relationships and the foundation upon which people form community.

Level III attachment: transcending

Most discussions of attachment and social support end with the secular concept inherent in level II attachment. That is, social support is seen as an exchange occurring within human relationships. But is there the possibility of a higher level of social support which transcends human relationship, which also has a positive influence on health and well-being? In its original form, attachment theory is an instinctual theory. Is it instinctual to transcend human attachments to form a secure attachment with God? Ornish[42] suggests transcending feelings of isolation by "Opening Your Heart to a Higher Power." "If God is everywhere, and if there is only one God, then we are not separate from God."[43]

Level III attachment, although it focuses on transcending human attachments, does not suggest that one transcend relationship. In the context of many spiritual faiths, the believer has a personal relationship with the higher power, be that Adonai for the Jew, the Holy Trinity for the Christian, or Allah for the Muslim. Hence, the communicant in a personal relationship with God is not isolated. The person of faith always has access to God as a secure attachment figure because of God's omnipresence.[42] A key consequence of secure attachments is the experience of felt security and spiritual faith may be a pathway for that felt security.

If level III attachment represents an inferred source of social support, what is the nature of this support? Pargament and associates[44] identify three faith-related coping styles, each of which suggests a different form of support relationship: self-directing, deferring, and collaborative. These styles differ in the assumed locus of responsibility and level of activity in the coping process. The self-directing or self-efficacy style places the responsibility for action with the individual, but sees God as providing positive appraisal for individual problem-solving.[45] The deferring style or outcomes-are-in-God's-hands style sees God as the source of solutions.[45] Individuals with a deferring style wait for solutions to appear through God's efforts.

Pargament and associates[44] assert that the most common coping style is collaborative, in which both God and the individual are seen as active partners. This view is reflected in the Apostle Paul's letter to the Philippians (4:13),[46] "I can do all things through Christ who strengthens me" and Benjamin Franklin's maxim, "God helps those who help themselves."

Faith and belief: ground for transcending attachment

To this point we have proposed that the healthy attachment between a parent and a child (level I attachment) forms the foundation for healthy attachments throughout adulthood (level II attachments), both important forms of social support characterized by mutual interdependence and self-reliance. Self-reliance characterizes people who accept responsibility for their own well-being, yet know with confidence that others are available and willing to help as needed.[8]

According to attachment theory, the attachment figure serves two critical functions: safe haven and secure base. As a safe haven, a mother (level I) or a trusted loved one (level II) acts as a protection against predators, or as a refuge during periods of distress. As a secure base the attachment figure acts as base for exploring the environment, assuring the child of attention and availability. According to Bowlby[5] these attachments are instinctive in nature, by which he meant what is inherited is a potential to develop certain sorts of systems, termed here as behavioral systems, not the instinctive behavior itself.

Levels I and II attachments as discussed here are horizontal, human attachments to another person(s). However, a third level of attachment is also possible, even necessary, for healthy development and support. This third level of support is vertical in nature: the attachment to God through faith. As Kirkpatrick and Shaver[47] point out, "the God of most Christian traditions seems to correspond very closely to the idea of a secure attachment figure."

In using illustrative examples from our reformed Christian faith tradition, we recognize the inherent risk of exclusion of other faith traditions for which we cannot speak. We believe the concepts of Transcending Attachment are universal and suggest each to examine these ideas in the context of their own faith traditions. For example, Radhakrishnan[48] may be an excellent source for the Hindu and David-Neel[49] one for the Buddhist. From our tradition, Old and New Testament writers saw God as a protective parent figure who was readily available to His children in time of need, yet provided individual freedom for exploration of their environment. This freedom was such that the "child" was even allowed to stray from and break the fellowship with their God, yet was welcomed back. Examples of this reception of prodigal children are found in both the Old Testament (see Hosea) and New Testament (see Luke 15).

Certainly the biblical writers believed this desire to form an attachment with God is instinctive in the sense defined by Bowlby.[5] In the Judeo-Christian tradition (though many others have a parallel), man is seen to have been created in need of relationships: "it was not good for the man to be alone" (Genesis 2:18). Women and men need horizontal relationships, and they need the vertical relationship with their creator. According to Paul, this need for relationship with God was "evident within man . . . who knew God" (Romans 1:19, and 21).

The image of God as a safe haven runs throughout the Psalms, where God is described as a rock, a stronghold, a shield, a fortress, a refuge, and the salvation of the Psalmist (Psalms 18:2, 62:1, 62:2, 3:3, 18:2, 7:1). This theme is continued through the New Testament and is particularly clear in Jesus' prayer to His Father for His followers in John 17 where he asks not "to take them out of the world, but to keep them from the evil one" (John 17:15).

The availability of God as a secure base to those who seek Him is also a recurring theme throughout the Bible, with recurrent reassurance to "be strong and courageous for the LORD your God will be with you" (Joshua 1:1–9). The apostle Paul reflects both the safe haven and the secure base images of God in his instruction concerning anxiety in Philippians 4: "Be anxious for nothing . . . And the peace of God, which surpasses all comprehension, shall guard your hearts and your minds in Christ Jesus" (Philippians 4:6–7). Experiencing God as a safe haven and secure base provides those who relate to Him through faith with the potential to view distressful life events in a different light. Specifically, integrated faith enables the believer to engage in transformational coping (i.e., actively changing a distressful event into something subjectively less stressful by viewing it in a broader life perspective) to avoid distress. This process may include altering the course and outcome of the event through action and/or by achieving a greater understanding of the process.[50] When faced with distressful events, people of faith see God's hand at work to create a higher good or to help them cultivate a deeper relationship with Him. Certainly the apostle Paul had this view when he wrote "And we know that God causes all things to work together for good to those who love God, to those who are called according to His purpose" (Romans 8:28).

We have argued that faith in a personal God who acts as both a safe haven and a secure base provides the basis for the transformational coping. Empirical support for this position has been explored by Sethi and Seligman,[51] who looked at the optimism of three different religious faiths: Orthodox Judaism, Calvinism, and Islam. They reported that the fundamentalist in these faith groups were significantly more influenced by and more involved in their religion than those categorized as moderates or liberals. Additionally, the fundamentalists were more hopeful than the others and more optimistic than the moderate and liberal groups. This optimism stemmed from the hope the religion engendered and the daily influence of their faith.

The key element in this analysis is hope. Hope allows the faithful to view circumstances in a different light and with a teleological view of a greater good to come. This theme was echoed by the apostle Paul when he wrote "If we have hoped in Christ in this life only, we are of all men most to be pitied" (I Corinthians 15:19). If hope is the active component of transformational coping, faith activates hope. In fact it may be impossible to separate the two concepts in the biblical tradition: "Now faith is the assurance of things hoped for, the conviction of things not seen" (Hebrews

11:1). The writer to the Hebrews goes on to explain that it is by faith that we "understand that the worlds were prepared by the word of God" (Hebrews 11:2), that it was by faith that the Old Testament saints were justified, and that it is impossible to please or have relationship with God without faith (Hebrews 11:6). Thus, through faith we form an attachment to God which meets the criteria set forth by Bowlby.[5] God as the "attachment figure" in this relationship fulfills the dual functions of safe haven and secure base. Additionally, this relationship forms the basis for the hope required to cope transformationally when faced with distressful life events.

Empirical evidence for the role of religion

If level III attachment, as manifested in religiousness, is accepted as a form of social support, then the question remains whether there is a relationship between this form of social support and health. Research in this area has used various measures of religiousness, including church attendance, frequency of prayer, religious category (fundamentalist, moderate, liberal), and self-reported religious involvement, religious motivation, religious hope, or religious influence in daily life.[44,45,51]

Sethi and Seligman[51] cite studies dating back 100 years that suggest an association between religious belief and well-being, both physical or mental. Durkheim[52] found fundamentalist groups such as Catholics had much lower suicide rates than liberal groups. Ross[45] reviews studies showing associations between greater religiousness and lower levels of psychological distress, better adjustment, higher life satisfaction, lower levels of depression, and better physical health. But in a meta-analysis of the 24 studies, Bergin[53] found a positive association between religion and mental health in only about half.

Variations in demonstrated associations between belief and well-being may reflect differences in methodology or complexities in the way these elements interact. Ross,[45] for example, found that the degree of psychological distress is inversely related to strength of religious belief; the stronger the religious belief of respondents, the lower the psychological distress. But those who had no religious belief expressed the same low level of psychological distress. Ross suggests that this U-shaped association between religiousness and psychological distress argues for a causal relationship and against the notion that very distressed people seek support in religious belief.

Developing social support and preventing distress

There are three implications of the research on social support and health for developing social support to prevent distress. The first are individual initiatives, the second are organizational initiatives, and the third concern the emerging international workplace.

Individual initiatives

Individuals can be encouraged to serve as secure attachments and sources of social support for others, either in organizational or nonorganizational settings. There are several means through which organizations can encourage these forms of individual behavior, such as through newcomer socialization efforts, mentoring systems, and networking programs. For example, the American Academy of Management instituted a cross-organizational mentoring program in 1994 for people of color. People must recognize the emotional and time-related costs of providing support, and returns of these investments may not come quickly. Organizations and associations may help by rewarding those willing to give to others in this way. Too often social support is encouraged in principle, yet not recognized with tangible rewards that reinforce providing support to others.

Organizational initiatives

Organizations can strive to encourage self-reliance among individuals. Employees can be trained to evaluate work situations, rely on their own resources when appropriate, and ask for support from others when it is needed. Too often, organizations emphasize the value of independence to the extent that employees are afraid to seek support. To counter this, leaders can send a message that seeking assistance from others and developing relationships at work are valued activities. Educating employees about the health risks of social isolation and the benefits of social support encourages self-reliant behavior.

Team building at all levels of the organization promotes the establishment of interdependent relationships. Another way to foster self-reliance among people is to help establish support systems. Special attention can be paid to high-risk groups such as newcomers, those who travel frequently, and people whose work requires them to be isolated from others. Organizations can also provide lists of resource people who may be consulted in times of special need, such as downsizing, re-engineering or other major structural change.

The international workplace

The influence of international work environments on social support must be recognized by organizations. Expatriate work assignments break down established social support systems, thus requiring special attention in developing social support. Efforts can be made to help expatriates build new social support systems consisting of multiple sources and multiple forms of support. Further, collectivist or group-oriented cultures may be more adept at providing social support and encouraging interdependent behavior, while individualistic cultures may foster more counterdependent behavior. International work environments thus offer the advantage of learning about social support from a diverse work force, but they also pose risks in terms of overseas assignments and the potential for disruption in existing support networks.

Organizations and individuals have a shared responsibility to develop social support and to manage stress preventively. Too often the burden of managing stress is shifted to the individual. There are opportunities for organizations to intervene by providing professional support when an individual's own social resources become inadequate or fail. Social support is one of a host of effective intervention points. Using social support as a means of preventing distress and encouraging health become most effective if both parties share joint responsibility.

Future directions for research

There is much still to learn about the relationship between social support and health. The developmental framework presented in Table 2 may be one guide for future studies. Previous research has concentrated on the first two levels of attachment, receiving and exchanging. Comparatively little is known about the third level, transcending. This opens a new line of inquiry for researchers interested in social support and attachment. There are four basic lines of research we advocate for expanding our knowledge of social support as a method of preventive stress management.

First, further research is needed on gender differences and social support. Current research indicates that women report more social supports than men, and more positive effects from support than do men.[54] Further, women are more likely to be called upon as providers, and tend to become more emotionally involved in the problems of others.[55] Women, thus, are more likely than men to experience both the positive and negative aspects of social support. While these results suggest gender differences in the provision and receipt of support, gender differences in the social support and health relationship require further investigation. Are certain types of support and sources of support more effective for men or women? Do the specific health consequences of support differ by gender? Are there gender differences concerning individuals' progression in the three-stage developmental attachment framework? There are many unexplored questions.

Second, do individuals with strong personal faith relationships heal faster or live longer than others? The association between faith and health is complex, and provides many opportunities for research. What is it about faith that produces health benefits? Preliminary evidence indicates a relationship between faith and optimism.[51] Perhaps individuals with strong belief systems cope better with the stress of living. In particular, religious individuals may use transformational coping, which allows them to reframe stressors and cope with them constructively. Further, the combination of self-reliance and faith may produce the greatest health benefits.

Third, what are the health effects of being a provider of social support? Our review has argued that providing support to others is an essential part of healthy adult behavior; however, the specific health consequences, both positive and negative, can be studied. Some relationships, for example, are characterized by one individual providing all the support while the other individual fails to reciprocate. This leaves the provider drained, and facing an absence of potential resources for the support he/she needs. The specific benefits and risks of serving as a support provider require further exploration. Further, we need to know more about the characteristics of good support providers. Based on the evidence so far, we suggest that those individuals who are self-reliant are also good providers of support.

Finally, what are the limitations of social support? Are there conditions under which social support is simply not effective? Or, are there situations in which the provision of social support is more of a hindrance than a help in managing stress? Sometimes a provider may attempt to calm the distressed individual by minimizing the stressful situation, and in so doing may actually create additional stress for the individual. Studies need to address these questions in order to better understand the boundaries of social support.

Consideration should be given to varied methods of investigation in future research. Though randomized trials of club membership, improved peer relationships at work, or religious fervor are unlikely, prospective interrupted time series analysis and other quasi-experimental designs offer feasible methods for exploring cause-effect relationships in the social support-health relationship.[56]

Acknowledgments

The authors thank Stanislav Kasl, the Reverend Elizabeth Pense, Joseph Rosenstein, Lawrence L. Schkade, and Jerry C. Wofford for their critical reviews of earlier drafts of this chapter. Thanks go to James S. House and Marie Klatt for help to complete Table 1 and to Abdul Rasheed for Hindu and Buddhist references.

References

1. House, J. S., Landis, K. R., and Umberson, D., Social relationships and health, *Science*, 241, 540–545, 1988.
2. Ainsworth, M. D. S. and Bowlby, J., An ethological approach to personality, *Am. Psychol.*, 46, 333–341, 1991.
3. House, J. S., *Work Stress and Social Support*, Addison-Wesley, Reading, MA, 1981.
4. Cobb, S., Social support as a moderator of life stress, *Psychosom. Med.*, 38, 300–314, 1976.

5. Bowlby, J., *Attachment and Loss, Vol. I: Attachment* (Rev. ed.), Basic Books, New York, 1982.
6. Bowlby, J., *A Secure Base*, Basic Books, New York, 1988.
7. Shumaker, S. A. and Brownell, A., Toward a theory of social support: closing conceptual gaps, *J. Soc. Issues*, 40(4), 11–16, 1994.
8. Quick, J. C., Nelson, D. L., and Quick, J. D. *Stress and Challenge at the Top: The Paradox of the Successful Executive*, John Wiley & Sons, Chichester, England, 1990.
9. Zey, M. G., *Winning with People*, Jeremy P. Tarcher, Los Angeles, 1990.
10. Bloom, J. R., The relationship of social support and health, *Soc. Sci. Med.*, 30, 635–637, 1990.
11. Callaghan, P. and Morrissey, J., Social support and health: a review, *J. Adv. Nurs.*, 18, 203–210, 1993.
12. House, J. S. and Wells, J. A., Occupational stress, social support, and health, in *Proc. Reducing Occup. Stress Conf. (DHEW (NIOSH) Pub. 78–140)*, McLean, A., Black, G., and Colligan, M., Eds., U. S. Government Printing Office, Washington, D.C., 1978, 8–19.
13. Fleury, J., An exploration of the role of social networks in cardiovascular risk reduction, *Heart Lung*, 22, 134–144, 1993.
14. Kulik, J. A. and Mahler, H. I. M., Social support and recovery from surgery, *Health Psychol.*, 8, 221–238, 1989.
15. Gerin, W., Pieper, C., Levy, R., and Pickering, T. G., Social support in social interaction: a moderator of cardiovascular reactivity, *Psychosom. Med.*, 54, 324–336, 1992.
16. Connell, C. M., Davis, W. K., Gallant, M. P., and Sharpe, T. A., Impact of social support, social cognitive variables and perceived threat on depression among adults with diabetes, *Health Psychol.*, 13, 263–273, 1994.
17. Revenson, T. A. and Majerovitz, S. D., The effects of chronic illness on the spouse, *Arthritis Care Res.*, 4, 63–72, 1991.
18. Spiegel, D., Effects of psychosocial support on patients with metastic breast cancer, *J. Psychosoc. Oncol.*, 10, 113–120, 1992.
19. Horman, S., The role of social support on health throughout the lifecycle, *Health Educ.*, 20, 18–21, 1989.
20. Hibbard, J. H. and Pope, C. R., Women's employment, social support, and mortality, *Women Health*, 18, 119–133, 1992.
21. Falk, A., Bertil, S. H., Isacsson, S., and Ostergren, P., Job strain and mortality in elderly men: social network, support, and influence as buffers, *Am. J. Public Health*, 82, 1136–1139, 1992.
22. Greller, M. M., Parsons, C. K., and Mitchell, D. R. D., Additive effects and beyond: occupational stressors and social buffers in a police organization, in *Stress and Well-being at Work*, Quick, J. C., Murphy, L. R., and Hurrell, J. J., Jr., Eds., American Psychological Association, Washington, D.C., 1992, chap. 3.
23. Kobasa, S. C. O., Maddi, S. R., Puccetti, M. C., and Zola, M. A., Effectiveness of hardiness, exercise and social support as resources against illness, *J. Psychosom. Res.*, 29, 525–533, 1985.
24. Cohen, S. and Edwards, J. R., Personality characteristics as moderators of the relationship between stress and disorder, in *Advances in the Investigation of Psychological Stress*, Neufeld, W. J., Ed., John Wiley & Sons, New York, 1989, 235–283.

25. Frankenhauser, M., The psychophysiology of workload, stress, and health: comparison between the sexes, *Ann. Behav. Med.*, 13, 197–204, 1991.
26. Vinokur, A. D. and van Ryn, M., Social support and undermining in close relationships: their independent effects on the mental health of unemployed persons, *J. Personality Soc. Psychol.*, 65, 350–359, 1993.
27. Auslander, G. K. and Litwin, H., Social networks, social support, and self-ratings of health among the elderly, *J. Aging Health*, 3, 493–510, 1991.
28. Shumaker, S. A. and Hill, D. R., Gender differences in social support and physical health, *Health Psychol.*, 10, 102–111, 1991.
29. Romano, P. S., Bloom, J., and Syme, S. L., Smoking, social support, and hassles in an urban African-American community, *Am. J. Public Health*, 81, 1415–1421, 1991.
30. Evans, G. W., Palsane, M. N., Lepore, S. J., and Martin, J., Residential density and psychological health: the mediating effects of social support, *J. Personality Soc. Psychol.*, 57, 994–999, 1989.
31. Cohen, S. and Wills, T. A., Stress, social support, and the buffering hypothesis, *Psychol. Bull.*, 98, 310–357, 1985.
32. Reifman, A., Biernat, M., and Lang, E. L., Stress, social support, and health in married professional women with small children, *Psychol. Women Q.*, 15, 431–445, 1991.
33. Wilcox, V. L., Kasl, S. V., and Berkman, L. F., Social support and physical disability in older people after hospitalization: a prospective study, *Health Psychol.*, 13, 170–179, 1994.
34. Revicki, D. A. and Mitchell, J. P., Strain, social support, and mental health in rural elderly individuals, *J. Gerontol.*, 45, S267–274, 1990.
35. Sprecher, S., Investment model, equity, and social support determinants of relationship commitment, *Soc. Psychol. Q.*, 51, 318–328, 1988.
36. Cummins, R., Locus of control and social support: clarifiers of the relationship between job stress and job satisfaction, *J. Appl. Soc. Psychol.*, 19, 772–788, 1989.
37. Linden, W., Chambers, L., Maurice, J., and Lenz, J. W., Sex differences in social support, self-deception, hostility, and ambulatory cardiovascular activity, *Health Psychol.*, 12, 376–380, 1993.
38. Hazan, C. and Shaver, P., Love and work: an attachment-theoretical perspective, *J. Personality Soc. Psychol.*, 59, 270–280, 1990.
39. Quick, J. C., Joplin, J. R., Nelson, D. L., and Quick, J. D., Behavioral responses to anxiety: self-reliance, counter-dependence and overdependence, *Anxiety, Stress Coping*, 5, 41–54, 1992.
40. Cooley, C. E., *The Distress Vulnerable Child*, Fourth Street Project, Arlington, Texas, Undated.
41. Vaillant, G. E., Attachment, loss and rediscovery, *Hillside J. Clin. Psychiatry*, 10, 148–164, 1988.
42. Ornish, D., *Dr. Dean Ornish's Program for Reversing Cardiovascular Disease*, Random House, New York, 1990, chap. 9.
43. Ornish, D., *Dr. Dean Ornish's Program for Reversing Cardiovascular Disease*, Random House, New York, 1990, p. 232.
44. Pargament, K. I., Olsen, H., Reilly, B., Falgout, K., Ensing, D. S., and Van Haitsma, K., God help me. II. The relationship of religious orientations to religious coping with negative life events, *J. Sci. Study Religion*, 31(4), 504–513, 1992.

45. Ross, C. E., Religion and psychological distress, *J. Sci. Study Religion*, 29(2), 236–245, 1990.

46. All Old and New Testament Biblical references come from the New American Standard Bible.

47. Kirkpatrick, L. A. and Shaver, P. R., Attachment theory and religion: childhood attachments, religious beliefs, and conversion, *J. Sci. Study Religion*, 29(3), 315–334, 1990.

48. Radhakrishnan, S., *The Hindu View of Life*, Macmillan, New York, 1975.

49. David-Neel, A., *Buddhism*, Mandala Books, London, 1939.

50. Borysenko, J., *Minding the Body, Mending the Mind*, Bantam, Toronto, 1987.

51. Sethi, S. and Seligman, M. E. P., Optimism and fundamentalism, *Psychol. Sci.*, 4, 256–259, 1993.

52. Durkheim, E., *Suicide: A Study in Sociology*, Free Press, New York, 1951 (Original work published 1897).

53. Bergin, A. E., Religiosity and mental health: a critical reevaluation and meta-analysis, *Professional Psychol. Res. Pract.*, 14, 170–184, 1983.

54. Rodin, J. and Ickovics, J. R., Women's health: review and research agenda as we approach the 21st century, *Am. Psychol.*, 45, 1018–1033, 1990.

55. Trobst, K. K., Collins, R. L., and Embree, J. M., The role of emotion in social support provision: gender, empathy and expressions of distress, *J. Soc. Personal Relationships*, 11 45–62, 1994.

56. Cook, T. D. and Campbell D. T., *Quasi-Experimentation: Design & Analysis Issues for Field Settings*, Houghton-Mifflin, Boston, 1979.

Stress, health, and families

chapter fifteen

Destiny of hope: immigrant couples coping with multiple stresses

Lea Baider, Bella Kaufman, Pnina Ever-Hadani, and Atara Kaplan De-Nour

Background

As part of an ongoing interest in the study of coping with stress, we studied 166 couples who were new immigrants to Israel from the former Soviet Union and in whom one of the partners had cancer. The main focus of the present study was to understand how people cope with two severe stresses—immigration and cancer disease.

The psychological distress of the patients was very high and that of the spouses just a little lower. The adjustment of the couples to the new country was, as they reported, very poor. One is inclined to link the two findings, suggesting that the extremely high distress of the subjects is due to the additive impact of the two stresses—immigration and cancer disease. However, we did not find a significant relationship between the distress and any of the specific "immigration" factors studied: length of time in Israel, additional family in Israel, and the subjects' assessment of their employment or of their social situation. The only factor that had a protective effect was employment, but only in the groups of male patients and their wives.

Thus, we are inclined to suggest that the stress of immigration does make the subjects, and especially the patients, more vulnerable to extreme psychological distress. However, we could not pinpoint any specific causal factors.

We did not find a difference in the level of psychological distress of male and female patients (controlling for age and medical condition). Male patients had, as one could expect, higher distress than their wives. Contrary to the expected husbands' distress, it was not significantly lower than that of the female patients.

0-8493-2908-6/96/$0.00+$.50
© 1996 by CRC Press, Inc.

As in previous studies, a significant relationship was found between the distress of patients and spouses. Furthermore, it seems that we found a partial answer about directionality: the female patients' coping (Intrusiveness on the Impact of Events Scale, IES), contributed substantially and significantly to the distress of the husbands. It seems that the women coping with disease affects not only their own psychological distress but also that of their husbands. At the same time, the men coping with their disease does not affect the emotional welfare of their wives.

Another major gender difference was found with family support, which had no significant protective effect only on the female patients.

These findings strongly suggest that there are, indeed, gender differences in coping with stress. The findings also suggest that specific interventions, which take these gender differences into account, could be more effective (e.g., reducing the intrusiveness of disease in female patients should improve the emotional welfare of their husbands, too, while supplying more support to female patients might do only little to benefit the couples. On the other hand, supplying support to male patients could be very effective for the couple interaction).

Introduction

The epic migration of Jews from the former Soviet Union to Israel has given researchers a rare opportunity to study the human condition from a wide variety of perspectives.

Between the end of 1989 and June 1992, 380,152 Soviet citizens swelled Israel's population by nearly 10%. The waves of immigrants came from an array of ethnic backgrounds. The newcomers were highly diverse, not only in terms of age, education, customs, and beliefs, but also in the prevalence of a number of diseases (Bar-Zuri and Hendels, 1993; Fishman, 1994; Rosen and Ottenstein, 1994). This historic migration, unlike most others, was not economically motivated: many were forced to flee because of danger, hardship, and discrimination.

The demographics of this particular immigration differed substantially even from preceding Soviet-Jewish migrations. Educational and professional levels were higher and the average age was higher as well, proportionally exceeding that of Israel's general population: the over-65s comprised 11.8% of Russian immigrants in 1990 and 12.3% in 1991, compared with 10.7% in the general population (Gitelman, 1992; Statistical Abstract of Israel, 1993).

Although immigration is a worldwide phenomenon, its complex influence on health and quality of life has not been sufficiently explored or understood. Several studies have investigated the relationship between immigration and mental health, chiefly by examining psychiatric disturbances among immigrants. Hertz (1993), Popper and Horowitz (1992), and Shemesh et al. (1993), consistently found that immigrant populations exhibit greater psychological distress than nonimmigrants.

The psychopathology of immigration, which may result from the intense anxieties inherent in the process, has been examined also by Grinberg and Grinberg (1984) and Lerner and Zilber (1991). Individual common symptoms include depression, anxiety disorders, somatic complaints, and a sense of helplessness.

To our surprise, only scattered information has been reported on physical illness. With few exceptions, the implications of illness behavior and medical care in this population have been almost ignored or referred to only tangentially. For older immigrants, the medical realities of aging and chronic illness—compounded by the cultural differences—make the health care system a natural vehicle where stress of immigration is expressed.

When these people left their homeland, they lost not only their natural environment but also their role within the extended family, their professional status, and their familiar culture, language, and idioms. From the start, they found themselves handicapped by often insurmountable cultural barriers. Frailty and age-related illnesses underscored their losses.

Studies of illness behavior among immigrants reveal a dimension of interaction with the environment that is not readily explained in terms of culturally distinct beliefs, values, or customary practices.

For newcomers, cultural dynamism in their adopted country is of particular importance. Changes in economic, social, and medical customs force old and familiar routines to reorganize and reacculturate—which could affect health. Intercurrent illnesses can be influenced directly and indirectly through diet, sanitary habits, environment, and climatic factors such as humidity and temperature. Social behavior, lifestyle, and system of beliefs may be inappropriate, maladaptive, or even pathogenic in the host country; and that, too, can affect health, though usually at a slow rate (Althausen, 1991; Hull, 1979).

In a recent survey of new immigrants from the former Soviet Union, Rosen and Ottenstein (1994) selected a sample of 1200 individuals from a pool of 181,000 newcomers aged 25 to 65 years. Almost half of the interviewees said that at least one family member was chronically ill, and 20% indicated that they themselves were suffering from some kind of chronic illness.

Naon and King (1993), using the same population of 181,000, found that elderly immigrants reported a significant deficiency in their physical health, at a much higher rate than that of comparable Israelis: some 89% of new immigrants aged 65 or older assessed their health as bad or not good, as compared to only 64% of Israelis of the same age bracket. Data from the Israel Cancer Registry have shown that 1% of the early arrivals (December 1989 to December 1991) had neoplastic disease—an age- and sex-adjusted cancer rate of 350/100,000 versus 225/100,000 for native Israelis. The additional 3500 cases would account for the flooding of the oncology centers around the country with Russian immigrants (Fishman, 1994).

Our study comprises a sample of 166 Soviet immigrant couples, with one of the partners having been diagnosed as suffering from cancer. There is vast clinical and research evidence that cancer puts severe distress both on the affected individual and the family. This psychological byproduct of the disease has concerned clinicians and researchers, and many have attempted to describe and delimit the psychological and social sequelae of cancer and its treatment (Cella, 1987; Cooper, 1984; Cooper and Watson, 1991; Noyes et al., 1990).

Cancer diagnosis and treatment are powerfully negative stressful events that often alter the victim's physiological and psychological homeostasis. The sufferer requires maximum adaptive response to reduce the effects of these stresses, in order to return a harrowingly disrupted life to some degree of normalcy.

The new immigrant who suffers from cancer has to deal with two highly demanding stress situations, which could well overtax an individual's capacity to adapt. This report investigates the lives of new immigrants who must deal with the double stress of living with a chronic illness in a new and unfamiliar culture.

Subjects and methods

Our study sample was drawn from the medical records at the Institute of Oncology at Hadassah University Hospital in Jerusalem. Each medical record provides data on sociodemographic background, including country of origin and date of immigration.

We collected the names of all cancer patients registered at the Institute who arrived in Israel between October 1989 and February 1992 and who had settled, at least temporarily, in Jerusalem. The selection criteria within this population were: being a Russian immigrant with a stable partner or spouse who was also a newcomer, being registered as an outpatient at Hadassah's Oncology Department, and being in relatively good physical condition with a minimal Karnofsky rating of 60.

One hundred eighty-one ambulatory married patients were identified. However, 11 patients could not be located, and another 4 refused to be interviewed because they were suspicious of our motives. This reduced the final sample to 166 cancer patients (123 women and 43 men) and their partners.

Table 1 presents the sociodemographic background of the group. This is a group of elderly people who have been in Israel an average of 2.5 years and who have a higher level of education than the national average. About 40% of them had left family behind when they emigrated, and only about 25% of them had family in Israel.

Initial contact with the patients was done by phone by a research assistant, also a new immigrant from the former Soviet Union. Patients and spouses were interviewed at their homes by the same assistant. After sign-

Table 1   Sociodemographic Background

	Male patients	Wives	Female patients	Husbands
Number	43	43	123	123
Age mean years	64.0	61.0	57.0	59.6
Education mean years	15.0	14.1	14.0	14.5
Mean months in Israel	28.7	28.7	28.1	28.7
% have family in former USSR	44	35	48	44
% have family in Israel	28	33	24	25

ing a consent form (written in Russian), a semistructured interview took place. Information was gathered about their social background, absorption, and assessment of their life in Israel. They assessed their employment, economic, and social situations as better, not changed, or worse than in their country of origin. As no one answered "better", it was later decided to record the answers in two categories of "no change" and "worse."

Following the interviews, the patients were administered three and the spouses two self-reports translated into Russian:

1. Family support was assessed according to the Perceived Family Support (PFS) questionnaire (Procidano and Heller, 1983), which consists of 20 questions with scores ranging from 0 (no support) to 20 (maximal support).
2. Psychological distress was assessed by the Brief Symptom Inventory (BSI) questionnaire (Derogatis, 1982), an abbreviated form of the SCL90, composed of 53 questions. The BSI provides a global score of distress (GSI), as well as information about nine specific dimensions of distress, such as somatization, depression, anxiety, and hostility. The raw scores were later transformed to a T score along the American norms for nonpatients (there are no Israeli norms) to enable comparison between males and females.
3. The patients were also administered the Impact of Events Scale (IES) (Horowitz et al., 1979), a 15-item questionnaire that measures to what extent an event (cancer in this study) is intrusive and how much the respondent tries to cope with the stress of avoidance.

Medical information on each patient was acquired from their medical records and is presented in Table 2. Female patients had significantly higher Karnofsky scores ($p = 0.05$). No significant difference was found between

Table 2   Medical Information

	Male patients	Female patients
Number	43	123
Months from		
diagnosis	30/31.8	31/32.4
Breast		73
Uterus		20
GIT	20	11
Lymphomas	7	3
Lung	3	1
Others	13	15
Karnofsky	82/16.0	89/11.8
Stage		
I	3	12
II	12	56
III	16	25
IV	5	15
Still unknown	4	3
Russian diagnosis	3	12
Active Disease		
Active	16	53
Not Active	8	32
Follow-Up	19	38

male patients and female patients for stage and active disease. Note that less than 10% of the patients were diagnosed before emigrating, that is, a population of new immigrants who have had to cope with cancer diagnosed only shortly after their arrival.

Results

Table 3 presents the adjustment and the reported distress of the subjects for the four groups: male patients, their wives, female patients, and their husbands.

Most of the subjects were unemployed, which was only partly related to their age. They assessed their economic and social situation as greatly deteriorated compared to pre-immigration: about 60% stated that their employment situation is worse now than it had been, and over 70% assessed their economic and social situations as worse. Thus, both patients and spouses described very poor adjustment.

On the Perceived Family Support, most of the subjects reported high perceived family support. Nonetheless, they also reported extreme psychological distress. The definition of "caseness" is a GSI score of 63 or higher. Only the group of wives fell below that level for "psychopathol-

Table 3   Adjustment and Psychological Distress

	Male patients	Wives	Female patients	Husbands
Number	43	43	123	123
% Working	14	19	11	37
Employment worse %	65	60	65	56
Economic worse %	81	81	73	76
Social worse %	77	74	79	72
Perceived family support (PFS)	17.5	16.5	16.5	16.4
Psychological distress (GSI)	67.5	62.0	64.2	63.1
Somatization	68.9	62.1	66.4	60.7
Obsessive-compulsive	63.9	61.6	60.3	62.2
Interpersonal sensitivity	59.3	60.9	61.1	57.1
Depression	62.3	57.8	59.4	60.8
Anxiety	65.3	60.0	62.1	60.9
Hostility	63.9	59.6	61.1	59.7
Phobic anxiety	60.6	56.0	59.2	58.9
Paranoid	54.1	56.2	53.6	53.6
Psychoticism	61.8	60.5	61.7	58.8

ogy". The husbands were at the cut-off point, the female patients above it, and the male patients far above it (Razavi and Stiefel, 1994).

On the IES, the patients have mobilized a great deal of avoidance, yet the disease was still intrusive. Males scored 14.5 (SD 6.99) on Avoidance and 11.7 (SD 8.26) on Intrusiveness. Female scores were not much different: 13.9 (SD 4.75) on Avoidance and 12.7 (SD 8.00) on Intrusiveness.

The four groups were compared to each other using paired *T*-tests when comparing patients to spouses and *T*-tests when comparing patients or spouses by gender (Table 4). No statistically significant difference was found between the groups in the assessment of life in Israel as compared to the former Soviet Union. In other words, both patients and spouses perceived similar amounts of deterioration in employment, economic, and social conditions.

In the category of perceived family support, the only notable difference was that male patients reported higher support than their wives. This expected difference was not found in the female group; i.e., the female patients did not report having more support than their husbands.

Table 4 Comparison of Background and Adjustment

	Male/ Female patients	Male patients/ Wives	Pearson correlation	Female patients/ Husbands	Pearson correlation	Wives/ Husbands
Number	M-43 F-123					W-43 H-123
Age	0.002	0.000		0.000		—
Employment %	—	—		—		0.020
Psychological distress (GSI)	0.050	0.000	.76	—	.42	—
Somatization	—	0.000	.74	0.000	.49	—
Obsessive-compulsive	—	—	.58	0.050	.47	—
Interpersonal sensitivity	—	—	.49	0.000	.23	0.030
Depression	—	0.003	.71	—	.21	—
Anxiety	—	0.000	.73	—	.41	—
Hostility	—	0.005	.48	—	NS	—
Phobic anxiety	—	0.020	.31	—	.28	—
Paranoid	—	—	.59	—	.45	—
Psychoticism	—	—	.52	0.009	.34	—

Nonrelated groups compared by t-test and couples by paired t-test;— nonsignificant.

The female patients reported significantly lower psychological distress than the male patients. However, the two groups differed in age and Karnofsky score. Once these two variables were controlled (ANCOVA), the main effect of gender on psychological distress became nonsignificant.

Female patients and their husbands did not differ on psychological distress, but male patients reported much higher distress than their wives. This latter finding was maintained when the groups were subdivided into three age categories, and, again, when subdivided into three levels of support. Thus, one can say that in all age groups and in all levels of support, the male patients expressed higher distress than their wives.

We sought further understanding into the factors that influence the psychological distress in each of the four groups of subjects. Some variables have no relation to the GSI in any of the groups, including how long they had been in Israel, how long they had been sick, whether they had family in Israel, as well as their assessment of employment and social situation. Table 5 summarizes the univariate analysis—significant Pearson correlations for the continuous variables and the ANOVA for the dichotomous variables—of the factors that related significantly to the GSI. (The variables in the spouses' analysis are those of the spouses, except for the IES which are only the patients' scores.) Being employed had a relation to the GSI in all the groups. The spouse's education did not reduce his or her psychological distress. It should also be noted that patients' scores on the intrusion subscale of the IES correlated not only with their own distress but also with that of their spouses.

Table 6 summarizes the multiple regressions based on the data from Table 5. Note that the factors studied explain more of the variance in the

Table 5 Variables Related to GSI

	Male patients	Wives	Female patients	Husbands
Number	43	43	123	123
Significant				
Pearson correlation				
Age				0.28
Education	−0.46		−0.27	
Karnofsky			−0.21	
IES-Intrusion	0.49	0.31	0.64	0.34
IES-Avoidance	−0.36			
PFS	−0.44	−.032	−0.26	−.026
ANOVA				
Significant results				
Employed	0.0011	0.0031	0.0319	0.0094
Economic situation		0.0800	0.0028	0.0500

Table 6 Factors Influencing Psychological Distress

Male Patients

$F = 11.50\ p = .0000$ Multiple R .740 R^2 .548

Variable	T	sig. T
IES-Intrusion	2.696	.0104
PFS	−2.895	.0063
Education	−2.113	.0413
Employment	−2.289	.0277

Not in equation: IES-Avoidance, Karnofsky

Wives

$F = 7.18\ p = .0022$ Multiple R .514 R^2 .264

Variable		
PFS	−1.954	.0577
Employment	−2.838	.0071

Not in equation: IES-Intrusion (patient), economic situation

Female Patients

$F = 32.32\ p = .0000$ Multiple R .670 R^2 .449

Variable		
IES-Intrusion	8.108	.0000
Education	−1.742	.0840
Economic situation	2.613	.0096

Not in equation: Karnofsy, PFS, employment

Husbands

$F = 15.95\ p = .0000$ Multiple R .539 R^2 .290

Variable		
IES-Intrusion (Patient)	3.023	.0031
PFS	−4.594	.0000
Age	2.866	.0049

Not in equation: employment, economic situation

patients' groups than in the spouses' groups, even though the physical condition (Karnofsky score) lost its significant influence on the psychological distress.

Education maintained its protective influence in the patients' groups but not among the spouses (Cella et al., 1991). Being employed maintained its influence on the male patients and wives but not on the female patients and their husbands.

Of special interest is the finding that only among the female patients did perceived family support have no protective effect. Furthermore, only among the husbands did the intrusion of the sick partner have a very significant impact on the husband's psychological distress.

Discussion

It is argued that a multitude of factors influence the ability to manage chronic illness. For the chronically ill immigrant, the difficulties are exacerbated by the experience of uprooting from the homeland and resettling in a new country.

It is well documented in the health care literature that ethnicity patterns our behavior in ways both subtle and obvious. Ethnicity plays a major role in determining how we feel about health and illness and how we manage treatment (Helman, 1984; Sachs, 1983; Waxler-Morrison, et al., 1990).

Findings of various studies have led to a sharper focus on how illness is affected by the total circumstances of a person's life. It is acknowledged that cultural categories confer specific meaning on illness and that the meaning and experience of illness are not static but are reorganized through social interaction within a new country's environment (Althausen, 1991).

We may ask, then, what the effects are of chronic stress, such as migration, on coping with an additional crisis, such as cancer. Is coping with a new trauma more difficult when one is already under stress, or are individuals strengthened with each crisis and become more capable of dealing with subsequent stresses?

Theorists have offered conflicting answers. Research suggests that various types of prior stresses may influence subsequent coping very differently—sometimes with a positive effect and at other times proving deleterious. The first view contends that repeated stresses strengthen the ability to cope and promote resilience in the face of future adversity (Coleman et al., 1980; Gibertini et al., 1992). However, there is more consistent evidence that people who undergo severe stress are left more vulnerable and more sensitive to future adversity (Baider et al., 1993; Silver and Wortman, 1980; Solomon and Prager, 1992).

Christenson et al. (1981) examined the reactivation of stress reactions among elderly American World War II combat veterans. The study found that stressful life events such as retirement, relocation, loss of job, and death of a loved one served as triggers that accelerated and unmasked latent post-traumatic stress disorders.

We studied a group of 166 couples who had to cope with two severe stresses: immigration and cancer. The subjects emigrated from the former Soviet Union and have been in Israel an average of 2.5 years. They were elderly, well-educated, and only about 25% of them had relatives in Israel. One partner had cancer (43 men and 123 women) which, in over 90% of the cases, was diagnosed after immigration.

Integration in Israel was poor: the great majority were unemployed and assessed their employment, economic, and social situations as worse than before immigration. Psychological distress of the patients was extremely high and that of the spouses nearly as high. Distress of patients was much higher than in most groups we have studied in the past (Baider and Kaplan De-Nour, 1988) and similar to that found in cancer patients who had referred themselves for intervention (Baider et al., 1994).

It seems in our study, however, that only little of this severe distress can be attributed to immigration. Even in univariate analysis, life situations, such as length of time in Israel, having family in Israel, or having left family behind, had no significant relation to psychological distress.

The same lack of relationship was found between the subjects' psychological distress and their assessment of social and employment situations. Only having or not having a job had a notable effect on psychological distress, and in the multivariate analysis, it remained significant only for couples in which the man was ill. Economic situation only maintained a significant relationship in the female patients' group.

Our study stresses similar findings by other reports. For example, Bultena (1969) evaluated the effects of a voluntary migration of elderly people from northern American states to retirement areas in the south. Bultena studied the role of health in the decision to move, as well as the effects of health on adaptation. People in poor health fell disproportionately in the lower socioeconomic status and scored lower on the Life Satisfaction Scale. Better socioeconomic status and success in finding employment were directly related to better health status and were positively associated with rapid adaptation to the new environment, especially for women.

In the present study, the specific immigration variables studied did not explain the severe psychological distress. Yet, we would like to suggest that the upheaval of immigration must have made them vulnerable, resulting in the very high psychological distress we observed, especially in the patients. Klinger (1977) and Raphael (1983) maintain that individuals facing an overwhelming set of problems are likely to find their coping capacities beyond normal adaptive capacities. Weisman (1979) found that cancer patients who exhibited higher levels of emotional distress either had marital problems, were unemployed, came from lower socioeconomic strata, or had marginal resources.

No gender differences were found in psychological distress on either the patients or the spouses. In the past, we did report gender differences (Baider et al., 1989, 1993), with female patients reporting higher distress than male patients, and husbands reporting more distress than wives. However, that was when only one diagnosis was studied.

The patients had high scores both on Avoidance and on Intrusion. In this sample, Avoidance seemed to be a "good" mechanism in decreasing distress, but the relationship was not statistically significant (in multivariate analysis). On the other hand, the contribution of Intrusion was very substantial. One could suggest, therefore, that patients with high intrusiveness should be regarded as vulnerable and that psychological intervention should aim to reduce this mechanism.

Significant correlation was found between distress of the patients and that of their partners, as reported in earlier studies (Baider and Kaplan De-Nour, 1988), suggesting a "transmission" of distress within the couple but saying nothing about directionality.

We see as important the findings that the patient's score on Intrusion contributed to the husband's psychological distress. We have often speculated about the directionality of transmission of distress within the couple. The present finding strongly supports the suggestion that the ill woman and her coping with the disease influence the psychological welfare of her healthy husband. That was not found in couples in which the man was sick. The intrusion scores of the male patients did not influence the psychological distress of their healthy wives.

Another point we would like to make concerns family support. The female patients reported notably less (perceived) family support. Furthermore, in multivariate analysis, family support had no significant protective effect in the female patients, though it did in all other groups: male patients, healthy wives, and healthy husbands.

Studies on social support stressed the importance of the family as the most intimate and natural environment of support. It is, however, a major source of emotional stress as well as social support, both of which affect health. The most important source of social support appears to be the spouse (Bloom, 1982; Winefield and Neuling, 1987; Wortman, 1984).

Our results suggest that the male patient feels more supported than the female patient. It seems, however, that there is also gender difference in the importance of support; i.e., that it is more important for the emotional well-being of the male patient than of the female patient.

The last point we would like to make is about the lack of relationship of physical condition (as expressed by the Karnofsky score) and psychological distress. None of the patients had very low scores, which suggests that in such patients the distress is probably more connected to being a cancer patient than to actual physical condition.

The immigrant's experience of illness, the mediating circumstances that influence quality of life, the emotions, fears, and difficulties of dealing with a totally new environment and system of health care, all have a bearing on how illness is managed. Yet, these aspects of a person's life are often not seen as an integral part of cancer management.

Health-care personnel could contribute at least partially. Counseling might decrease the stress of "being a cancer patient" and thus decrease the psychological distress.

Acknowledgment

This research project was supported by the Dr. Esther Haar Award.

References

Althausen, L., (1991). Reflections on working with elderly Soviet immigrants. *Jewish Soc. Work Forum*, 27, 46–55.

Baider, L. and Kaplan De-Nour, A. (1988). Breast cancer—a family affair. in *Stress and Breast Cancer* (Ed. C. L. Cooper), John Wiley & Sons, New York, 155–170.

Baider, L. and Kaplan De-Nour, A. (1993). Impact of cancer on couples. *Cancer Invest.*, 11, 706–713.

Baider, L., Peretz, T., and Kaplan De-Nour, A. (1989). Gender and adjustment to chronic disease: a study of couples with colon cancer. *Gen. Hosp. Psychiatry*, 11, 1–8.

Baider, L., Peretz, T., and Kaplan De-Nour, A. (1993). Holocaust cancer patients: a comparative study, *Psychiatry*, 56, 349–355.

Baider, L., Uziely, B., and Kaplan De-Nour, A. (1994). Progressive muscle relaxation and guided imagery in cancer patients, *Gen. Hosp. Psychiatry*, 16, 340–347.

Bar-Zuri, R. and Hendels, S. (1993). *Needs and priorities of Russian immigrants.* Institute of Economic and Social Research, General Trade Unions Organization Publication, Tel-Aviv, Israel (Monograph in Hebrew).

Bloom, J. R. (1982). Social support, accommodation to stress and adaptation to breast cancer. *Soc. Sci. Med.*, 16, 1329–1338.

Bultena, G. L. (1969). Health patterns of aged migrant retirees, *J. Am. Geriatr. Soc.*, 17, 1127–1131.

Cella, D. F. (1987). Cancer survival: psychosocial and public issues, *Cancer Invest.*, 5, 59–67.

Cella, D. F., Orav, J. E., Kornbilt, A. B., Holland, J. et al. (1991). Socioeconomic status and cancer survival, *J. Clin. Oncol.*, 9, 1500–1509.

Christenson, R. M., Walker, J. I., Ross, D. R., and Maltbie, A. A. (1981). Reactivation of traumatic conflicts. *Am. J. Psychiatry*, 138, 984–985.

Coleman, J. C., Burcher, J. N., and Carson, R. C. (Eds.) (1980). *Abnormal Psychology and Modern Life*, 6th ed., Scott Foresman, Glenview, IL.

Cooper, C. L. (Ed.) (1984). *Psychosocial Stress and Cancer*. John Wiley & Sons, New York.

Cooper, C. L. and Watson, M. (Eds.) (1991). *Cancer and Stress*, John Wiley & Sons, New York.

Derogatis, L. R. (1982). *The Brief Symptom Inventory (B.S.I.) Administration, Scoring and Procedures Manual*, Clinical Psychometric Research, Baltimore, MD.

Derogatis, L. R., Morrow, G., Fetting, J., Penman, D. et al. (1983). The prevalence and severity of psychiatric disorders among cancer patients, *JAMA*, 249, 751–757.

Fishman, R. H. B. (1994). Russians and unhealthy migrant effect in Israel, *Lancet*, 343, 966.

Gibertini, M., Reintgen, D. S., and Baile, W. F. (1992). Psychosocial aspects of melanoma. *Ann. Plast. Surg.*, 28, 17–21.

Gitelman, Z. (1992). Recent demographic and migratory trends among Soviet Jews: implications for policy. *Post-Soviet Geography*, 33, 139–145.

Grinberg, L. and Grinberg, R. (1984). A psychoanalytic study of migration: its normal and pathological aspects, *J. Am. Psychoanal. Assoc.*, 32, 13–38.

Helman, C. (1984). *Culture, Health and Illness: An Introduction for Health Professionals*, Wright and Sons, London.

Hertz, Dan G. (1993). Bio-psychosocial consequences of migration: a multidimensional approach. *Isr. J. Psychiatry*, 30, 204–212.

Horowitz, M. J., Wilner, N., and Alvarez, W. (1979). Impact of event scale: a measure of subjective stress, *Psychosom. Med.*, 41, 209–218.

Hull, D. (1979). Migration, adaptation and illness: a review, *Soc. Sci. Med.*, 13A, 25–36.

Klinger, E. (1977). *Meaning and Void: Inner Experiences and the Incentives in People's Lives*, University of Minnesota Press, Minneapolis.

Lerner, Y. and Zilber, N. (1991). *Psychological distress and help seeking behavior among Soviet immigrants*. Presented at the National Conference on Soviet Immigrants: Health and Mental Health, Chicago. Falk Institute, Publication No. 17. Research Report, J.D.C., Israel (Monograph).

Naon, D. and King, I. (1993). *Survey of elderly immigrants from the Soviet Union*, Brookdale Institute of Gerontology, J.D.C., Jerusalem, Israel (Monograph in Hebrew).

Noyes, R., Kathol, R. G., and Enemark, D. P. (1990). Distress associated with cancer as measured by the illness distress scale, *Psychosomatics*, 31, 321–330.

Popper, M. and Horowitz, R. (1992). *Immigrants in psychiatric hospitalization in Israel: Trends in 1988–1990*. Ministry of Health, Department of Information and Evaluation in Mental Health Services, Jerusalem. Statistical Report No. 7 (Monograph in Hebrew).

Procidano, M. E. and Heller, K. (1983). Measures of perceived social support from friends and from family: three validation studies, *Am. J. Community Psychol.*, 11, 1–24.

Rafael, B. (1983). *The Anatomy of Bereavement*, Basic Books, New York.

Razavi, D. and Stiefel, F. (1994). Common psychiatric disorders in cancer patients, I. *Supportive Care Cancer*, 2, 223–232.

Rosen, B. and Ottenstein, N. (1994). *Immigrants, Health and Health Care*. Brookdale Institute of Gerontology, J.D.C., Jerusalem, Israel (Monograph in Hebrew).

Sachs, L. (1983). *Evil Eye on Bacteria: Turkish Immigrant Women and Swedish Health Care*. Stockholm Studies in Social Anthropology. Stockholm Press, Stockholm.

Shemesh, A. A., Horowitz, R., Levinson, D., and Popper, M. (1993). Psychiatric hospitalization of immigrants to Israel from the former U.S.S.R: assessment of demands in future waves of immigration, *Isr. J. Psychiatry*, 30, 213–222.

Silver, R. L. and Wortman, C. B. (1980). Coping with undesirable life events, in *Human Helplessness* (Eds. J. Garber, and M. E. Seligman,), Academic Press, New York, 279–340.

Solomon, Z. and Prager, E. (1992). Elderly Israeli Holocaust survivors during the Persian Gulf war: a study of psychological distress, *Am. J. Psychiatry*, 149, 1707–1710.

Statistical Abstract of Israel 1993, No. 44, Central Bureau of Statistics, Jerusalem, Israel.

Waxler-Morrison, N., Anderson, J., and Robertson, E. (Eds.) (1990). *Cross-Cultural Caring: A Handbook for Health Professionals in Western Canada*, University of British Columbia Press, Vancouver.

Weisman, A. D. (1979). *Coping with Cancer*, McGraw-Hill, New York.

Winefield, H. R. and Neuling, S. J. (1987). Social support, counselling and cancer, *Br. J. Guidance Counselling*, 15, 6–16.

Wortman, C. B. (1984). Social support and the cancer patient, *Cancer*, 53, 2339–2360.

chapter sixteen

Social support and well-being in HIV disease

John Green and Agnes Kocsis

It is generally agreed that social support is an important factor in maintaining well-being in individuals affected by HIV/AIDS (human immunodeficiency virus/acquired immunodeficiency syndrome). It is much less clear why social support is important, what aspects of social support are important, which aspects of well-being social support affects, and how social support and its effects should be measured. These problems have created enormous confusion in the literature which, probably fortunately, have not been reflected in the efforts of service providers on the ground. The very extensive networks of social support provided in developed countries, and in many places in developing countries, for those affected by HIV/AIDS are an unusual, perhaps unique, aspect of this disease.

It is worthwhile considering some of the fundamental issues in the area before looking at the published research and considering some of its implications, and gaps.

Why social support is important

If social support is, in fact, useful to the individual, it is not at all clear why it is useful. One explanation might be that man is a social animal, we have an innate need for the contact of others, we seek to meet this need, and a failure to do so leaves us in a state of deprivation and distress. However, this is a static model; presumably our need is likely to be the same when we are ill as when we are well. What might change in illness would be our ability to obtain social support. However, simple though the explanation is, it is only likely to be one part of a wider picture. Social contact with other people provides us with a number of very tangible gains.

Firstly, other people provide the basis for many sorts of pleasurable leisure activities. It is difficult to have a party or play squash or engage in amateur dramatics on your own. Conversation, which provides stimulation and interest to most people, is rather limited if you have no one to talk to except yourself.

Secondly, social support often provides practical as well as emotional help. If you are ill your friends may go shopping for you, your family may help you out financially, you may have someone to call upon if you become ill during the night.

Other people also provide feedback and advice on problems the individual is facing and it may well be that simply talking to others about problems allows the individual to put some structure to what is happening to them. If this is not so, it is hard to see why so many people seek formal counseling and therapy. There is no reason to suppose that such help is provided only by formal counselors and therapists; indeed, it would be suprising if more than a tiny proportion of such help was provided formally.

Other people can also provide factual information about HIV/AIDS and that information may well be positive, as when a person with AIDS is told that a particular symptom is not serious, and this, too, can be a form of support. Clearly a lot of such information is likely to be provided by health care professionals and voluntary organizations, but a lot of it may well come informally from others with HIV/AIDS.

What aspects of social support are important?

The measurement of social support has always been an area of considerable disagreement. In part the problem is methodological, but in large part it is conceptual. In order to measure social support effectively, it is necessary to know which aspect of social support is important. There are several possible dimensions of social support.

The amount of social support may be important. The size of the social network, how many friends and contacts one has, may be the key issue. The more people you have available the more likely it is that one of them will be able to help if you are in difficulties or simply want to find someone to go out with for the evening.

On the other hand, it may be the quality, rather than the quantity, of social support that matters. One close friend may be more likely to meet someone's needs than five acquaintances. So closeness may be a key factor. Particularly in the case of HIV/AIDS, a stigmatized disease, individuals may be unwilling to reveal their infection to people they are not close to and therefore may be unable to obtain support from them.

Or it may be that satisfaction with social support may be the critical factor. It is possible to have close friends but to feel that they are not meeting all one's needs. Particularly early in the HIV/AIDS epidemic many of our patients who had extensive networks of friends, and sufficient close friends, felt that only others who were infected themselves could properly understand the situation they found themselves in. The same situation applies to many patients in the U.K. today, particularly heterosexual patients who may know no one else with HIV infection.

The source of social support may also be important. The interactions between someone infected with HIV/AIDS and friends, family, sexual partner, and professional caregiver are likely to be different. It is striking that patients often seek to guard and protect family members, particularly parents, from the more unpleasant aspects of HIV/AIDS. Many patients do not wish to discuss their possible death with their parents (although there are exceptions), at least until they are *in extremis*. Different sources of social contact may fulfill different roles for an individual and it may be the balance of these different sources of contact, rather than overall volume, that matters.

In order to illuminate the issue of social support through research it is important to know what to measure. Measuring everything all at the same time is seldom possible, and even if it is, there still has to be some way of weighting the relative importance of different elements. Part of the confusion in the literature is the result of uncertainties about what to measure.

What aspects of well-being might be influenced by social support?

If social support does influence well-being there is a question about what aspect of well-being it influences. There are various possibilities. Firstly, it might in principle affect physical well-being. It might do so through some direct influence on the immune system, perhaps through helping to reduce stress. Psychological influences on immune functioning in HIV/AIDS are particularly difficult to identify (Green and Hedge, 1992); however, the possibility is there. On the other hand, social support might have an indirect effect on physical health. An individual with better social support might eat better, exercise more, look after themselves better, or be better looked after. Such an outcome would not be surprising.

An influence of social support on behavior, particularly risk behavior, would also be possible. Individuals who had greater support might feel more constrained by the norms of those around them, which might either lead to more or less risk behavior, depending on what those norms were. There might be other influences; for instance, sex can be a means of meeting other people. An individual with a wide range of social contacts might have less need to use this particular route to social contact and so might be able to modify risky sexual behaviors more easily. An individual with many social contacts might have more potential sexual partners and so be able to select those who were more positive about safer sex. At a very simple level, individuals with a permanent sexual partner might find implementing safer sex and reducing the number of sexual contacts easier than someone with no permanent partner.

However, the area in which almost all researchers would expect to see an effect of social support is in the area of psychological well-being. It is more difficult to decide which areas of psychological functioning might be affected. There is evidence on non-HIV infected individuals that those who have more supportive social networks are less prone to depression and so an effect on depression might be expected. This might or might not affect the rate of suicide. The effects on anxiety, obsessional problems, or on the incidence of major mental illness are less easy to predict. However, simply looking for an effect of social support on symptoms of mental ill-health is rather a narrow perspective. One might equally expect individuals with better social support to be happier or to have a higher "quality of life." Mental well-being cannot simply be reduced to an absence of psychiatric symptoms (Green and Henderson, 1993).

In looking for the effects of social support on well-being, it is important to be clear what the outcome measures or expected correlates of "better" social support might be. There is often a profound lack of clarity in the HIV/AIDS literature about this issue and it is hard to escape the conclusion that too few researchers give it much thought, relying all to often on the scales and questionnaires they happen to have to hand.

Individual differences

It would be a reasonable working hypothesis that, just as some people need more food than others or are less tolerant of high ambient temperatures, so individuals might differ in the sorts and amount of social support that they might require or like. It is not obvious that, if X amount of social support is good then 2X amount of social support is twice as good. Not only are there likely to be differences between individuals in their needs and requirements, but it is possible that the relationship between social support and other variables is not always linear. Indeed, it would be surprising if it were. Most people need some privacy and beyond a certain point they might find additional social contact or support overintrusive or positively aversive.

Social support and physical health

It might be thought that HIV/AIDS is an ideal area in which to test out the links between various physical aspects of immune functioning and disease and psychological factors. In fact a moment's reflection suggests that a disease that itself directly attacks the immune system is probably a poor model on which to test such ideas (Green and Hedge, 1992). Any effect of psychological factors on immune functioning is likely to be more difficult to pick up against the background of the persistent viral attack on the immune system seen in this disease.

There are other difficulties. It is a problem to know what measure of physical health to use as an outcome measure. There are several possible measures. The level of CD4+ lymphocytes is frequently used as a measure of immune functioning in AIDS. There is a broad trend towards individuals who are in worse health having lower levels of CD4+ cells, as these are one of the main targets of HIV, and the loss or impairment of such cells is a major factor in the disease process in HIV disease. However, CD4+ levels in the individual are naturally subject to large fluctuations and the links between absolute CD4+ levels and overall physical health in the individual are a good deal less close than they are when averaged for large groups.

At best, CD4+ levels are a crude measure of worsening immune functioning subject to large apparently random variance. Some antiviral treatments appear to elevate CD4+ levels independently of any noticeable effect on the underlying disease process. Where CD4+ levels are used as an outcome measure, large samples and considerable caution in interpretation have to be used.

More direct measures of outcome can be used. For instance, measures of the number of symptoms individuals have can be used. However, many individuals with HIV infection have few or no symptoms. It can be difficult to tell the difference between some of the direct physical symptoms of HIV disease and physical symptoms of depression. Anxiety and mood state may influence readiness to report symptoms and the importance attached to them by patients. This is obviously an important potential confound in studies of the effects of social and psychological factors.

Progression to frank AIDS can also be used as an outcome. However, AIDS is an arbitrary point on the continuum of HIV disease, dependent usually on the individual developing one of many diseases on an arbitrary list of opportunistic infections and tumors and, in the U.S., on their CD4+ level. The list of diseases changes from time to time and there is a considerable degree of chance in the point in HIV disease at which an individual develops an AIDS-defining illness. Individuals with Kaposi's sarcoma only at the point of diagnosis, for instance, tend to be in better health and to have a better prognosis than those with cytomegalovirus retinitis only. This almost certainly reflects the fact that Kaposi's sarcoma can develop earlier with lower levels of immune system damage.

Death is the obvious ultimate outcome. The ideal study might use death rate or time to death as an outcome measure. However, time to death can be many years, there is plenty of time for social support to fluctuate wildly in those years, and it takes a long time to assemble a suitable size sample if death is the only outcome measure used.

Given these difficulties in determining a suitable outcome measure, it is not surprising that some of the data on social support and physical health are difficult to interpret. Some studies have reported a relationship between physical health and social support; others have failed to find such a relationship. The extent to which this is related to differences in methodology, method of measuring social support, different outcome measures, sample differences, and effectiveness in eliminating artefacts is difficult to assess.

Starting with those studies that have failed to find any relationship between physical health and social support, Perry et al. (1992) found no relationship between baseline levels of social support or 21 other psychological variables to CD4+ levels at 6 months or 12 months in HIV+ subjects. However, emotional distress was related to reported symptom severity. Coates et al. (1989) failed to find any relationship between disease progression and social support over a 2-year period in HIV+ men. Blaney et al. (1992) reported that negative life events, but not social support, predicted number of symptoms experienced by HIV+ individuals over a 6-month period. Nokes and Kendrew (1990) reported that loneliness in persons with AIDS was not related to the rate of development of infections over a 1-year period.

On the other hand, several studies have found a relationship. In a study of 63 HIV+ men, Evans et al. (1992) reported that the number of social supports, but not satisfaction with social support, was related positively to the number of CD4+ cells and negatively to the level of CD8+ lymphocytes. Interestingly, it is difficult to specify whether lower CD8+ lymphocytes is a good or a bad sign. In HIV– controls there were no associations. Fletcher et al. (1989) reported in a small sample that those who progressed to AIDS were lower in social support offering reassurance and higher in loneliness. Solano et al. (1993) found that social support was linked to clinical evolution of HIV disease when CD4+ levels were corrected for, but not to CD4+ levels per se. In a study by Persson et al. (1992) the size of the social network and the amount of social support were linked to CD4+ levels cross sectionally in HIV+ individuals. Canmartin et al. (1991) reported that, in the large MACS cohort, longer survival times in persons with, or developing, AIDS over a 2-year period were associated with greater involvement with the gay community and with lower levels of depression, although other measures of social support were unrelated. The effect was independent of AZT use (currently the most commonly used anti-HIV drug), CD4+ levels, or disease of diagnosis of AIDS.

It is difficult from these studies to decide whether there is, or is not, an effect of social support on physical health. The evidence either way is balanced. It needs to be borne in mind that simply demonstrating an association between physical health and social support is not sufficient. Individuals who are less well or more prone to fatigue (a common symptom in HIV disease) are likely to find maintaining social support networks more difficult, if only because they may not feel much like socializing. Moreover, patients who feel less well are likely to be more prone to depression and this may cause them to reduce their level of social contacts. More good prospective studies are required if the links, if any, are to be teased out.

Social support might not only affect health but also treatment. Katz et al. (1992) reported that those with lower levels of social support were slower to seek treatment after an HIV+ test result. Those with smaller social networks have been reported to make greater use of hospital services (Hoffman and Winiarski, 1989). Todak et al. (1992) found that those who declined AZT had lower levels of social support, although the effect was a small one statistically. On the other hand, Nannis et al. (1992) did not find a relationship between social support and discontinuing AZT once started, or patient-initiated changes in dosage, although there were relationships with other psychosocial variables. The possibility that social support may be linked to physical health through willingness to seek, or compliance with, treatment needs to be borne in mind in any study of the links between social support and physical health in HIV/AIDS.

Social support and mental health

Many investigators have looked at the links between mental health and social support. Interestingly, most have looked at the negative aspects of mental health, either psychiatric symptoms or anxiety or depression or distress. There have been few studies looking at positive aspects of mental well-being. In other words, researchers have tended to ask questions like "do people with more social support have lower levels of depression?"; rather than "are people with more social support happier?" Happiness and lack of depression or distress are not necessarily the same thing.

Many of the studies that have looked at social support have looked at it as one of many different measures rather than targeting the specific issue of social support itself. Consequently, many researchers have only included a few questions on the subject and, given the many different aspects of social support that can be measured, there is great disparity in the ways they have measured social support. In the negative studies it is sometimes difficult to assess whether some other measure of social support might not have given different results. It is also difficult sometimes to assess precisely what aspect of social support is the important one.

Very few studies have failed to find at least some association between social support and mental health. Storosum et al. (1990) did not find any correlation between seeking social support and mood disturbance in 119 seropositive men. Adinolfi et al. (1989) failed to find a relationship between depression and social support in 22 individuals with AIDS. However, the number of subjects was extremely low. On the negative side one should perhaps include Fleishman and co-workers (1990), who reported that depression was related to the number of tasks for which an individual believed that he was very likely to receive support from others, but the relationship was a very weak one.

Another study suggesting a weak relationship between mental health and social support, at least the sort of social support most researchers look at, was that of Grace and colleagues (1990). They reported that among those with HIV infection in the military overall social support was strongly inversely related to depression but most of the variance was accounted for by self-esteem relative to others with availability of material help, availability of others to discuss problems with, and having people with whom to do things contributing little to the association. The unusual social circumstances in the military and the fact that most subjects were asymptomatic may have influenced the results obtained. On the other hand, it may simply be that they chose to try to break down social support in a way that most researchers do not do.

Set against these studies are the very large number of studies that have found a relationship, although the strength and nature of the relationship is highly variable. Lackner et al. (1993) found that subjective social isolation predicted significantly worse mental health at 6 months in 520 men at risk for HIV infection. O'Brien et al. (1993) reported that depression and anxiety were lower where social support was higher. Social conflict tended to increase anxiety and depression. Dew and co-workers (1989) reported that in hemophiliacs, distress and mental health problems were associated with low social support from spouses and friends. Kelly et al. (1993a) found that depression was related to lower perceived social support. Ritchie et al. (1992) reported that, in 55 HIV+ military personnel, depression was associated strongly with divorce but less strongly with not telling friends or family and with a feeling that either significant others or the military were unsympathetic. Fishman et al. (1989) studied individuals seeking an HIV test. Perception of social support was strongly related to distress at the time of testing and 9 weeks later.

These studies are essentially correlational in nature. They are open to a greater or lesser extent to the argument that lower social support is an *effect* rather than a *cause* of depression. However, there are a number of studies which suggest that lower social support may be a cause of lowered mood rather than just an effect.

Hays et al. (1992) reported that, in 508 gay men, the number of HIV-related symptoms predicted depression at baseline and 1 year. Men who were more satisfied with their social support at baseline were less likely to have become more depressed at 1 year. The amount of information available to patients was important in reducing the stress associated with increased HIV symptoms. Clearly this sort of predictive study is crucial in trying to establish the direction of the arrow of causation. However, there are other possible approaches. If poor social support leads to reduced psychological well-being, then increasing social support should reduce adverse mental health. Kelly et al. (1993b) looked at the effects of two types of intervention, cognitive therapy groups and social support groups, in comparison with controls in depressed HIV+ men. Both interventions led to reductions in depression. The social support group condition led to decreased overall psychiatric symptoms and some reduction in interpersonal anxiety and in risky sexual behavior.

A number of studies have looked at the sources of social support that individuals with HIV infection use and the perceived benefits of these different sources of support. Hays et al. (1993) looked at 163 HIV+ men. They found that they were most likely to disclose their HIV status to their lover or close gay friends but not to colleagues or relatives until they started to develop symptoms. The more helpful and sympathetic others were, the lower the levels of anxiety and depression. Catania et al. (1992) reported that HIV+ men with symptoms and HIV– men were more likely to seek social support from family than asymptomatic HIV+ men. Symptomatic individuals were more likely to seek formal medical and psychological help than men in the other groups. Hays et al. (1993) found that gay men with AIDS sought support from a wide range of sources, both formal and informal, whereas seropositives tended to seek support mainly from peers. For both groups peer support was most highly rated among possible sources of support. The study was conducted in San Francisco where there is a well-developed gay community with extensive peer support mechanisms in place.

A few authors have looked at specific areas of distress and the effects of social support on these. For instance, Sciolla et al. (1992) reported that men who had failed to come to terms with bereavement were likely to have lower levels of social support. This is of importance because of the very high number of bereavements that many individuals with HIV face among friends, partners, and close contacts. Catania et al. (1992) found that both asymptomatic and symptomatic patients tended to seek support in dealing with anxieties about death mainly from friends and partners, rather than from families and other caregivers.

Some researchers have looked at risk behaviors and their relationship to social support. Kennedy et al. (1993) looked at 106 couples in which one was infected with HIV and the other not. Greater condom usage in women was associated with being in employment. Abdul-Quader et al. (1990) reported that reduced sexual risk behavior in injecting drug users was related to having a friend who had made changes in their sexual risk behaviors and having someone available with whom to discuss problems. Wanting to have another child was significantly related to risk reduction in women only. Peterson et al. (1992) reported that in gay and bisexual black Americans, unprotected anal sex was related to perceived lower levels of social support among peers for risk-reduction behaviors. The possibility that this may have been *post hoc* rationalization cannot be excluded.

Most studies of social support and HIV have concentrated on gay men living in the U.S. It is by no means a foregone conclusion that issues to do with social support will be the same in other populations, or that the same findings even apply to subsets of the gay U.S. population. Wilson et al. (1991) reported that social support was linked to risk-reduction behavior in 300 people in an area of relatively high heterosexual HIV prevalence in Africa. Ostrow et al. (1991) reported that there were differences in social support and in the nature of the relationship between distress and social support between black and white HIV+ men in the U.S.

Just as there may be differences between different populations in the links between social support and mental well-being or risk behaviors, so there may be individual differences. A commonsense view might suggest that different individuals would differ in the extent and nature of social support that they desire or find helpful. Much effort has gone into looking at coping strategies or coping approaches, but rather less into differences in needs. Gala et al. (1989) found an interaction between the effects of social support on distress and the characteristics of the individual (in this case internal versus external locus of control). While their data were limited the point is an interesting one which deserves further investigation.

Finally it is worth noting that, while there is a good deal of information on the effects of social support on the individual with HIV, there is relatively little information on the effects of the individual with HIV on their social supporters. There has been a fair amount of work on formal caregivers (i.e., doctors, nurses, volunteers, etc.), but little on informal caregivers, who are likely to carry the main burden of caring in most cases. Church et al. (1989) looked at the informal caregivers of persons with HIV infection, in other words, friends, relatives, and significant others identified by the patient with AIDS as being their primary caregiver. They found that for caregivers social support was negatively related to anxiety and depression levels. Some were in worse shape psychologically than the individuals they were caring for. This is clearly an area that merits much greater attention than it has received so far.

So what conclusions can be drawn from all this? Several issues come out of the available literature. First, there would appear to be a reliable correlation between social support and mental well-being. The evidence supports the view that better social support is linked to lower levels of depression and, possibly, anxiety. The nature and direction of causal links need to be established.

Second, available research suggests that individuals actively seek out social support from a range of different sources and the sources they seek support from may differ with how ill they are. In order to get support specifically for HIV-related issues an individual has to be willing to tell others that they have HIV. At least among gay men there seems to be a tendency to tell partners and friends but to be less likely to tell family and others about HIV infection. It would appear that gay men with HIV infection are more likely to tell their families, specifically parents and siblings, that they are infected when they start to become ill. Perceptions about the likely reactions of others may also play a part in who gets told and when. Differentiating between different sources of social support is important for future research.

Third, there is a need to look in more detail at other populations than gay men in the U.S. Getting peer support in a West Coast U.S. city with a large gay population, many gay men with HIV, a thriving gay scene, and many HIV peer support organizations is not likely to be the same proposition as a drug user looking for social support in a small British city or a hemophiliac looking for social support in Germany, or a heterosexual man looking for social support in the Middle East. This is not to say that social support is not important to such individuals in such settings, nor that they will be unable to find it. However, the number and nature of available sources of support may be quite different. In the Caribbean region and in parts of Africa, for instance, it is our experience that the family, including the extended family, is a much more important source of primary social support than it is for San Francisco or London gay men.

Fourth, there is a need to look at individual differences in the need for social support and what factors determine who needs social support, how much they need, and what sources they seek support from. These issues have an important practical as well as theoretical element in planning services for person with HIV.

Finally, if social support is important, there is a need to evaluate much more carefully the effectiveness and impact of interventions aimed at improving it, otherwise we shall never turn theory into practice.

Speculations

The picture presented above is like a jigsaw with half (or more) of the pieces missing. It is, perhaps, worth trying to go beyond the published data and guess what the full picture looks like. Like all guesses this one is likely to be wrong in many respects. We present it, therefore, in the most tentative of fashions, as a story that may touch the truth at some points.

In people with HIV better social support has some protective effect against distress. At the same time poor mental health, particularly depression, leads to people having worse social support. The worse someone's physical health, the less they are able to harness available social support, and poor physical health makes people more prone to depression. So the links between social support and mental state are complex and, sometimes, circular.

It is not clear whether social support affects physical health and, if it does, how it does so. A direct effect on immune functioning, while not impossible, seems unlikely and an effect through how well the individual looks after themselves or gets looked after, or even their use of physical treatments, looks more plausible.

People seek their social support from different sources according to the situation they find themselves in and according to their disease staging. For both gays and heterosexuals, if they have a partner, that partner is *likely* to be their most important source of support. Gay men who are fairly well and move in circles where being gay is acceptable get a great deal of their social support from their peers and even when they are ill, peers play a key part. Once they get ill, by the nature of things, the importance of other sorts of support grows, for instance that provided by health professionals. They are unlikely to get great support from their families early on because they tend not to tell them, partly through concerns about their reactions, partly because they do not want to worry them. A whole host of other caregivers who are neither other gay men nor their families also play a role, but who such caregivers will be less predictable.

Other groups of people with HIV may have different patterns of support-seeking. Hemophiliacs and heterosexuals rely much less on their peers and more on the support of their families. They usually have no comparable peer reference group to that available to gay men. Also they are more likely to live with their family. "Family" means something different in these groups. It is likely to include the partner and is more likely to include the individual's own children as well as siblings and parents. Where peers are likely to be less sympathetic, as in the military, peer support is unlikely to be sought out. Gay men in areas where they face great prejudice and gay men linked into communities that have negative attitudes to being gay find similar problems. Models of augmenting social support developed for gay men in San Francisco may not be directly transferable to London drug users or Nairobi heterosexuals.

Social support can either help or hinder risk reduction. If people around one are implementing risk reduction and support safer sex, then being better integrated with one's peers is helpful. If one's peers favor risk-taking then risk reduction is hindered.

For those who have poor social support, increasing the amount and quality of that support is valuable. Because individuals draw their support from a range of sources and have varied needs, there needs to be a range of support mechanisms available.

Whether this picture is correct only time, and further research, will tell.

References

Abdul-Quader, A. S., Tross, S., Friedman, S. R., Kouzi, A. C., and Des Jarlais, D. C. (1990). Street-recruited intravenous drug users and sexual risk reduction in New York City, *AIDS*, 4, 1075–1080.

Adinolfi, A., Suarez, E., Dideriksen, P., and Bartlett, J. A. (1989). Psychological and sociological correlates of depression, Int. Conf. AIDS, June 4–9, Abstract No. D.670.

Blaney, N. T., Goodkin, K., Feaster, D., Morgan, R., Baum, M., Wilkie, F., Szapocznik, J., and Eisdorfer, C. (1992). Life events and active coping predict health status in early HIV disease, Int. Conf. AIDS, July 19–24, Abstract No. PUB 7213.

Catania, J. A., Turner, H. A., Choi, K. H., Coates, T. J., and George, R. D. (1992). Coping with death anxiety: help-seeking and social support, *AIDS*, 6, 999–1005.

Canmartin, S., Joseph, J. G., and Chmiel, J. (1991). Premorbid psychosocial factors, Int. Conf. AIDS, June 16–21, Abstract MC3105.

Church, J., Kocsis, A. E., Vearnals, S. F., and Green, J. (1989). A longitudinal study examining the impact of AIDS and HIV on carers, Int Conf AIDS, June 4–9, Abstract No. E.509.

Coates, T. J., Stall, R. D., Ekstrand, M., and Solomon, G. F. (1989). Psychosocial predictors as co-factors for disease progression, Int. Conf. AIDS, June 4–9, Abstract No. MA049.

Dew, M. A., Ragni, M. V., and Nimorwicz, P. (1990). Infection with human immunodeficiency virus and vulnerability to psychiatric distress, *Arch. Gen. Psychiatry*, 47, 737–744.

Evans, D. L., Perkins, D. O., Murphy, C., and Folds, J. D. (1992). Relationship of social support and immunity in AIDS, Int. Conf. AIDS, July 19–24, Abstract No. PC 4384.

Fishman, B., Perry, S., Jacobsberg, L., and Frances, A. (1989). Psychological factors predicting distress after HIV testing, Int. Conf. AIDS, June 4–9, Abstract No. T.D.P.66.

Fleishman, J., Piette, J., and Mor, V. (1990). Correlates of depressive symptomatology among people with AIDS, Int. Conf. AIDS, June 20–23, Abstract No. S.B.391.

Fletcher, M. A., Ironson, G., LaPerriere, A., Simoneau, J., Klimas, N., and Schneiderman, N. (1989). Immunological and psychological predictors of disease progression, Int. Conf. AIDS, June 4–9, Abstract No. WBP 181.

Gala, C., Martini, S., Pergami, A., Rossini, M., Russo, R., and Durbano, F. (1989). Locus of control, social supports and depression among HIV, Int. Conf. AIDS, June 4–9, Abstract No. W.B.P.219.

Grace, W. C., Rundell, J. R., and Oster, C. N. (1990). Types of social support and their relationships to depressive symptoms, Int. Conf. AIDS, June 20–23, Abstract No. S.B.379.

Green, J., Hedge, B., (1992). Psychological factors in HIV disease progression in: *Cancer and Stress*, Cooper, C., (Ed.), Oxford University Press, Oxford.

Green, J. and Henderson, F. (1993). Quality of life and social function, in *Social Function in Psychiatry*, Tyrer, P. and Casey P., Eds., Wrightson, Petersfield, 140–152.

Hays, R. B., Catania, J. A., McKusick, L., and Coates, T. J. (1990). Help-seeking for AIDS-related concerns, *Am. J. Community Psychol.*, 18, 743–755.

Hays, R. B., Turner, H., and Coates, T. J. (1992). Social support, AIDS-related symptoms, and depression among gay men, *J. Consult. Clin. Psychol.*, 60, 463–469.

Hays, R. B., McKusick, L., Pollack, L., Hilliard, R., Hoff, C., and Coates, T. J. (1993). Disclosing HIV seropositivity to significant others, *AIDS*, 7, 425–431.

Hoffman, X. and Winiarski, M. (1989). Relationship between social support and loneliness and hospital usage, Int. Conf. AIDS, June 4–9, Abstract No. D602.

Katz, M., Bindman, A. B., Komaromy, M. S. (1992). Coping with HIV infection: why people delay care. *Annals of Internal Medicine*, 117, 797.

Kelly, J. A., Murphy, D. A., Bahr, G. R. et al. (1993a). Factors associated with severity of depression, *Health Psychol.*, 12, 215–219.

Kelly, J. A., Murphy, D. A., Bahr, G. R., et al. (1993b). Outcome of cognitive-behavioral and support group brief therapies, *Am. J. Psychiatry*, 150, 1679–1686.

Kennedy, C. A., Skurnick, J., Wan, J. Y., Quattrone, G., Sheffet, J., Quinones, M., Wang, W., and Louria, D. B. (1993). Psychological distress, drug and alcohol use as correlates of condom use in HIV-serodiscordant heterosexual couples, *AIDS*, 7, 1493–1499.

Lackner, J. B., Joseph, J. G., Ostrow, D. G. et al. (1993). A longitudinal study of psychological distress in a cohort of gay men, *J. Nerv. Ment. Dis.*, 181, 4–12.

Nannis, E., Temoshok, L. Noncompliance with Zidorudine (1992). *Int. Conf. AIDS,* July 19–24, Abstract No. PuB 7377.

Nokes, K. M. and Kendrew, J. (1990). Loneliness in veterans with AIDS and its relationship to the development of infections, *Arch. Psychiatr. Nurs.,* 4, 271–277.

O'Brien, K., Wortman, C. B., Kessler, R. C., and Joseph, J. G. (1993). Social relationships of men at risk for AIDS, *Soc. Sci. Med.,* 36, 1161–1167.

Ostrow, D. G., Whitaker, R. E., Frasier, K., Cohen, C., Wan, J., Frank, C. and Fisher, E. (1991). Racial differences in social support and mental health in men with HIV infection, *AIDS Care,* 3, 55–62.

Perry, S., Fishman, B., Jacobsberg, L., Frances, A. (1992). Relationship over 1 year between lymphocyte subsets and psychosocial variables. *Arch. Gen. Psychiatry,* 49, 396–401.

Persson, J. L., Hanson, B. S., Ostergren, P. O., and Moestrup, T. (1992). Social network, social support and the amount of CD-4 lymphocytes, Int. Conf. AIDS, June 16–21, Abstract MC3176.

Peterson, J. L., Coates, T. J., Catania, J. A., Middleton, L. H. B. and Hearst, N. (1992). High-risk sexual behavior and condom use among gay and bisexual African-American men, *Am. J. Public Health,* 82, 1490–1494.

Ritchie, E. C., Radke, A. Q., and Ross, B. (1992). Depression and support systems in male army HIV+ patients, *Milit. Med.* 157, 345–349.

Sciolla, A., Patterson, T., Atkinson, J., Chandler, J., and Grant, I. (1992). Psychosocial characteristics of grief in HIV-infected men, Int. Conf. AIDS, 8, July 19–24 Abstract No. PoD 5474.

Solano, L., Costa, M., Salvati, S., Coda, R., Ainti, F., Mezzarona, I., and Bertini, M. (1993). Psychosocial factors and clinical evolution in HIV-1 infection, *J. Psychosom. Res.,* 37, 39–51.

Storosum, J., Van den Boom, F., Van Beuzekom, M., and Sno, H. (1990). Stress and coping in people with HIV-infection, Int. Conf. AIDS, June 20–23 PG Abstract No. S.B.365.

Todak, G., Kertzner, R., Remien, R. H., Lin, S. H., Williams, J. B., Friedman, R., Ehrhardt, A. A., and Gorman, J. (1992). Psychosocial factors in the decision to decline zidovudine (AZT), Int. Conf. AIDS, July 19–24, Abstract No. PoD 5582.

Wilson, D., Dubley, I., Msimanga, S., and Lavelle, L. (1991). Psychosocial predictors of reported HIV-preventive behaviour, *Cent. Afr. J. Med.,* 37, 196–200.

Wolf, T. M., Dralle, P. W., Morse, E. V., Simon, P. M., Balson, P. M., Gaumer, R. H., and Williams, M. H. (1991). A biopsychosocial examination of symptomatic and asymptomatic HIV, *Int. J. Psychiatry Med.,* 21, 263–279.

chapter seventeen

Dealing with stress: families and chronic illness

Coleen Shannon

Introduction

According to the Bureau of the Census, approximately 110 million people in the U.S. suffer from chronic illness.[1] In fact experts believe that currently, chronic illnesses are the dominant health care problem.[2] As a consequence, 110 million families are affected by stress related to dealing with ongoing medical conditions. Medical providers tend to agree that illness of one family member invariably impacts the entire family, causing family disruption and leading to changes in roles and financial status, as well as altering the family's social and emotional life.[3] Chronic illness affects the entire family system.

Although a number of articles have addressed the importance of family adjustment in relation to the chronically ill family member's adjustment and ability to manage his or her illness, relatively little literature has been devoted to the discussion of family functioning. The purpose of this chapter is to address the impact of chronic illness on families, explore family coping, and to discuss methods to strengthen families. This discussion is not limited to medical conditions of one age group or one illness category, since the stressors seem to be generic to most chronic illnesses. Included in the first section is a discussion of stressors and problems faced by caregivers and family members, along with methods that have been used for coping and adapting. The second section gives personal viewpoints from interviews with three families who have severely chronically ill children. The next section discusses community services and resources available to families in a large urban area. A fourth section is a discussion of programs and methods to strengthen families. The concluding section gives some thoughts for development of services for families dealing with the stress of chronic illness.

Families, stressors, and problems

Chronic illness is generally defined as an illness that continues for 6 months or longer and requires ongoing medical management. The differentiation of chronic illness from acute illness is explained through several dimen-

0-8493-2908-6/96/$0.00+$.50
© 1996 by CRC Press, Inc.

sions. For example, the likelihood of cure is low, social support is usually given to the patient, and adaptation rather than cure is the medical goal.[4] Without a doubt, the family, as well as the patient, is required to make many adaptations.

Families living with a chronic illness face a wide range of physical and social changes which are viewed as stressors. Those identified as impacting families include financial difficulties, role changes, uncertainty and unpredictability, and the burden of constant care.[5] When levels of stress have been measured, results strongly indicate that the demands associated with chronic illness lead to high subjective ratings of stress by family members. For example, in studies of hemodialysis patients researchers have found that spouses report moderate to excessive levels of subjective stress.[6,7] In an extensive study of the children and spouse caregivers of Alzheimer's disease patients, Pearlin and co-workers[8] identified primary and secondary stressors. Primary stressors are durable over time and can produce other stressors, referred to as secondary. Specific primary stressors include the cognitive status of the patient and problematic behavior requiring surveillance and control. Secondary stressors are seen as role strain found in roles outside the caregiving situation, as well as a variety of intrapsychic strains.[8] Additional studies report problems including feelings of anxiety, anger, guilt, frustration, blame, spousal depression, marital dissatisfaction, lower levels of life satisfaction, nervousness, fatigue, sadness, grief, altered family relations, modification of family activities, isolation, and worry about the future.[9-12]

Several authors, including Phillips[13] and Warda,[14] discuss chronic sorrow as a common reaction families have to chronically ill and disabled children. Chronic sorrow is described as a continuous sense of sadness that, unlike grief, does not exhibit stages such as shock, anger, and guilt. Although chronic sorrow is not considered to be an abnormal feeling for parents, it is not found in all families of chronically ill children. Preliminary studies indicate that it may be more likely to develop in the face of hopelessness regarding progress and when the condition is seen as permanent. Current studies do not distinctly indicate whether chronic sorrow is a response to stress or if it is a coping strategy.

Clearly, families are confronted with constant, ongoing stressors related to caring for and living with chronic illness. Some families develop varying degrees of problems while others seem to exhibit well-being. Critical to well-being is the family's ability to cope.

Coping and adapting

According to Monat and Lazarus, research related to coping in general has increased rapidly over the last few years.[15] As defined by Folkman and Lazarus, "Coping consists of cognitive and behavioral efforts to manage specific external and/or internal demands that are appraised as taxing or exceeding the resources of the person".[16] In order for a cognitive process to be considered coping it must involve purposeful effort. In other words, an individual engages in coping when he or she expends effort to master demands that are perceived as being larger than current resources.

Adapting is not the same as coping. Adaptation is considered to be an automatic process in reaction to one's environment. According to early work by Feldman, the process of adaptation is coming to terms with the reality of chronic illness.[17] For the family it may include letting go of false hope and hopelessness, as well as engaging in a process of restructuring the environment. In a model of psychosocial adaptation developed by White and co-workers, life events and health status are considered stressors, with coping strategies and social support as predictor variables leading to outcome that is defined as adaptation.[18] Consequently, coping is seen as a component or subset of adapting.

In regard to outcome related to coping strategies, Folkman and Lazarus point out that "the best coping is that which changes the person-environment relationship for the better".[19] However, no strategy can in itself be considered good or bad, because the context must be taken into account. Since chronic illness is a specific context that has been identified as highly stressful for families, researchers have attempted to determine which coping strategies have been used and to understand their effectiveness.

Although research concerning coping strategies employed by individuals are numerous, there are far fewer studies utilizing the family as a unit. One reason for the lack of research is that there are very few models of coping with chronic illness that consider the family as the unit of study or assessment. The most comprehensive family-based model for understanding families living with chronic illness comes from Patterson and Garwith.[20] In their Family Adjustment and Adaptation Response (FAAR) Model, the family is seen as attempting to maintain homeostasis through using its capabilities to meet its demands. Families cycle through times of adjustment, crisis, and adaptation, with outcomes that can range from good to poor. According to the model, coping is "a specific effort by an individual or family that is directed at maintaining or restoring the balance between demands and resources".[20] In general, research has been related to families dealing with specific conditions such as Alzheimer's disease or cystic fibrosis. Since most of the studies of families are exploratory, and not generalizable across illnesses, theoretical explanation is in an early stage.

In their study on well- and poorly adjusted families, Hough et al.[21] identified coping strategies used by both types of families. The study was concerned with developing a model of family coping and adaptation to a mother's chronic illness. Results indicated that "the wife's illness affected her spouse's view of how the family coped".[21] How the family experienced various demands of the mother's illness was related to the family's use of a type of coping behavior referred to as "familial introspection". This type of introspection is a process by which the family looks inward and reflects on its performance. Families using familial introspection on a frequent basis were found to have better adjusted marriages and better parent-child relations.

Two additional distinguishing factors were found to differentiate well- and poorly adjusted families. The first was that all well-adjusted families constructed some positive meaning out of the illness experience. According to the authors, these families commonly reported "a greater appreciation of life, of living in the here and now and achieving a better balance between work and other aspects of one's life." Other positive meanings include a positive evaluation of competence and self-efficacy, and an increase in sensitivity and empathy with others. In contrast to the well-adjusted families, poorly adjusted families reported no positive effects or meanings related to the illness experience. This negative view was so strong that it was extended to experiences that had the potential of being positive.

A second distinguishing factor was the perception of social support available to the family. All adjusted families discussed their experiences of support from family and friends. Consequently, support emerged as a highly important and highly valued aspect of the illness experience. Poorly adjusted families, on the other hand, showed persistence in their global negative view of the illness by complaining about a lack of social support. This perceived lack of support from family and friends was mentioned by all of the poorly adjusted families.

In conclusion, the authors suggest that it is possible for families as a unit to engage in the process of developing positive meanings through introspection. This ability to construct positive meanings related to a mother's chronic illness can lead families to higher levels of functioning than might be expected.

Another group of researchers, Seaburn et al.,[22] used ethnographic methods to explore the process implemented by families to develop chronic illness meanings. Through their discussions with families, the authors found that families faced with the task of giving meaning to the illness experience used storytelling, narrative, and language that is transgenerational to develop meanings for current experiences. These meanings are then shaped to support the family's way of dealing with the demands of illness. How a family copes can be greatly enhanced by giving the illness experience a personally significant meaning.

The authors conclude with four organizing ideas. The first is that families must give their illness experience meaning. For example, a family's view that the illness is a challenge may bring order and direction to daily living. A second idea is that family meanings are passed from one generation to another and are continually evolving. These historical meanings can guide families and may contain spiritual, political, or cultural elements. The third idea is that storytelling is a vehicle through which families pass on illness meanings. Stories from the past create a structure for current experiences. The fourth and final idea is that meanings resulting from stories told by families provide influences and guides for daily functioning. Those families who construct meanings from stories of strength and triumph find chronic illness to be less burdensome.[22]

According to the Patterson and Garwick FAAR Model, family meanings are constructed on three levels that are dynamically interrelated. Situational meanings are the most concrete and can increase the family's perceived resources and competencies. Family identity defines boundaries and guides family relationships. The third and most abstract level is the family world view relating to the family's orientation to the world and the way reality is interpreted. All three levels of meanings shape the family's response to the chronic illness.[23]

A second component in adapting that has received attention from researchers is social support, which is related to positive adaptation in a number of areas, including physical health, mental well-being, and social function. Although the effects of social support have been well researched in relation to individuals facing illness, little is known about social support as a stress buffer for families of the chronically ill. As stated earlier, all well-adjusted families in the study reported by Hough et al.[24] perceived that they had a high level of social support available to them. According to the authors, "It was obvious that for these families, the love, concern, and support they felt they had received from people was extremely important."[24]

Parents of children with cystic fibrosis (CF) responded that social support was an important and needed resource. Spouse and family support was most frequently reported as helpful. In fact, the husband's support was rated as important in the mother's ability to cope with caregiving demands.[25] A second source of support identified was the multidisciplinary CF clinic team that helped parents understand the medical information needed for caregiving. The third and final source of support was the CF Foundation that offered groups to parents aimed at sharing ideas among families.[26]

When individual and group support interventions were compared several factors related to group outcomes were important. Results indicated that both modalities can lead to changes in knowledge, attitudes, and behaviors. However, groups provide "greater positive changes in social support, both informal and formal."[27] Participants increased the size of their informal support networks and increased their knowledge of community resources. Both individual and group support increased feelings of personal control of difficult caregiving situations. However, individual support was more helpful with psychological issues.

Communication is another coping strategy recommended but not analyzed by several authors.[28,29] However, Canam[30] reported on a study of the ways in which parents communicate about feelings and the type of guidance received. Subjects were 24 families of children with epilepsy and 12 families of children with cystic fibrosis. Findings indicated that 56% of the respondents did not talk about their feelings to anyone. When asked about their feelings, most (72%) said that they felt some degree of fear. Parents also said that they did not talk with their children about their feelings (81%). Comments by parents indicated that they did not talk to their children because they did not have answers and did not want to make the child feel worse.[30] Although communication is recommended as important in coping, results in this study indicate a lack of communication. More research is needed to bring the concept into clear focus.

In the words of families

Another way to understand families dealing with the stress of chronic illness is to use grounded theory and qualitative methods, as described by Strauss and Corbin.[31] In an ongoing qualitative study of families with chronically ill children, parents were asked to tell their stories related to their illness experience.[32] These experiences were then compared with previously reported findings regarding family stress. Three representative families are presented here. All three families had severely disabled children with multiple physical problems. Two of the families lived in rural areas and one in a large metropolitan area. They were asked to discuss their views of the illness, stressors, and resources.

The M. family

The M. family lives in a rural area and consists of two parents and their son, B. who is diagnosed with infantile neuronal-ceriod-lipfuscinosis (NCL). He is almost 4 years old, blind, hearing impaired, and severely retarded. He also has frequent seizures, is highly sensitive to touch, and needs to be held constantly.

Outside stressors included difficulties in locating and accessing educational and developmental programs, long complicated application procedures for programs, long waiting lists, long travel distances to needed resources, and financial burdens.

B.'s need for constant care is a primary concern for the family. They have received some assistance with care through a state-funded program that supplies a few hours of nursing care per week. Other services are early childhood intervention through another state agency and physical therapy from the public school system. Accessing these needed services involved a long and difficult process. In fact, the mother commented that if their social worker had not been an advocate for them, they would have given up.

Both parents said that they went through a short grief process at the time doctors confirmed the seriousness of B.'s condition. However, the pressing need to care for B. has taken precedence over most personal feelings. They simply do not have much time for grief. The burden of care is ongoing, to the extent that lack of sleep is a major concern for the parents.

When B. has a bad night, it usually means that he will also have a bad day the next day and will need extra attention.

In addition to sleep deprivation, the parents have experienced marital problems. Although they can usually discuss problems, exhaustion and lack of sleep places increased pressure on their relationship. The mother also reports feelings of depression and low self-esteem.

On the other hand, the parents express a sense of accomplishment due to the fact that they have been able to care for their child and see to it that he has received the best services available. In addition, each feels support from the other which they link to their ability to communicate. They also receive support from family, friends, and from their social worker.

The G. family

The G. family lives in a rural area and consists of two parents, two teenage daughters, and a severely disabled grandson, J. Custody of the 3-year-old grandson was given to the G.s after he was severely abused by his mother. J. received severe brain damage during his abuse and is mentally retarded, has a large number of seizures every day, and is blind. He receives all nutrition and medication through a feeding tube. His condition requires constant care.

Services for J. and his family have been difficult to obtain. For example, when J. needed a wheelchair, paper work delayed delivery for so long that he outgrew the two wheelchairs before they could be delivered. Other resources for services have been accessed but the family views the struggle to get their needs met as a major stressor. Other stressors include financial concerns, since medical insurance for J.'s care is not covered by the family's medical insurance.

Responsibility for the burden of care rests on the grandmother, because the grandfather's job frequently takes him out of town. However, she receives a great deal of help from her family and from a few close friends. Emotional and spiritual support also comes from members of her church, who are highly involved with the family.

The S. family

The S. family lives in a large city and consists of two parents and two children. The youngest son, M., is 10 years old and has a very rare debilitating condition. He is severely retarded, has frequent seizures, and requires constant care. He has outlived his expected survival age.

Although urban areas have more resources available than rural areas, the process of access is often so complicated that the mother commented that she has not pursued some services. She explained that she has had to be assertive to get information from medical doctors, to get appropriate educational plans, and to find out what might be available for her son.

Stressors for the family have been the demand for constant care for M., lack of time for the parents, constant fear of M.'s death, and financial concerns. In spite of medical insurance, care for M. is quite expensive for the family.

On the other hand, the family has exhibited a high level of coping. Each parent is supportive of the other and they both say that they receive a lot of support from other family members and from friends. The mother has actively pursued a demanding career path while assuming the major responsibility for caregiving. Although time, money, and energy are all problems, the family feels a sense of appreciation for M. and believes that he has enriched their lives.

Common experiences

These three families are representative of families with chronically ill children who participated in an ongoing qualitative study. As families tell their stories, common themes such as type of stressors, meanings of the illness experience, coping strategies, use of resources, and support systems emerge.

Stressors

As stated by Pearlin, et al.,[33] stressors may be primary or secondary. Primary stressors are usually seen as coming directly from the needs of the patient, in this case, the child. In the above examples, the needs of chronically ill children lead to other stressors, which are considered secondary stressors. Obviously, the burden of constant care of these very disabled children creates a number of additional stressors for the families.

Several secondary stressors were discussed by the families. One mentioned by all families is the financial strain created by medical services. Without a doubt, insurance was viewed as helpful but it does not solve all financial problems. Families without insurance are completely dependent on public assistance and publicly supported health care services. Such services are often inconveniently located, inadequate, and difficult to obtain. Even when a family has medical insurance, health care costs thousands of dollars each year in addition to high premiums and deductibles.

Another secondary stressor mentioned by all families is the difficulty in accessing resources. Often families are unaware of the resources available, do not know how to apply for services, and are confused by rules, regulations, and paper work. Families reported that even after resources are located, they are confronted by long waiting lists and the requirement to travel long distances. A result of all of these barriers can lead to such discouragement that families will give up the pursuit. Additional secondary stressors mentioned by families are lack of personal time as well as time with one's spouse, and marital conflict.

Problems resulting from stress

The most commonly related problem reported by the families is fatigue. Since the children need 24-hour constant care, families are always on call, with very little "down time." Sleep deprivation results in fatigue, irritability, and feelings of depression. Other emotional reactions frequently mentioned are moodiness, low self-esteem, feeling alone or isolated, chronic anxiety, and fear of the child's death.

Family coping

As the families told their stories, several coping strategies emerged. All of the families reported here developed meanings related to the illness experience that were positive. The children were viewed as valuable and important human beings who enriched the family. Both parents and siblings spoke with affection concerning the ill child, commenting that although care giving was exhausting it was also rewarding. Families generally believed that life was good and that the chronically ill child was a part of life.

A second coping strategy was communication among family members. Communication in this context refers to discussion of problems, expression of feelings, and making plans. Several family members commented that communication was not only a stress reliever but also a source of strength. One of the mothers said that communication, "is like the cement that makes us stronger." Another said that sometimes, "we try to protect each other but that takes energy away." In addition, communication facilitates other coping strategies, such as support within the family and problem solving.

A third coping strategy found in all of the families is support. Families want and seek support. They seem to look first to their immediate family and secondly to the extended family, and finally to the community. Interestingly, some families do not find officially defined support groups to be helpful. Factors that may influence the helpfulness include location, how far does the family have to travel to attend meetings, and does the family have access to other support networks such as extended family, friends, or church groups. Also, one family said that the support of their social worker was extremely helpful. Others commented that locating a supportive person in the medical or social service system made a difference for them.[34]

When families tell their stories, many of the concepts reported in previous research come alive. Some observations from these families are noteworthy and suggest areas for further exploration. For example, the way a family views the child and the chronic condition is important to family functioning. Families who see the child as a person, not as illness, seem to be able to find joy and fulfillment in family life. This process of developing meanings seems more comprehensive and complex than a cognitive appraisal of events.

A second area of interest for exploration arising out of the family stories is the idea of social support. Certainly the need for social support has been recognized and addressed by a number of authors. In addition, many organizations have developed groups for the purpose of providing education and support to both patients and families. However, little is known about which groups are the most beneficial for families.

Community-based support groups

According to both families and researchers social support is important for mediating stress, as well as for a coping strategy. In a 1994 survey of support groups in a large U.S. metropolitan area, 75 groups addressing specific diseases were identified.[35] These groups ranged from nationally incorporated nonprofit agencies that address common illnesses, such as the American Heart Association, to small grassroots groups that address less well known illnesses, such as Tourette syndrome. The illnesses ranged from life threatening to nonterminal but all dealt with chronic conditions that affect daily living. The purpose of the study was to explore the way various groups work with families of the chronically ill.

Forty-five groups were selected to receive the survey, including 23 national disease organizations, 8 hospital-based groups, 3 groups for caregivers of the elderly, and 11 grassroots self-help groups. Twenty-six (58%) returned the mailed questionnaires. Completed surveys were received from groups involved with the following diseases or conditions: leukemia, cancer, lupus, diabetes, heart and lung disease, strokes, cerebral palsy, epilepsy, Parkinson's, AIDS, Alzheimer's, multiple sclerosis, burns, elderly care, pediatric care, and neurofibromatosis.

The first topic of concern was to determine, from the viewpoint of the groups, the nature of stressors experienced by the families. When groups were asked to identify family stressors, financial burden was the most frequently named. This burden is associated with decreased income resulting from job loss or absence, expenses for medical care, special equipment, and transportation. The second category of frequent stressors included time demands associated with care giving and medical care, and the burden of care giving. Other stressors mentioned were social isolation/stigma, accessing resources, transportation problems, and conflicting needs of family members.

A second section of the survey explored the services provided by the groups. Most groups provide education and resource information (77%). All respondents offer support groups, about half are exclusively for patients and half include both patients and family members. Community referrals to services are provided by 50% of respondents. Direct services such as in-home service, financial aid, and respite care are provided by 15% of respondents. Additionally, special family counseling and home health equipment are provided by 8% of respondents.

The last part of the survey concerned the needs of families as perceived by the groups. Fewer respondents commented on this section than on others. However, those who responded most frequently cited low cost or free respite care (26%) and transportation assistance (19%) as the services most needed by families of the chronically ill. Further service needs identified included financial assistance, family counseling, in-home services, and adult day care. A few respondents defined a need for case management, improved access to services, positive support groups, disease education, and family networking.

The results of this study confirm that in large urban areas there are numerous existing groups formed to address specific diseases and conditions but they focus primarily on the patient and on the disease rather than on the family system. In addition, the groups most frequently meet needs through disease education, referrals to community resources, and positive support groups for patients.

Although respondents recognized that families function with varying amounts of stress resulting in problems such as fatigue, mood disorders, communication difficulties, and worry, none of the respondents reported that their organizations offer any information regarding stress or coping strategies. Information concerning coping with stress involved in the burdens of care giving is passed along from one family to another through informal conversations. These groups and organizations offer the potential of providing families with valuable tools for stress management.

Strengthening families

Several methods of enhancing the coping strategies of families facing the stress of chronic illness have been identified. Important roles can be played by medical staff, social service personnel, volunteers, self-help groups, and friends. This section explores innovative approaches and ideas for strengthening these families.

As seen in the previously cited studies, family meanings, perceptions, and belief systems are important to the family's ability to cope. In addition, social support, communication, respite care, and generally healthy lifestyles can increase the family's adaptation. Organizations, groups, and medical professionals have developed programs for patients and families in a variety of ways. For example several programs have offered a comprehensive package of services. Meyerstein[36] described a program, the Family Asthma Program, involving the school system, public health nurses, American Lung Association, physicians, family therapists, volunteers, and self-help groups. Goals were defined as: "1) outreach; 2) education; 3) support; 4) provision of coping skills; and 5) fostering self-help for families of children with asthma."[36] The program was structured to offer up to four 2-hour sessions. Parents and children were involved in activities simultaneously so that children could learn through experiences with other children and parents had time to be with other parents to engage in both structured learning and sharing experiences. Of the 17 families enrolled in the program, 13 participated in an evaluation of the program. The two items ranked as the most helpful were the provision of information of pathophysioloy, treatment, and equipment, and psychosocial aspects of coping with asthma. This comprehensive effort involving both professionals and volunteers was particularly appreciated by the parents who said that they liked the exercises related to communication and that the information given was practical.

Another program targeting the whole family rather than just the patient was carried out at the Soroka Medical Center in Beer Sheva, Israel.[37] Goals were to improve the family's coping ability and increase the cooperation between the medical and family system. The family systems model was used to structure the program, which was developed by a multidisciplinary team. An intervention group consisting of 18 asthmatic children and their parents participated in six psychoeducational sessions. Results indicate that as the families progressed through the program, children were encouraged by their parents to become more independent and more responsible for their own care. In fact parents tended to view their child less as suffering unfortunates. Families demonstrated an increase in competence in dealing with asthma and an opening of communication pathways. Family members learned about feelings and perceptions from each other and from other families. The authors concluded that the model could easily be adapted to other chronic diseases in order to improve the lives of families.

Other programs and recommendations for helping families cope with chronic illness have tended to concentrate on one aspect of coping. For example, a modern "high tech" program called ComputerLink was described as a method to "deliver social support to home-based caregivers."[38] According to Brennan, et al.,[38] ComputerLink's advantage to a group of Alzheimer's patient caregivers was the 24-hour availability. In addition, caregivers using a terminal, modem, and telephone line could choose the amount of time they wanted to be on-line, as well as topics of interest. During 1 week, on-line usage of 47 subjects was passively monitored. Results from the data indicated that the most frequently used component was the Forum, which functioned like a support group. Caregivers used the Forum to read and post messages to each other. Through these messages they shared information, expressed feelings, and gave and received support. Other services available were an e-mail system, an encyclopedia, and questions and answers.

Although this was a small experimental program, the growth of commercial on-line services along with media attention given to the information superhighway, access to other people and to information is expected to grow rapidly in the next few years. In fact, user groups related to various illnesses are already found on both Internet and on commercial services. For some individuals and families electronic communication may be a valuable tool to provide social support and to break down isolation.

Another type of program often requested by families and recommended by professionals is respite care. The combination of technological advances and hospital cost containment efforts are increasing the need for families to care for more chronically ill children and adults. Experts agree that the burden of constant care of a chronically ill child or adult can lead to burnout, fatigue, health problems, and other signs of stress. Respite care can, at least for a short time, relieve these symptoms.[39] In addition, Miller reported that using respite care before family members become completely exhausted can prevent premature institutional placement of elderly patients.[40] However, respite care is not readily available. A California survey revealed that although the population of chronically ill and/or technology-dependent individuals maintained at home has increased in the last few years, the number of programs offering respite care has not increased in relation to the need.[41] As more medical care in general is shifted from institutions and hospitals to homes, respite care, like home health care services, may increase in availability.

Conclusions

Observations made by Dohrenwend and Dohrenwend[42] in 1974 concerning individuals still applies to families today. As they commented, "A major question, and for some investigators the central problem concerning the effects of stressful life events, grows out of the observation that one individual may become ill and another remain healthy after both experience the same life event."[42] All families who live with and care for a chronically ill member are affected by the illness experience. Chronic illness is considered to be a chronic life stressor involving the entire family system. However, this continual burden of caregiving does not necessarily lead to symptoms of distress. Ample evidence suggest that families may experience satisfactions and psychological well-being. A family's coping abilities, along with social support, are major mediating factors in the adaptation to chronic illness.

Consistent with the stress and coping model, families who develop positive meanings from the illness experience report lower stress and higher levels of well-being. They are also seen as better adjusted by researchers. Since the process of appraisal involves the development of meanings through open communication within the family, story telling, and transgenerational attitudes, health care professionals as well as self-help programs could facilitate families in their efforts to understand the illness experience. Positive meaning is also related to self-efficacy, competence, and an increased sense of mastery, which can be taught to families. Programs related to health care facilities such as hospitals, clinics, and/or community-based support groups could focus on development of stress-resistant families through psychoeducational instruction.

Social support, the second major mediating factor for families, comes from both internal and external sources. For example, within the family, spouse support along with support from extended family is important.[43] Other sources of support include medically based and community-based support groups. Although these groups function very well as providers of information, forums for information exchange, and vehicles for sharing experiences, very few offer purposeful guidance on stress reduction. In addition, according to our family stories, if the group is geographically inconvenient, the family will not attend meetings. Perhaps new informational technology will make social support more accessible to isolated families, particularly in rural areas.

In addition to the need for expanded services focusing on the family as a unit, more research is needed to understand how families living with chronic illness cope and adapt over time. In order to increase the generalizability of findings longitudinal studies along with studies of various types of chronic illness are needed. Lastly, if we are going to effectively strengthen families, new programs must include good outcome studies.

Acknowledgment

The author gratefully acknowledges the research assistance of Barbara Collie, Julia Easley, and Sherry Schusterman, graduate students in social work, in the preparation of this manuscript.

References

1. White, N. E., Richter, J. M., and Fry, C., Coping, social support, and adaptation to chronic illness, West. J. Nurs. Res., 14, 211, 1992.
2. Forsyth, G. L., Delaney, K. D., and Gresham, M. L., Vying for a winning position: management style of the chronically ill, Res. Nurs. Health, 7, 181, 1984.
3. Piening, S., Family stress in diabetic renal failure, Health Soc. Work, 9, 134, 1984.
4. Kotarba, J., Chronic Pain: Its Social Dimensions, Sage, Beverly Hills, 1983, 13.
5. Smeltzer, S. C., Use of the trajectory model of nursing in multiple sclerosis, Schol. Inquiry Nurs. Pract. Int. J., 5, 219, 1991.
6. Brown, D. J., Craick, C. C., Davies, S. E., Johnson, M. L., Dawborn, J. K., and Heale, W. F., Physical, emotional and social adjustments to home dialysis, Med. J. Aust., 1, 245, 1978.
7. Farmer, C. J., Beweick, M., Parsons, V., and Snowden, S. A., Survival on home hemodialysis: its relationships with physical symptomatology, psychosocial background and psychiatric morbidity, Psychol. Med., 9, 515, 1979.
8. Pearlin, L. I., Mullan, J. T., Semple, S. J., and Skaff, M. M., Caregiving and the stress process: an overview of concepts and their measures, Gerontologist, 30, 583, 1990.

9. Doherty, E. S. and Power, P. W., Identifying the needs of coronary patient wife-caregivers: implications of social workers, *Health Soc. Work*, 15, 291, 1990.

10. Toseland, R. W., Rossiter, C. M., Peak, T., and Smith, G. C., Comparative effectiveness of individual and group interventions to support family caregivers, *Soc. Work*, 35, 209, 1990.

11. Hough, E. E., Lewis, F. M., and Woods, N. F., Family response to mother's chronic illness: case studies of well and poorly adjusted families, *West. J. Nurs. Res.*, 13, 568, 1991.

12. McCubbin, M. A., Family stress and family strengths: a comparison of single and two parent families with handicapped children, *Res. Nurs. Health*, 12, 101, 1989.

13. Phillips, M., Chronic sorrow in mothers of chronically ill and disabled children, *Issues Comprehensive Pediatr. Nurs.*, 14, 111, 1991.

14. Warda, M., The family and chronic sorrow: role theory approach, *J. Pediatr. Nurs.*, 7, 205, 1992.

15. Monat, A. and Lazarus, R. S., Introduction: stress and coping—some current issues and controversies, in *Stress and Coping: An Anthology*, Monat, A. and Lazarus, R. S., Eds., Columbia University Press, New York, 1991, 5.

16. Folkman, S. and Lazarus, R. S., Coping and emotion, in *Stress and Coping: An Anthology*, Monat, A. and Lazarus, R. S., Eds., Columbia University Press, New York, 1991, chap. 10.

17. Feldman, D., Chronic disabling illness: a bibliography, *J. Chronic Dis.*, 27, 16, 1974.

18. White, N. E., Richter, J. M., and Fry, C., Coping, social support, and adaptation to chronic illness, *West. J. Nurs. Res.*, 14, 211, 1992.

19. Folkman, S. and Lazarus, R. S., Coping and emotion, in *Stress and Coping: An Anthology*, Monat, A. and Lazarus, R. S., Eds., Columbia University Press, New York, 1991, chap. 10.

20. Patterson, J. M. and Garwick, A. W., The impact of chronic illness on families: a family systems perspective, *Ann. Behav. Med.*, 16, 131, 1994.

21. Hough, E. E., Lewis, F. M., and Woods, N. F., Family response to mother's chronic illness: case studies of well- and poorly adjusted families, *West. J. Nurs. Res.*, 13, 568, 1991.

22. Seaburn, D., Lorenz, A., and Kaplan, D., The transgenerational development of chronic illness meanings, *Family Systems Med.*, 10, 385, 1992.

23. Patterson, J. M. and Garwick, A. W., The impact of chronic illness on families: a family systems perspective, *Ann. Behav. Med.*, 16, 131, 1994.

24. Hough, E. E., Lewis, F. M., and Woods, N. F., Family response to mother's chronic illness: case studies of well and poorly adjusted families, *West. J. Nurs. Res.*, 13, 568, 1991.

25. Gibson, C., How parents cope with a child with cystic fibrosis, *Nurs. Papers Perspect. Nurs.*, 18, 31, 1986.

26. Gibson, C., Perspective in parental coping with a chronically ill child: the case of cystic fibrosis, *Issues Comprehensive Pediatr. Nurs.*, 11, 33, 1988.

27. Toseland, R. W., Rossiter, C. M., Peak, T., and Smith, G. C., Comparative effectiveness of individual and group interventions to support family caregivers, *Soc. Work*, 35, 209, 1990.

28. Blasio, P. D., Molinari, E., Peri, G., and Taverna, A., Family competence and childhood asthma: a preliminary study, *Family Systems Med.*, 8, 145, 1990.
29. Adams, T., Dementia and family stress, *Nurs. Times*, 85, 27, 1989.
30. Canam, C., Coping with feelings: chronically ill children and their families, *Nurs. Papers Perspect. Nurs.*, 19, 9, 1987.
31. Strauss, A. and Corbin, J., *Basics of Qualitative Research*, Sage Publications, Newbury Park, 1990, chap. 1.
32. Shannon, C., unpublished data, 1994.
33. Pearlin, L. I., Caregiving and the stress process: an overview of concepts and their measures, *Gerontologist*, 5, 583, 1990.
34. Shannon, C., unpublished data, 1994.
35. Shannon, C., unpublished data, 1994.
36. Meyerstein, I., Creating a network of volunteer resources in a psychoeducational family asthma program, *Family Systems Med.*, 10, 99, 1992.
37. Tal, D., Gil-Spielberg, R., Antonovsky, H., Tal, A., and Moaz, B., Teaching families to cope with childhood asthma, *Family Systems Med.*, 8, 135, 1990.
38. Brennan, P. F., Moore, S. M., and Smyth, K. A., Alzheimer's disease caregivers' uses of a computer network, *West. J. Nurs. Res.*, 14, 662, 1992.
39. Larkin, J. P. and Hopcroft, B. M., In-hospital respite as a moderator of caregiver stress, *Health Soc. Work*, 18, 132, 1993.
40. Miller, D. B., Perceptions of caregivers about special respite services for the elderly, *Gerontologist*, 29, 498, 1989.
41. O'Connor, P., Plaats, S. V., and Betz, C. L., Respite care services to caretakers of chronically ill children in California, *J. Pediatr. Nurs.*, 7, 269, 1992.
42. Dohrenwend, B. S. and Dohrenwend, B. P., Overview and prospects for research on stressful life events, in *Stressful Life Events: Their Nature and Effects*, Dohrenwend, B. and Dohrenwend, B. P., Eds., John Wily & Sons, New York, 1974, chap. 18.
43. Borden, W., Stress, coping, and adaptation in spouses of older adults with chronic dementia, *Soc. Work Res. Abstr.*, 27, 14, 1991.

Preventing and treating stress-related illnesses

chapter eighteen

Theories and practices of mobilizing support in stressful circumstances

Benjamin H. Gottlieb

Introduction and overview

During the past 20 years the concept of social support and its bearing on health have been vigorously researched by investigators in the health and social sciences. Epidemiologists and sociologists have scrutinized how the structure and composition of people's social relationships, as well as the ties they have to the institutions of the community, reduce both morbidity and mortality.[1,2] Meanwhile, psychologists have delved into social support's role in the stress process, principally striving to identify how people's perceptions of and interactions with their close associates modify their reactions to time-limited life events and role transitions, as well as to chronic hardships.[3,4] In addition, social support has captured the attention of policy makers in the health and social services fields because mutual aid and informal care are indispensable complements to the programs provided by local and federal governments. Without the contributions made by family caregivers and by the natural systems of service delivery that take shape among family members and friends, institutional resources would be overwhelmed and indicators of health and well-being would decline precipitously.

The topic of social support is of special interest to practitioners who serve clients and patients with stress-related disorders. This is because many of these disorders arise in the wake of life events that have weakened the client's social network or made demands that outstrip the network's coping resources. Practitioners are therefore keen to gain instruction about ways they can reweave, strengthen, or enrich the social fabric to optimize its responsiveness and its durability. Moreover, many practitioners are more sanguine about the prospects for successful intervention through effecting change in the social environment than through person-centered psychotherapeutic efforts. They recognize that a social interven-

0-8493-2908-6/96/$0.00+$.50
© 1996 by CRC Press, Inc.

tion is called for when distress is an expression of absent, lost, or disordered social relationships. In addition, many professionals acknowledge that their clients' feelings of control, efficacy, and self-worth depend far more strongly on the messages they receive from their personal communities than on those communicated by professionals.

This chapter identifies several types of interventions involving the mobilization and augmentation of social support among populations that are at risk by virtue of their actual or potential exposure to stressful events, chronic strains, and role transitions. It begins by addressing the theoretical underpinnings of support interventions, reviewing literature that bears on the stressful circumstances that warrant the introduction of support, the psychological mechanisms implicated in support's ameliorative effects, and the social psychological conditions that promote the utilization of support programs. The next section presents an overview of dyadic and group interventions, distinguishing between those that optimize the support of preexisting relationships and those that introduce new social relationships. The chapter concludes with a discussion of the risks and the challenges that surround the conduct and evaluation of support interventions.

Theoretical grounding of support interventions

Support interventions are theoretically grounded in three bodies of literature. The first offers a framework for understanding the stressful circumstances that call for the mobilization of support, and the types of support that may be required to meet the stressful demands. The second offers several theoretical viewpoints on social support's mechanisms of action, thereby supplying ideas about how social support ameliorates stress. The third source of theory addresses the social psychological conditions that are most hospitable to the intended beneficiaries of the intervention. Here, attention focuses on ways of structuring the program to make it an attractive social intervention. Collectively, these three sets of literature are united by a common proposition, namely that the feedback, companionship, guidance, and sense of reliable alliance which people gain from their close associates serve health protective ends, and that rends and losses occurring in the social fabric dispose toward maladjustment and illness.

Stressful circumstances and types of support

The first body of literature that provides the theoretical foundation for the mobilization of support testifies to the health risk resulting from the loss of significant attachment figures or of the resources they typically provide.[5-7] It follows that support interventions are called for on those occasions when people sustain such losses. Examples include programs for recent widows,[8,9] for bereaved children,[10] and for children whose parents have separated,[11] for elderly persons whose spouses have recently been placed in long-term care,[12] and for single parents.[13] Evidence of the risk attendant upon the loss of support has also spurred the creation of primary prevention programs, targeting persons who are imminently undergoing events that threaten to deplete the resources of their networks. For example, retirement planning programs typically focus on the social repercussions of this transition, encouraging employees to participate in volunteer activities and other leisure pursuits that afford opportunities for affiliation. Similarly, many hospice programs have introduced family support groups to facilitate the anticipatory grief process. Moreover, institutional policies that historically prevented individuals from gaining needed support at times of stress have been abandoned and replaced by practices that encourage greater and more regular access to sources of support. For instance, many hospitals and nursing homes now welcome family members as partners in patient care, while numerous schools have redefined the teacher's role in a way that emphasizes a closer mentoring relationship with students, and created more intimate schools within schools.

The theoretical import of these studies for the planning of support interventions is that they offer rich information about the nature of the support that is communicated and needed in close relationships. For example, in an effort to understand the onset of depression in adulthood, Brown and colleagues[5] have observed that parental loss in itself is not predictively implicated. Instead, they discovered that it is the loss of affectionate care, demonstrated by both the imposition of control and the expression of affection and attention, that results in adverse mental health sequelae. Drawing on this evidence, Sandler et al.[10] designed a support intervention for recently bereaved children that sought to enhance these dimensions of the child's caretaking environment. Weiss[14] has proposed an equally rich theoretical formulation of the provisions of social relationships on the basis of his inquiries among single parents and bereaved persons. He maintains that supportive relationships provide attachment and opportunities for nurturance, while affording a sense of reliable alliance and social integration. In addition, they provide guidance and reassurance of worth. Weiss also calls attention to the distinction between social losses that occasion feelings of emotional isolation and those that engender feelings of social isolation. This distinction has important implications for intervention. For example, it suggests that people's needs for empathic understanding cannot be met by programs that concentrate exclusively on providing them with companionship.

In a recent effort to develop theoretical guidelines for designing support interventions, Cutrona and Russell[15] reviewed a large number of studies examining the relevance of different functional components of support to different types of stressful events and transitions. Their goal was to determine whether adjustment to different types of stressors is predicated upon the availability or receipt of specific kinds of support.[16] Although their theoretical model received only partial support, it underscores the importance of crafting support interventions in ways that address the major demands and threats imposed by particular stressors. For example, Cutrona and Russell[15] state that: "For medical illness, not only physical capacity but also income, contact with others, and a sense of achievement may be lost, and consistent with this broader view of resulting social needs, tangible support, social integration, and esteem support predicted more positive outcomes" (p. 359). Whereas Cutrona and Russell's[15] "theory of optimal matching" mainly addresses the goodness of fit between supportive provisions and stressful demands, a comprehensive theoretical framework for intervention would also include information about the most relevant sources of certain kinds of support[17] and both the timing and duration of their support.[18] To extend the previous example of medical illness, intervention would be more fully informed by knowledge of who (e.g., physicians, family, friends, work associates) is best equipped to provide the tangible esteem and emotional support that are called for, and when their support should be introduced (e.g., prior to the formal diagnosis, immediately thereafter, during the period of recovery or convalescence).

Table 1 provides an overview of these and other issues that require consideration in the planning of support interventions. It is noteworthy that characteristics of the intended support recipient must also be taken into account. Persons who present themselves in ways that are highly threatening to potential providers of support,[19] as well as those whose social skills or attitudes toward help-seeking make it more difficult for them to accept support,[20] are less likely to be reached and to benefit from these interventions.

Social support: mechanisms of action

The second body of literature provides the theoretical bases for understanding how social support accomplishes its much-heralded stress buffering function. It addresses the behavioral, physiological, and perceptual processes that mediate the social environment's impact on health, morale, and well-being. For example, research on the social comparison process reveals that social support is based in part on feedback that is gained through contact with peers undergoing comparable stressful events. Early experimental research on the "psychology of affiliation" demonstrated that anxiety arouses the motive to affiliate in order to gain information about the appropriateness of the thoughts and feelings engendered by the stressful situation. In a series of classic studies, Schachter[21] observed that, even when subjects were prevented from verbally communicating with one another, they still wished to share one another's company, and in doing so, gained emotional relief. Equally important, Schachter discovered that his subjects preferred to share the company of persons facing the same stressful predicament, leading him to conclude that misery loves miserable company in particular. As discussed later, this social psychological phenomenon attesting to the calming effects of exposure to similar peers has provided the theo-

Table 1   A Framework for Planning Stress-Related Support Interventions

Nature and demands of the stressor
    Chronic or acute
    Changes in demands during phases of the stress process

Supportive needs aroused by the stressor
    Emotional support
    Tangible support
    Esteem support pertaining to self-worth and performance
    Social integration, including companionship and belonging

Sources of support
    Existing social network ties
    New ties grafted onto the social network
    Group of dyadic intervention

Characteristics of support
    Duration of support (reliability, commitment, continuity)
    Quantity or intensity of support (dosage, frequency)
    Symmetry of supportive interaction (mutuality)
    Coverage of supportive needs (social, emotional, practical)
    Specialization of support (prescribed activities or general befriending)

Characteristics of recipient of support
    Relationship needs, motivation, and skills
    Coping behavior (receptiveness to support)
    Nature and extent of visible distress that threatens others
    Cultural beliefs about and attitudes toward help-seeking

Goals of intervention
    Support as an end in itself (measures focus on the formation of
        relationships, changes in network size or composition, frequency of social
        interaction, quantity and satisfaction with actual and perceived support,
        loneliness)
    Support as a means to other ends (measures focus on psychiatric
        symptomatology, morale, life satisfaction, adherence to prescribed
        regimens, adjustment, use of services, subjective burden)
    Distinguishing between short-term and long-term outcomes

retical foundation for both dyadic and group interventions composed of fellow sufferers.

Recently, more specific social psychological phenomena have been implicated in the support process that unfolds when similar peers have opportunities to compare their stressful experiences. Principally, they center around the stress-moderating impact of empathy, normalization, and validation. For example, based on their analysis of a number of support groups, Coates and Winston[22] concluded that emotional ventilation mitigated feelings of deviance and depression, producing a normalizing effect that could not have occurred through the members' interactions with associates who had not been subjected to the same stressful encounter. Similarly, Thoits[23] underscores the role that similar peers play in validating new social roles and consolidating personal identities during major life transitions. For example, as couples pass through the transition to first-time parenthood, they gradually form new ties to other new parents and reduce their involvement with childless couples.[24] Other social psychological mechanisms that underlie the protective effects of peer support include the sense of control and personal efficacy that are gained from a reciprocal helping process.[25] In addition, since mutual aid is exchanged, the parties alternate between the roles of helper and help recipient, gaining a sense of self-worth at the same time as they communicate esteem to others. Additional theoretical views concerning the stress reducing impact of peer support include Pennebaker and O'Heeron's[26] and Silver and Wortman's[27] formulations concerning the positive impact of emotional ventilation on mood states, and Janoff-Bulman's[28] ideas about the ways in which support groups can assist people to find meaning when life crises have shattered their assumptions about the world.

Conditions conducive to the exchange of support

The third body of literature draws largely on social psychological theories to inform particular contours of the program design that affect its acceptability to its intended beneficiaries, rates of participation, and the self-perceptions that the program conditions. Specifically, social psychological research on recipients' reactions to the receipt of help suggests that program planners must avoid casting people strictly in the role of help recipients, but should concentrate on spurring the expression of mutual aid among peers.[29] For example, Lieberman and Videka-Sherman's[30] studies of self-help groups for bereaved widows and widowers revealed that the benefits derived from participation only accrued to those who formed new friendships characterized by mutual exchange. Similarly, the results of an intervention designed to establish friendships among elderly women through the creation of telephone dyads revealed that the telephone partners were not nominated as friends nor did their telephone contact result in any increase in their levels of perceived friend support. Commenting on this finding, Heller et al.[31] state: " . . . it is possible that telephone friendships were too limiting, and did not allow sufficient contact for the development of intimacy and mutual sharing" (p. 23).

When people are invited to participate in social programs that cast them exclusively in the role of recipient of support, their self-esteem is threatened and any feelings of deviance and incompetence they may have can be magnified. The help recipient can only draw pejorative implications regarding his/her inferior position relative to the helper. Moreover, feelings of dependency and indebtedness are heightened because there is no opportunity to reciprocate the support. Under such conditions, the possibility of friendship formation is precluded because the norm of reciprocity is violated. Finally, the recipient of aid is saddled with the extra burden of having to show gratitude to the provider, and having to feign acceptance of the aid, two gestures that may undermine feelings of self-efficacy.[32]

Three propositions are suggested by this theoretical foundation for creating program conditions conducive to the expression of support. First, efforts should be made to avoid the stigmatizing consequences of targeting programs to identified "at risk" or "red-tagged" populations. For example, by assigning mentors only to youth who are deemed likely to drop out of school, or by introducing home visitors only to parents who show early warning signs of abusing their children, programs are likely to arouse or reinforce negative self-perceptions among the intended program beneficiaries and bring stigma upon them. Universal recruitment strategies should be used, rather than targeted strategies that entail screening for pathology or disability.

Second, programs should operate in a style that places a premium on opportunities for reciprocity and mutuality, calling attention to the supportive resources that people bring to the program rather than to their deficiencies. Third, if there is any truth to the notion that unsolicited support confers greater value upon relationships than support that must be requested,[33] then conditions must be arranged that make help-seeking less salient and interdependence more prominent. By establishing a social context that blurs the distinction between the provider and the recipient of support, and is characterized by spontaneous and mutual exchanges, program planners can circumvent creating status hierarchies in which the helped are subordinate to those who render help.

A definition of support interventions

Elsewhere I have defined support interventions as *efforts to optimize the psychosocial resources which individuals proffer and/or receive in the context of relations with their primary social field.*[34] Before reviewing various types of support interventions, some preliminary comments regarding this definition are in order. First, psychosocial resources refer to various types of support, including esteem, emotional, and tangible support, as well as guidance and companionship (see Table 1). Empirically, these several dimensions of support are highly intercorrelated, reflecting the reality that people do not differentiate among these types of support in the course of their daily interactions with their close associates. Surely, when family members or friends lend a hand, or when they take the time to listen, they also communicate a sense of reliable alliance and esteem. From a practical perspective, then, it is doubtful that an intervention could influence one of these dimensions without also influencing other related aspects of support.

Second, support programs may concentrate on equipping providers with the skills, knowledge, or confidence to tender support, or on supplying the recipient with a higher quality, a greater amount, greater specialization, or lengthier periods of support. Support programs may also concentrate on both the provider and the recipient. For example, in self-help and support groups, each member assumes the support provider and recipient roles. In marriage, or at least in happy marriages, the spouses are continuously alternating between these two roles.

Third, the definition explicitly focuses on exchanges among primary group members, including family members, friends, and other close associates with whom they have or can develop emotionally important relationships. Support interventions involve lay persons who presently occupy or are likely to develop peer-like, kinship, or friendship relationships with one another. Although persons with professional training have occasionally served as support providers, in every instance the intervention aimed to instigate a process of befriending or to capitalize on some basis for identification between the provider and the support recipient. For example, Olds'[35] program for high-risk teenaged mothers assigned public health nurses to be home visitors, charging them with the task of educating the mothers about child development, and assisting the mothers to make better use of the resources of their informal support systems and of the community's health care institutions. However, their mandate also included befriending the young mothers and being available to them in ways typical of a close family friend. Similarly, in designing a bereavement program for families in which a parent had died, Sandler et al.[10] introduced a "family adviser" who had not only received training in working with bereaved families, but also had personally experienced an episode of grief. The authors explicitly describe the advisers as peers who " . . . provide the companionship, and nondirective, empathic support which bereaved adults often describe as particularly helpful" (p. 79).

Types of support interventions

The vast majority of support interventions can be organized along two dimensions. The first pertains to the social context in which support arises. It can be either a group or a dyadic, partner relationship. The second pertains to the intervention target. It can be either members of the existing network or one or more new relationships that are grafted onto the network. Naturally, there are combinations of these two dimensions, an example being Vachon et al.'s[9] "self-help intervention for widows". In this program a support group was convened only after each new widow had established a relationship with a veteran widow who offered practical help and emotional support. In other programs, the dyadic and group modes of support are provided concurrently rather than sequentially. An example from the public health field is the combined use of support groups and spousal/partner coaching in prenatal classes. It is also noteworthy that one type of intervention can have a range of social effects, an example being the way in which new relationships formed in a support group exert an impact on close relationships in the participants' natural networks.

Support groups

Support groups are by far the most widely adopted strategy of delivering supplemental or compensatory support to populations at risk. These groups are typically composed of eight to ten members who are trying to adjust to a life crisis, transition, or chronic exigency by sharing their experiences, swapping ways of coping, gaining and expressing empathic understanding, and taking comfort in the company of "fellow sufferers". Typically, the group meets in an agency or institutional setting for a fixed number of sessions, guided by a professional who supplements the participants' experiential knowledge with expertise about the group's process, the stressors members face, and relevant coping strategies. Unlike many self-help groups that have a dual focus on coping and advocacy, support groups tend to focus exclusively on the former. Examples include support groups for the bereaved,[9] for parents at risk of abuse and neglect,[36] for the divorced[12,37] and their children,[10,38] and for persons who experienced two or more recent life changes of any sort.[39]

The diversity of the goals of support groups, their format, intensity, duration, leadership, programming, and composition preclude comparative and cumulative evaluation of their short- and long-term impacts on participants. However, two recent reviews of several support group programs in one particular stress domain spotlight some of their limitations as well as some of the challenges associated with evaluating the impact of support groups. Specifically, Toseland and Rossiter[40] examined 29 studies, and Lavoie[41] examined 23 studies of support groups implemented for family members who provide daily care to physically or cognitively impaired elderly relatives. Both reviews conclude that, despite high levels of consumer satisfaction, the groups have relatively little impact on mental health, life satisfaction, or morale, as measured by psychometrically robust instruments. Toseland and Rossiter[40] state that: " ... existing studies do not indicate whether support groups can help caregivers to cope with or alleviate stress from specific problems they experience in providing care, prevent, diminish, or alleviate common psychological disturbances such as depression; increase access to and use of informal social support systems and community resources; or improve caregivers' ability to care for themselves" (p. 446).

There are numerous reasons why objective measures of the results of caregiver support groups may be so disappointing, and they may generalize to the evaluation of support groups in other stress contexts. First, since these support groups typically meet for only 6 to 8 weeks, the intervention is probably too brief to effect changes in such affective states as depression and anxiety, and in global indicators of life satisfaction. In fact, as Table 1 suggests, it is important to match the duration of the intervention to the participants' stress exposure. Simply stated, family caregivers are more likely to require ongoing support than crisis support. Second, unrealistic outcome measures may have been selected. There is little reason to believe that the support of similar peers would moderate either the objective burdens shouldered by caregivers or their feelings of sadness or anxiety regarding the health and functioning of their elderly relatives. Moreover, the caregivers may have joined the groups for entirely different reasons, suggesting a set of goals that were unmeasured by the researchers. For example, they may have come to the group looking for support for their identity as caregivers since such support may have been lacking in their natural networks. They may have come with expectations that they would learn about community services or about new, more effective and less taxing ways of coping with their relatives' impairments. Or they may have come to the group seeking information that might help them to adopt a more sanguine life outlook, or gain the ability to accept their relative's illness, and find a new framework for rebuilding their assumptions about the world. The accomplishment of these ends may account for the positive subjective reports of the participants, but they have yet to be gauged more rigorously by researchers.

Aside from the possibility that inappropriate outcomes have been measured, support groups may fail to ameliorate stress because they have not been composed in a way that optimizes the expression of support. Although social comparison theory suggests that misery loves miserable company, the challenge facing those who compose these groups is to determine the exact basis for perceptions of similarity in stressful circumstances. For example, it is unlikely that middle-aged daughters who are caring for their fathers at home would identify with elderly spouses who have already placed their husbands in long-term care. Fundamental differences in the life stage of these two groups of caregivers, in their relationship with the recipient of care, and in the locus of care would preclude them from identifying with one another. Similarly, in composing groups for persons with particular medical diagnoses and conditions, victims of domestic abuse, parents of children with developmental disabilities, or single mothers, it is critical to first determine the dimensions along which they perceive others to be "in the same boat" as themselves. And once similar peers are identified, groups should be composed in a way that fosters comforting social comparisons with respect to the members' progress in coping and stressor severity.[42] More generally, there is a need for studies that systematically vary group composition along these latter two dimensions, examining how the resulting social comparisons mediate group cohesion, the formation of relationships, and both actual and perceived social support.

Whereas the support group introduces a new set of social ties, a complementary but less widely practiced approach is to optimize support through altering the structure or interactional dynamics of the natural network. Adopting the entire social network as the unit of analysis and change,

Gottlieb and Coppard[43] and Lugtig and Fuchs[44] outlined a set of activities designed to alter the structure of the social networks of chronic mental patients and high-risk parents, respectively. For example, social network therapy for the chronically mentally ill entails "coaching" certain central figures in the patient's social network to express less criticism and hostility, convening "network sessions" designed to foster greater consistency in the kinds of support provided to the patient by key associates, and fostering the formation of new peer ties through "network construction". Network interventions such as these begin by mapping the intended beneficiary's social ties, and proceed to the tasks of identifying sources of stress and support, planning structural changes, such as altering the density of the network or gaining direct contact with a network member rather than depending on another person for access to that member, and increasing the specialization or reciprocity of supportive interactions.

Essentially, these network-centered interventions aim to build more supportive personal communities on behalf of populations whose risk stems either from chronically stressful circumstances or from personal vulnerability. For example, families in which there is a child who has Down's syndrome or who suffers from a chronic medical condition such as cystic fibrosis, or families that render daily care to an elderly relative suffering from dementia, require continuous supplies of emotional support, tangible aid, and respite. These situations call for interventions that create more durable and reliable support networks composed of both kith and kin as well as volunteer and paid helpers. Yet as potentially valuable as these interventions may be, they also pose ethical dilemmas. There is the risk that structural changes in the network will backfire and deplete or overtax its fund of support, and because neither firm principles nor guidelines for effective intervention yet exist, network members must be full collaborators in the process.

Support dyads

Two additional types of interventions center on the support communicated in dyadic or partner relationships, one entailing the mobilization of a new social tie and the other the optimization of support from an existing tie. The former is epitomized by such programs as Big Brothers/Sisters, in which a child is introduced to a community volunteer who assumes a surrogate family role. The latter is best illustrated by the Lamaze method of childbirth in which the husband or another close associate offers specialized support during the prenatal, labor, and delivery periods.[45] Moreover, both types of interventions may vary in the degree of specialization of the support to be provided. For example, in the mental health field, general support and befriending are often provided to persons with chronic mental illness by volunteer companions and to elderly persons by friendly visitors.[46] In contrast, there are highly specialized support programs such as those designed to prevent relapse among persons suffering from schizo-phrenia by teaching the principal family caregivers exactly how to extend support to the patient. These latter programs aim to reduce the caregivers' levels of "expressed emotion", principally the expression of criticism, and to substitute less threatening and more supportive messages.[47] Similarly, in the smoking cessation, weight loss, and alcoholism fields, "partner manu-als" have been developed that prescribe exactly how to help a close asso-ciate who is attempting to quit smoking, shed weight, or moderate alcohol consumption.[48] Moreover, many treatment programs in the addictions field create buddy systems whereby fellow sufferers are matched and instructed in ways of supporting one another's efforts to maintain resolve and to com-ply with the recommended treatment regimen.

Programs that offer general support are predicated on the assump-tion that people's needs for companionship are unmet, or that they are lonely or socially isolated. In contrast, programs that are highly prescrip-tive in the support tendered by the partner are based on the assumption that the intended beneficiaries lack specific supportive provisions needed to cope with particular stressful demands. However, in practice, inter-vention is rarely informed by empirical data bearing on the target popu-lation's supportive requirements or on the relationship between pre-intervention sources, types and levels of support, and indices of morale and well-being. For example, Heller et al.[31] designed a support interven-tion for low-income elderly women that involved the creation of peer tele-phone dyads. Specifically, the intervention began with graduate students making friendly phone calls, and then entered a new phase in which the telephone dyads were composed exclusively of the elderly women them-selves. However, the decision was made to marshall support in this way before data were gathered which revealed that perceived family support, and not perceived friend support, was related to initial levels of mental health. Consequently, it appeared that the intervention failed to improve the women's mental health because it marshalled the more diffuse sup-port of peers instead of particular kinds of family support. Interestingly, Heller et al.[31] found that the telephone dyads did not even result in the formation of friendships among the elderly women, nor in a significant increase in their levels of perceived friend support. They speculate that this was due to the relative anonymity of the telephone as a medium for relationship formation, and for the development of the intimacy and mu-tuality that characterize friendship.

Both in schools and in the workplace, there is increasing recognition of the need for greater interpersonal support and guidance. For example, through an innovative program called "I Have A Dream" (IHAD), low-income, inner city grade school students who are deemed to be at risk of school failure and early leaving, are adopted by a company that agrees to provide extra tutoring, enrichment, and both advocacy and personal sup-port from a privately paid counselor who works at their school. In addition, employees of the sponsoring company take a personal interest in the IHAD children, inviting them to company offices and occasionally coaching them in their studies. In addition, as an extra incentive, the company agrees to pay for the entire post-secondary education of all students who stay in the program and graduate from high school. More generally, many schools have attempted to dispel students' feelings of anonymity and to shore up support by assigning students to small advisory groups convened by a teacher-mentor who they can get to know on a more personal basis. Similarly, in many corporate settings, initiatives involving the establishment of one-to-one mentoring relationships have been widely implemented to foster management and career development, to socialize new recruits into an organization's culture, and to promote upward mobility through the advocacy and championing offered by the mentor.[49]

In sum, whether programs involve the optimization of support from a central figure within the social network or from a peer or mentor who is recruited as a supportive ally, the goal of the intervention is to afford opportunities for more intimate communication, for gaining a sense of reliable alliance with another, and for securing supportive resources that are relevant to the particular stressful demands that may be at hand. Collectively, these dyadic interventions are predicated on evidence that a single intimate, confiding relationship is vital to health protection. Such relationships shore up valued identities, render practical and emotional support during times of stress, and provide individuals with the resilience that derives from a sense of social purpose and social self-worth.

Challenges in designing support interventions

Michael Rutter[50] has sagely pointed out that whatever protection is afforded by social support does not lie in the variable itself, but in the process. It follows that the challenge of designing effective support interventions is to create the social conditions in which people are most likely to exchange support and to perceive that support is available if needed. Some of the interventions reviewed in this chapter, such as support groups, seem to have been very successful in creating conditions that are highly favorable to the process of mutual aid. Through studies that systematically vary the structural properties of these groups (see Table 2) while monitoring the supportive processes that unfold, more knowledge can be gained about the conditions that are most conducive to the communication and perception of support.

At present, there is scant information to inform decisions about the types of support interventions that are called for in different stressful circumstances. When is it more advisable to intervene with people who already occupy central roles in the social network than to graft new ties onto the individual's network? When parents separate or divorce, should their children be invited to attend a support group or should efforts be made

Table 2   The Design and Processes of Support Groups

Design Features: The Structural Properties of the Support Group

Venue or setting
- Geographic proximity to participants
- Informal or agency/institutional setting sessions
- Total number, length, and duration of sessions
- Interval between sessions

Leadership and facilitation
- One or more professionals only
- Co-led by a participant and a professional
- Rotating professional leaders

Composition
- Number of participants
- Open or closed membership
- Geographic proximity of participants to one another

Criteria for matching, including
- Gender, age, socioeconomic, ethnic, racial, and verbal skill factors
- Severity of the stressor
- Stage of coping with stressor
- Intensity of distress and emotional expression
- Extent of mobilization of personal coping skills

Format
- Structured vs. unstructured agenda and allocation of time
- Balance between expert input and experience swapping
- Rotating or continuous leadership
- Use of contracts vs. no contract
- Homework assignments (e.g., skill practise) vs. none
- Prescribed extra-group contacts among participants or not
- Instructions regarding extra-group exchanges of support or not
- Occasional participation of network associates or not

Mechanisms of Action: Processes Linking Support to Outcomes

- Catharsis: emotional ventilation
- Normalization of emotions
- Validation: affirmation of valued role and identity
- Helper-therapy: helping others helps oneself
- Reduction of uncertainty in novel circumstances
- Modeling of coping strategies
- Hope and a positive outlook
- Making meaning of the adversity and consolidating a new or changed identity
- Predictability and anticipatory coping
- Social comparisons

---

to introduce a mentoring relationship or therapeutic partnership on behalf of these children? These questions require further research that addresses the supportive needs that are aroused in different stressful circumstances, as well as the coping preferences of the intended beneficiaries.[51]
Moreover, questions that concern the supportive needs of the target population are inextricably linked with questions that concern their relationship needs. For some individuals, stress moderation will be predicated
upon interactions that meet their needs for social integration and companionship, whereas for others it will result from meeting their needs for
intimacy and empathic understanding. More generally, because interactions derive their supportive meaning and impact from the character of
the relationship between the parties, the challenge is to design programs
that spur the formation of personal relationships. That is, the central intervention task should not be viewed as the creation of a storehouse con-
taining material aid, esteem, affection, and coping assistance, but the creation of relationships that offer such expressions of support on a mutual
basis.[52]

Although obvious, it is also important to acknowledge that well-
intentioned support efforts can miscarry, and that there are limits on the
amount, duration, and availability of support from even the closest relationships. Especially when one relationship partner is always providing
support or becomes a captive of the caregiving role, the burdens he or she
shoulders and the debt incurred by the recipient of aid can occasion severe
relationship tensions.[53] In addition, there is evidence suggesting that support is more likely to miscarry when the providers are distressed by the
emotions displayed by those they wish to help,[54] when the latter cope in
ways that deter others from providing support,[51] and when the providers
become emotionally overinvolved in efforts to improve potential recipients' feelings.[53]

Finally, we have only a dim understanding of the varied meanings and
expressions of support in social networks that vary along ethnic, racial,
and cultural lines.[55] Such information is needed to plan interventions that
show ecological fidelity in the ways they augment or shore up social support. In some communities, religious institutions play a crucial role in providing opportunities for developing support networks, whereas in others
labor, civic, and leisure organizations play this role. Equally important,
communities differ in the norms they have established regarding the occasions when it is legitimate to seek help and the responsibilities that kith
and kin have to render aid and support. Cultural beliefs also come into
play in the process of coping and in the distress occasioned by major life
events and transitions. For example, religious beliefs have a profound impact on such coping dimensions as acceptance, optimism, emotional ex-
pressiveness, and support seeking. It follows that programs that mobilize
support when major life events and transitions occur must comprehend
the varied cultural meanings of both distress and support.

References

1. Berkman, L. F., The relationship of social networks and social support to morbidity and mortality, in *Social Support and Health*, Cohen, S. and Syme, S. L., Eds., Academic Press, Orlando, FL, 1985, 241.
2. House, J. S., Landis, K. R., and Umberson, D., Social relationships and health, *Science*, 241, 540, 1988.
3. Cohen, S. and Wills, T., Stress, social support, and the buffering hypothesis, *Psychol. Bull.*, 98, 310, 1985.
4. Gottlieb, B. H., *Social Support Strategies: Guidelines for Mental Health Practice*, Sage, Beverly Hills, CA, 1983.
5. Brown, G. W., Harris, T. O., and BiFulco, A., Long-term effects of early loss of parent, in *Depression in Young People: Epidemiological and Clinical Perspectives*, Rutter, M., Izard, C. E., and Read, P. B., Eds., Guilford Press, New York, 1986, 251.
6. Osterweis, M., Solomon, F., and Green, M., *Bereavement: Reactions, Consequences, and Care*, National Academy Press, Washington, D.C., 1984.
7. Stroebe, M. and Stroebe, W., Who suffers more? Sex differences in health risks of the widowed, *Psychol. Bull.*, 93, 279, 1983.
8. Silverman, P. R., *Widow to Widow*, Springer, New York, 1986.
9. Vachon, M. L. S., Lyall, W., Rogers, J., Freedman-Letofsky, K., and Freeman, S., A controlled study of a self-help intervention for widows, *Am. J. Psychiatry*, 137, 1380, 1980.
10. Sandler, I. N., Gersten, J. C., Reynolds, K., Kallgren, C. A., and Ramirez, R., Using theory and data to plan support interventions: design of a program for bereaved children, in *Marshaling Social Support: Formats, Processes, and Effects*, Gottlieb, B. H., Ed., Sage, Newbury Park, CA, 1988, 53.
11. Kalter, N., Schaefer, M., Lesowitz, M., Alpern, D., and Pickar, J., School-based support groups for children of divorce: a model of brief intervention, in *Marshaling Social Support: Formats, Processes, and Effects*, Gottlieb, B. H., Ed., Sage, Newbury Park, CA, 1988, 135.
12. Fabiszewski, K. J. and Howell, M. C., A model for family meetings in the long-term care of Alzheimer's disease, *J. Gerontol. Nurs.*, 12, 113, 1986.
13. Warren, N. J. and Amara, I. A., Educational groups for single parents: the Parenting After Divorce programs, *J. Divorce*, 8, 79, 1984.
14. Weiss, R. S., The provisions of social relationships, in *Doing Unto Others*, Rubin, Z., Ed., Prentice-Hall, Englewood Cliffs, NJ, 1974, 17–26.
15. Cutrona, C. E. and Russell, D. W., Type of social support and specific stress: toward a theory of optimal matching, in *Social Support: An Interactional Perspective*, Sarason, B. R., Sarason, I. G., and Pierce, R., Eds., John Wiley & Sons, New York, 1990, 319.
16. Cohen, S. and McKay, G., Social support, stress, and the buffering hypothesis: a theoretical analysis, in *Handbook of Psychology and Health*, Baum, J., Singer, A. E., and Taylor, S. E., Eds., Erlbaum, Hillside, NJ, 1984, 253.
17. Dakof, G. A. and Taylor, S. E., Victims' perceptions of social support: what is helpful from whom?, *J. Personality Soc. Psychol.*, 58, 80, 1990.
18. Jacobson, D. E., Types and timing of social support, *J. Health Soc. Behav.*, 27, 250, 1986.

19. Silver, R. L., Wortman, C. B., and Cofton, C., The role of coping in support provision: the self-presentational dilemma of victims of life crises, in *Social Support: An Interactional View*, Sarason, B. R., Sarason, I. G., and Pierce, G. R., Eds., John Wiley & Sons, New York, 1990, 397.
20. Eckenrode, J., The mobilization of social supports: some individual constraints. *Am. J. Community Psychol.*, 11, 1983, 509.
21. Schachter, S., *The Psychology of Affiliation*, Stanford University Press, Palo Alto, CA, 1959.
22. Coates, D. and Winston, T., Counteracting the deviance of depression: peer support groups for victims, *J. Soc. Issues*, 39, 169, 1983.
23. Thoits, P. A., Coping, social support, and psychological outcomes, in *Review of Personality and Social Psychology*, Vol. 5, Shaver, P., Ed., Sage, Newbury Park, CA, 1984, 219.
24. Gottlieb, B. H. and Pancer, S. M., Social networks and the transition to parenthood, in *The Transition to Parenthood: Current Theory and Research*, Michaels, G. Y. and Goldberg, W. A., Eds., Cambridge University Press, New Rochelle, CT, 1988.
25. Taylor, S. E., Lichtman, R. R., and Wood, J. V., Attributions, beliefs about control, and adjustment to breast cancer, *J. Personality Soc. Psychol.*, 46, 489, 1984.
26. Pennebaker, J. W. and O'Heeron, R. C., Confiding in others and illness rate among spouses of suicide and accidental death victims, *J. Abnormal Psychol.*, 93, 473, 1984.
27. Silver, R. L. and Wortman, C. B., Coping with undesirable life events, in *Human Helplessness: Theory and Applications*, Garber, J. and Seligman, M. E. P., Eds., Academic Press, New York, 1980, 279.
28. Janoff-Bulman, R., *Shattered Assumptions*, The Free Press, New York, 1992.
29. Fisher, J. D., Nadler, A., and Whitcher-Alagna, S., Recipient reactions to aid, *Psychol. Bull.*, 91, 27, 1982.
30. Lieberman, M. A. and Videka-Sherman, L., The impact of self-help groups on the mental health of widows and widowers, *Am. J. Orthopsychiatry*, 56, 435, 1986.
31. Heller, K., Thompson, M. G., Trueba, P. E., Hogg, J. R., and Vlachos-Weber, I., Peer support telephone dyads for elderly women: was this the wrong intervention?, *Am. J. Community Psychol.*, 19, 53, 1991.
32. Fisher, J. D., Goff, B. A., Nadler, A., and Chinsky, J. M., Social psychological influences on help-seeking and support from peers, in *Marshaling Social Support*, Gottlieb, B. H., Ed., Sage, Newbury Park, 1988, 267.
33. Steinberg, M. and Gottlieb, B. H., The appraisal of spousal support by women facing conflicts between work and family, in *Communication of Social Support*, Burleson, B. R., Albrecht, T. L., and Sarason, I. G. (Ed.), Sage, Newbury Park, CA, 1994, 152–172.
34. Gottlieb, B. H., Support interventions: a typology and agenda for research, in *Handbook of Personal Relationships*, Duck, S., Ed., John Wiley & Sons, Chichester, England, 1988, 519.
35. Olds, D. L., The prenatal/early infancy project, in *14 Ounces of Prevention*, Price, R. H., Cowen, E. L., Lorion, R. P., and Ramos-McKay, J., Eds., American Psychiatric Association, Washington, D.C., 1988, 9.

36. Kline, B., Grayson, J., and Mathie, A., Parenting support groups for parents at risk of abuse and neglect, *J. Primary Prevent.*, 10, 313, 1990.

37. Bloom, B. L., Hodges, W., and Caldwell, R., A preventive program for the newly separated: initial evaluation, *Am. J. Community Psychol.*, 10, 251, 1982.

38. Kalter, N., Pickar, J., and Lesowitz, M., Developmental facilitation groups for children of divorce: a preventive intervention, *Am. J. Orthopsychiatry*, 54, 613, 1984.

39. Roskin, M., Coping with life changes—a preventive social work approach, *Am. J. Community Psychol.*, 10, 331, 1982.

40. Toseland, R. W. and Rossiter, C. M., Group interventions to support family caregivers: a review and analysis, *Gerontologist*, 29, 438, 1989.

41. Lavoie, J.-P., Support groups for informal caregivers don't work! Refocus the groups or the evaluations, Public Health Unit of Verdun Hospital, 4000 Lasalle Blvd., Verdun, Quebec, Canada, unpublished manuscript, 1994.

42. Wood, J. V., Taylor, S. E., and Lichtman, R. R., Social comparison in adjustment to breast cancer, *J. Personality Soc. Psychol.*, 49, 1169, 1985.

43. Gottlieb, B. H. and Coppard, A. E., Using social network therapy to create support systems for the chronically mentally disabled, *Can. J. Community Mental Health*, 6, 117, 1987.

44. Lugtig, D. and Fuchs, D., *Building on the strengths of local neighborhood social network ties for the prevention of child maltreatment*, Final Report of the Neighborhood Parent Support Project, Faculty of Social Work, University of Manitoba, Winnipeg, Manitoba, Canada, 1992.

45. Wideman, M. V. and Singer, J. E., The role of psychological mechanisms in preparation for childbirth, *Am. Psychol.*, 39, 1357, 1984.

46. Skirboll, B. W. and Pavelsky, P. K., The Compeer program: volunteers as friends of the mentally ill, *Hosp. Community Psychiatry*, 35, 938, 1984.

47. Goldstein, M. J., Ed., *New Directions for Mental Health Services: New Developments in Interventions with Families of Schizophrenics*, Vol. 12, Jossey-Bass, San Francisco, CA, 1981.

48. McIntyre-Kingsolver, K. O., Lichtenstein, E., and Mermelstein, R. J., Spouse training in a multicomponent smoking cessation program, *Behav. Ther.*, 17, 67, 1986.

49. Carden, A. D., Mentoring and adult career development, *Counselling Psychol.*, 18, 275, 1990.

50. Rutter, M., Psychosocial resilience and protective mechanisms, *Am. J. Orthopsychiatry*, 57, 316, 1987.

51. Dunkel-Schetter, C., Folkman, S., and Lazarus, R., Correlates of social support receipt, *J. Personality Soc. Psychol.*, 53, 71, 1987.

52. Gottlieb, B. H., Social support: a relationship process, not a commodity, *Can. J. Aging*, 11, 306, 1992.

53. Coyne, J. C., Wortman, C. B., and Lehman, D., The other side of support: emotional overinvolvement and miscarried helping, in *Marshaling Social Support: Formats, Processes, and Effects*, Gottlieb, B. H., Ed., Sage, Newbury Park, CA, 1988, 305.

54. Howes, M. J. and Hokanson, J. E., Conversational and social responses to depressive interpersonal behavior, *J. Abnormal Psychol.*, 88, 625, 1979.

55. Valle, R. and Vega, W., Hispanic Natural Support Systems: Mental Health Promotion Perspectives, State of California Department of Mental Health, Sacramento, CA, 1980.

chapter nineteen

Coping with the stress of cancer

Christina G. Blanchard and Gregory R. Harper

Introduction

Cancer presents patients and families with a multitude of demands. These range from the fear of dying and fears of treatment to concerns about emotional ramifications of the disease and disruptions in daily roles and routines. The impact of the demands on psychological well-being has been documented.[1] Investigators have also examined the ways adult cancer patients cope with these demands to reduce stress, improve psychological well-being, and possibly to influence disease progression. (The special needs of children and adolescents with cancer are beyond the scope of this chapter.)

This chapter begins with a current definition of coping as an active process involving an appraisal of the stressful event, a selection of coping strategies, implementation of these strategies, and reappraisal of the event. The most frequently employed instruments used to assess coping with cancer are reviewed. Predictors or determinants of coping responses (individual, disease-related, sociocultural) are discussed, and the impact of specific coping responses on outcomes, particularly mood, are explored. Several intervention studies are reviewed which were designed to improve outcomes, particularly psychological adjustment. A model is proposed (see Figure 1) which both represents our current understanding of the coping process and can serve as a guide for future research into coping mechanisms and outcomes.

Definition

Coping is a critical factor in the relationship between stressful life events and adaptation to these events. In early research Freud[2] conceptualized coping as a defense mechanism that was primarily an unconscious response of an individual to intrapsychic conflict. In the 1970s interest in the relationship between recent life events and stress led to the conceptualization of coping as an active, conscious process.[3]

0-8493-2908-6/96/$0.00+$.50
© 1996 by CRC Press, Inc.

The theoretical framework currently most commonly used was developed by Lazarus and Folkman, who defined coping as . . . "constantly changing cognitive and behavioral efforts to manage specific internal and external demands that are appraised as taxing or exceeding the resources of an individual" (p. 141).[4] According to this model, individuals appraise an encounter or transaction as representing harm, challenge, or the threat of harm (primary appraisal). If the encounter is perceived as stressful, coping resources and options are then evaluated in a process termed secondary appraisal. Coping responses are then implemented. If the threatening or harmful situation is appraised as having few possibilities for positive changes or outcomes, the person will use emotion-focused coping responses. On the other hand, if the situation is appraised as having the potential for improvement by action, problem-solving approaches are selected. This process is repeated as the individual interacts with the environment.

Somerfield and Curbow[3] suggested that three aspects of the Lazarus and Folkman model are relevant to a study of coping with cancer: (1) focus on what the individual does (behavioral) or thinks (cognitive) in a specific situation, (2) context-specific assessment, and (3) coping viewed as a dynamic process. Analysis is thus focused on the coping responses in a specific context rather than on coping responses used across many situations, i.e., a personality style or disposition. Thus, rather than asking "how are you coping with your cancer," questions focus on coping with specific issues such as pain, fear of dying, or communication with family. The coping process is therefore dynamic, not static, and changes as the context changes. It is also evident that a coping strategy may be adaptive in one context and maladaptive in another. For example, denial may be maladaptive if it prevents an individual from reporting new symptoms to the physician, but adaptive if it facilitates an individual's enjoying life as much as possible in the context of terminal illness.

A pragmatic advantage of the process/state approach for the design of intervention to assist coping of cancer patients is that it may be easier to change what people do (the process approach) than who they are (the dispositional approach).[5] The specific situation can then be targeted to ascertain if indeed the intervention was successful in improving coping effectiveness.

Instruments to measure coping

Several investigators have either modified standard coping instruments from the psychological literature to be relevant to the demands of cancer patients or developed new measures specifically targeted to cancer patients (see Table 1). As Somerfield and Curbow[3] cautioned, however, the potential benefits of standard instruments (strong psychometric properties and potential comparisons across studies/generalizability) may not

Table 1   Instruments Used to Measure Coping with Cancer

Instrument	Author(s)	Differentiating features
Ways of Coping (WOC)	Folkman et al.[8]	Problem-specific coping responses
Ways of Coping-Cancer (WOC-CA)	Dunkel-Schetter et al.[9]	Cancer problem-specific coping responses
Ways of Coping (WOC) modified and semi-structured interview	Jarrett et al.[10]	Comparison of fixed and open-ended responses
Ways of Coping (WOC) modified	Cooper and Faraher[11,12]	Personality traits and life events also assessed
COPE	Carver et al.[13,14]	Additional coping responses not included in WOC; Life Orientation Test (LOT) assesses optimism-pessimism
Ways of Coping (WOC) revised	Mishel et al.[16]	Mishel's Uncertainty in Illness Scale
Mental Adjustment to Cancer Scale (MAC)	Watson et al.[18]	Appraisal and coping responses in single instrument: global measure

be realized because of psychometric problems. For example, there is limited empirical support for coping subscales of these measures.[6] Additionally, differences in scoring of standard measures also limits the usefulness of these measures (see Reference 7).

One of the most widely used instruments to measure coping is The Ways of Coping (WOC) questionnaire designed and then revised by Folkman and colleagues.[8] It is a 51-item questionnaire which assesses the coping response a person selects to manage a particular stressful situation. Individuals are asked how often (never to very often) they used each of the listed coping responses to manage the specific problem. The instrument provides information on the frequency of each response. Two problem-focused subscales were found (planful problem solving and seeking social support). Six emotion-focused subscales were also reported (confrontive coping, distancing, self-controlling, accepting responsibility, escape avoidance, and positive appraisal). These categories have not been found in all studies using this instrument.[6]

The Ways of Coping questionnaire was modified for cancer patients by Dunkel-Schetter and colleagues (WOC-CA).[9] Following the model of Lazarus and Folkman[4] described earlier, the investigators selected four specific problem areas or demands confronting patients with cancer: fear and uncertainty about the future due to cancer, limitations in physical ability, appearance or lifestyle due to cancer; acute pain, symptoms, or discomfort from illness or treatment; and problems from family or friends due to cancer. They asked 603 cancer patients to select whichever one had been most stressful in the past 6 months and to rate how stressful it had been (primary appraisal).

Patients then were asked to indicate how often they had used each of a list of 52 possible coping responses to solve the identified problem (secondary appraisal). Factor analysis produced five coping factors: seeking and using social support (e.g., talked to someone about how I was feeling), focusing on the positive (e.g., rediscovered what was important in life), distancing (e.g., didn't let it get to me; refused to think about it), cognitive escape-avoidance (e.g., hoped a miracle would happen), and behavioral escape-avoidance (e.g., avoided being with people).

Several groups in Great Britain have modified the WOC for use with breast cancer patients. Jarrett et al.[10] eliminated 13 items considered inappropriate and found factor analysis did not correspond to the original factors reported by Lazarus and colleagues. A semistructured interview was included to provide patients the opportunity to describe coping strategies and also to express ambivalence in their responses resulting from the inherent uncertainty accompanying cancer and its treatment. Specific advantages of the WOC are the short amount of time required for completion and the elimination of observer bias. The advantage of the interview is the richness of responses while the disadvantages are length of time to administer and difficulty coding responses. The authors concluded that the two methods are complementary.

Cooper and Faragher[11,12] modified the WOC and studied women presenting for investigation of breast symptoms. The 36 most frequently cited coping strategies by patient volunteers were selected to use with their sample of 2163 women attending a breast screening clinic. Five factors were reported: denial (try not to think about it), internalize (sit and think), externalize (talk things over), emotional outlet (cry a lot much later), and anger (get angry with things to erase problem). The authors also explored the impact of life events and personality traits on the cancer diagnosis.

Carver et al.[13,14] used a self-report inventory called the COPE to assess coping responses to cancer. It measures a broad range of coping responses, some of which are not included in the WOC (e.g., denial, acceptance, behavioral disengagement, use of humor). The instability of the factor structure Carver et al. initially reported was addressed in their recent article in which they reported having to adjust several subscales due to problems with reliability.[14] These authors also contended that it is necessary to measure the individual's dispositional or personality style, i.e., the trait well-being and also the choice of coping responses. The personality variable measured was optimism-pessimism, chosen because it had been found to play an important role in both behavioral and psychological outcomes when people face negative life events (for a review see Reference 15). Optimism-pessimism was assessed by an eight-item instrument, the Life Orientation Test (LOT), which asks subjects how they generally respond to uncertain or ambiguous situations.

Mishel et al.[16] revised the WOC instrument to assess situation-specific coping. The authors contended that coping responses would be affected by the subject's sense of mastery or belief in their own ability to act to "mitigate the adverseness of events" (p. 237),[16] which was measured by a five-item form from Pearlin and Schooler.[17] Their model further viewed mastery as a response to the individual's assessment of the uncertainty of the situation, measured by Mishel's Uncertainty in Illness Scale. However, path analyses of the two studies testing this model have not provided clear support for this approach. The authors suggested that perhaps this was due to the fact that one sample was studied at home and the other in the hospital.

Another approach to measuring coping, developed by Watson et al.,[18] is the Mental Adjustment to Cancer Scale (MAC). Five adjustment styles were originally reported: anxious preoccupation, helpfulness, fatalism, avoidance, and fighting spirit. Unlike the versions of the WOC, it includes items measuring both appraisal (I see my illness as a challenge) and coping responses (I am trying to get as much information as I can about cancer) into one variable called mental adjustment to cancer. Rather than focus on a specific problem connected with cancer, cancer is viewed in a broad sense. The MAC was validated with patients in Great Britain and found to have reasonable psychometric properties, with the exception of the denial subscale. It may be useful as a global measure but lacks specificity to understand the specific problems with which the patient is dealing or the specific coping responses used.

In summary, there is no one instrument that is used to assess coping in response to the stress of cancer. With the exception of the MAC, there does seem to be agreement that whether measured by questionnaire or semistructured interview, the demands of cancer should be specified so that a coping response can be identified as relating to the specific context. There is disagreement regarding the need to examine dispositional factors such as optimism-pessimism, although even Lazarus recently[19] has concluded that the state and trait approaches are two sides of the same coin and both warrant investigation.

Predictors of coping responses

Rowland[5] discussed three categories influencing the patient's coping responses: disease-related, individual, and sociocultural. Disease-related variables include the nature of the illness, symptoms, type of treatment, and prognosis. These provide the context for the demands that the individual faces. A woman with stage I breast cancer who has a lumpectomy followed by radiation therapy faces different issues than does the woman with stage IV metastatic breast cancer who has failed conventional treatment and who is ineligible for a bone marrow transplant.

Individual determinants include the developmental stage of the individual (including age, skills), values and beliefs (including previous illness and cancer experience, religious beliefs), and social support. Using the above example, a young woman with breast cancer might be concerned about its impact on her desire for a family, a middle-aged woman might be concerned about her adolescent children or plans for retirement, and an older woman might worry about care of the spouse and financial issues. Values and beliefs also play a role in what the patient expects and fears. Social support provides an important assistance to coping; the absence of family and friends increases the psychological vulnerability of the patient.

Sociocultural factors include community attitudes and resources available. These help both to define the demands faced by the patient and the resources available to cope or manage the demands. For example, attitudes toward dying have changed over the past 25 years. These are reflected in changes in goals of care from cure to keep the dying patient comfortable. As a result, hospices developed to provide services to help the patient remain at home.

Disease-related variables

The complexity of the relationship between disease-related variables and coping responses can be seen in several studies. Gotay[20] interviewed patients with early-stage cervical cancer or pre-cancer ($N = 42$) and their mates ($N = 19$) and patients with advanced-stage breast or gynecological cancer ($N = 31$) and their mates ($N = 20$). The most common concern for each of the groups was fear of cancer itself; mates were more likely than patients to be concerned about the threat of the women dying. The most frequently used coping strategy was taking firm action; denial was not a predominant coping response. There were differences by stage of disease with the early-stage groups commonly employing information-seeking while those patients in advanced stages of disease often coped by using their religious faith.

Dunkel-Schetter et al.,[9] employing the WOC-CA on 603 cancer patients, found that time since diagnosis, type of cancer, and whether a person was in treatment had few or no relationships to the coping patterns used. The specific cancer-related problem also was not related to the coping pattern employed but perception of stressfulness was associated with significantly more coping through seeking and using social support and both cognitive and behavioral escape-avoidance.

Lerman et al.[21] conducted an intervention study of 48 cancer patients to examine the relationship of coping style to cancer chemotherapy side effects and then to determine whether coping style moderated the impact of a relaxation intervention on anxiety, depression, and nausea associated with chemotherapy. They used the Miller Behavioral Style Scale, which measures the respondents' characteristic mode of coping as "monitoring" or "blunting." A monitor is a person who copes by information seeking; a blunter copes by a tendency to use avoidance distraction techniques when under stress. They found the "blunting" coping style was associated with less anticipatory anxiety, less depression, and less nausea during and after chemotherapy. A "monitoring" style was associated with more anticipatory anxiety and more nausea before and during chemotherapy. The relaxation intervention was more effective in reducing anticipatory nausea among the "blunters" than among the "monitors," perhaps because the intervention was more similar to the distraction style of the "blunters".

Lewis[22] suggested that the results of these studies can be understood by examining coping responses in the context of the disease stage. Thus, an avoidant style may be inconsistent with the benefits of active information seeking which enhances control, but may be adaptive at certain points in the illness. For example, an avoidant style may allow a patient to undergo chemotherapy while an active information style might be more adaptive at the time of diagnosis. This may help to explain Lerman's study discussed above. Longitudinal studies are needed to examine more fully the relationship of coping strategy to the specific demands of each stage of the illness.

Individual determinants

Studies of the impact of individual variables on coping responses have generally focused on the issue of personality/dispositional style as a predictor of coping response. Scheier and Carver[23] suggested that one personality variable, dispositional optimism, affects how people will cope with stressful life events. This is based on their model of behavioral self-regulation, which predicts that people will persist in their efforts to attain desired outcomes only as long as those outcomes are perceived to be attainable. In a study of 59 breast cancer patients studied prospectively over 1 year from diagnosis, they found acceptance, positive reframing, and use of religion were the most common coping reactions. The least frequently used were denial and behavior disengagement. Three predominant relationships between optimism and coping responses were reported. Optimistic women were more likely than less optimistic women to accept the reality of the situation, and less likely to put the situation aside and thus refuse to deal with it. Optimists were also less likely to experience the feelings of giving up that characterize a helpless response to an uncontrollable or unmanageable situation.

In a study of 49 cancer patients with varied cancer diagnoses, Friedman et al.[24] also reported significant relationships between dispositional optimism and active-behavioral coping (measured by the Moos Coping Scale, Billings and Moos[25]). Avoidance coping was negatively related to optimism. Multivariate analyses showed gender and evidence of disease did not predict coping responses.

Hilton[26] built on the coping model described earlier by Lazarus and Folkman,[4] and investigated the relationships between coping responses measured by the revised WOC and (1) commitment, which she viewed as guiding people into or away from threatening situations, (2) perceptions of uncertainty, acknowledging difficulties in accurately appraising the situations, (3) perceptions of situational control, and (4) fears of recurrence. Two hundred twenty-seven breast cancer patients were studied.

Women who had low commitment and control together with high uncertainty and high threat of recurrence used escape-avoidance and accepting responsibility but not positive reappraisal strategies. Emotion-focused strategies were seen as trying to maintain hope in the face of situational ambiguity. Women with a high threat of recurrence and high control used social support, planful problem solving, escape-avoidance, positive reappraisal, and self-controlling strategies. These approaches would seem to be adaptive responses to a situation appraised as uncertain but also perceived as controllable. Using social support, planful problem solving, and self-controlling strategies may also reduce the helplessness of the situation while positive reappraisal may be used to make the best of the situation. Since the threat of cancer recurrence is never totally eliminated, the use of escape-avoidance seems understandable.

Sociocultural variables

To our knowledge there have been no empirical studies examining the relationship between sociocultural factors such as stigma attached to cancer and resources to help cope with specific coping responses with cancer. However, the findings by Mattlin et al.[27] of situational determinants of coping in a community sample suggest the importance of research aimed at comparing determinants of coping and coping effectiveness when the stressful event is cancer to determinants when the stressful events are not cancer related.

In summary, the predictors of coping responses that have been studied most frequently are disease severity or treatment and personality style, particularly optimism. To the best of our knowledge, there are no studies that have systematically investigated the relative importance of various predictors of coping. Furthermore, no longitudinal studies exist that follow individuals over the course of the illness to examine any changes in predictors over time. Finally, studies are primarily of breast cancer patients and thus the possible impact of gender and of disease site on coping responses is unknown.

Outcomes of coping responses

The initial short-term response to cancer may include significant depression, anxiety, and other symptoms of distress and reduced functioning. Yet, the majority of individuals adjust well over time and are no different on most psychological outcome measures from individuals with benign disease (see Reference 28). A number of studies have explored the relationship between coping responses and psychological distress to understand how this adaptation occurs and also to identify predictors of individuals at high risk for psychological distress. For example, Carver et al.,[14] in their examination of optimism, coping, and distress (measured by the Profile of Mood States), found optimism was inversely related to distress at each of the time periods studied over the year following diagnosis of breast cancer. This relationship held even when prior distress was controlled. They also found acceptance and the use of humor prospectively predicted lower distress; denial and disengagement greater distress. The authors suggested that optimists make every effort to remain engaged with goals giving their life meaning. Such an approach requires active coping and results in lower distress, in contrast to the passive approach of the pessimist.

Although optimism was not found to predict distress prospectively, Stanton and Snider,[29] in another study of breast cancer patients, did find that cognitive avoidance was an important predictor of high distress and low vigor. Similar results were reported by Dunkel-Schetter et al.[9] in their study described earlier. Coping through social support, focusing on the positive, and distancing were associated with less emotional distress, as measured by the Profile of Mood States (POMS). Using cognitive and behavioral escape-avoidance were associated with more emotional distress.

Several studies have examined the relationship between coping responses and another outcome measure, survival. Greer et al.[30] studied 69 women with breast cancer and found those responding to their illness by a fighting spirit or denial response were twice as likely to survive in the ensuing 5 years than were those responding with stoic acceptance or helplessness/hopelessness. Those with fighting spirit recognized the threat but were determined to cope as effectively as possible. How similar this is to the dispositional optimism described earlier, studied by Carver and colleagues,[14] remains to be examined, but both are clearly active coping responses. It is more difficult to understand why women employing denial fared better, but this pretense may have enabled the patients to "fight" in other areas of their lives. Stoic acceptance and helplessness responses represented doing little about the situation and giving up.

The search for personality correlates led to the conceptualization of a personality style, called type C. This involves the suppression of negative emotions (e.g., Cooper and Faragher[11]) and a reliance on the needs of others rather than oneself (Temoshak[31]). Temoshak reported that this style was common among cancer patients and that it predicted faster progression of malignant melanoma. On the other hand, Cassileth et al.[32] and Jamison et al.[33] did not find any significant relationships between personality variables and rate of disease progression or survival time.

Spiegel[34] suggested that, although their studies of breast cancer patients did not find personality variables predicted the rate of disease progression, they did find a "take charge" attitude of response to cancer seemed to be related to less anxiety and depression over the year the patients were studied. In his recent book, *Living Beyond Limits,* Spiegel advised cancer patients: "You cannot control everything, you cannot undo what has been done (like getting the disease), but you will benefit by taking hold of your current situation in whatever way is possible" (p. 62).[33] This is similar to the "fighting spirit" approach described earlier.

It should be noted that studies of the relationship between coping responses and outcomes have generally failed to assess outcomes in quality of life domains in addition to psychological distress. This is particularly surprising since there are studies showing different problem areas of life corresponding to stages of the disease. For example, Gordon et al.[35] followed 308 breast, lung, and melanoma patients through the first 6 months of their disease. At the time of initial hospitalization, the most frequently noted problems were the disease itself. After discharge, negative affect became the predominant worry. At 3 and 6 months later, problems were noted in many areas of life, including physical discomfort, concern about medical treatment, dissatisfaction with health care service, lack of mobility, financial concerns, family and social problems, worry about the disease, negative affect, and body image difficulties.

Additionally, there are a number of quality of life instruments that could be used as outcome measures. For example, Cella et al.[36] have developed the FACT (Functional Assessment of Cancer Scale), which produces subscale scores for physical, functional, social, and emotional well-being, as well as satisfaction with the treatment relationship. Another example is the CARES (Cancer Rehabilitation Evaluation System) developed by Schay and Henrich,[37] which assesses problems in a variety of areas: physical, psychosocial, medical interaction, sexual, and marital.

One study that has employed outcome measures of both positive and negative moods has been reported recently by Heidrich et al.[28] Outcomes measured were psychological well-being, assessed by three scales: measuring purpose in life; personal growth and positive relations with others; and psychological distress, assessed by the CES-D (Center for Epidemiological Studies Depression Scale). These authors suggested that discrepancies between actual and ideal conceptions of self influence adjustment and mediate the impact of disease-related variables on psychological well-being. Self-discrepancy was measured by a 20-item scale designed for this study of 108 cancer patients.

Cancer patients who reported more symptoms and worse functional status and who perceived their illness as chronic rather than acute had higher levels of self-discrepancy. A higher level of self-discrepancy was found to be a significant mediator of the effects of perceived health status on purpose in life and positive relations with others but not on depression, suggesting perceptions of physical health may have greater impact on psychological distress than on psychological well-being. They emphasized the importance of further studies of these variables, as clinical interventions would differ depending on the direction of causality found. If depression or well-being is increasing self-discrepancy, then interventions, such as problem-solving approaches, could focus on reducing depression. If, however, self-discrepancies are the causal variable, then interventions such as the provision of accurate information, which might change patients' capacity to deal with the illness and reduce self-discrepancy, would be indicated.

Selected interventions to assist coping and evaluate impact on adjustment and survival as outcomes

The most common forms of psychosocial interventions for cancer patients are education, behavioral training (e.g., relaxation training, guided imagery), individual support, and support groups. Interventions are generally designed to assist the patient to feel less hopeless and helpless and to be involved in active coping.

Although it is beyond the scope of this chapter to review all the intervention studies (see a recent review by Anderson[38] and a history of interventions by Fawzy and Fawzy[39]), the impact of support group interventions has received significant attention in the last few years in the lay and professional literature. Three studies are of particular importance. In a nonrandomized study, Gellert et al.[40] evaluated the impact of the widely publicized approach of Siegel employing weekly cancer peer support and family therapy in individual counseling and positive mental imagery. No significant differences were reported between the treatment group and others not in the program.

Spiegel and colleagues[41] randomly assigned 86 women with metastatic breast cancer to a no-intervention group or a group intervention consisting of supportive and expressive components. Thus, women were encouraged to care and support each other and to share their joys and fears. After a year of weekly meetings, women in the treatment group had significantly less anxiety, confusion, fatigue, and overall mood disturbance. Conversely, women in the control group showed increases in these areas. Women in the treatment group also used denial less, were able to face problems more directly, and were less frightened. It was suggested that the hypnosis component provided additional assistance to the other group treatment components. At 10-year follow-up, Spiegel et al.[42] reported a striking survival difference between subjects in the control group (18.9 months) and those in the treatment group (36.6 months) from study entry to death. This study's findings were viewed by the authors as unexpected and have generated much controversy. Spiegel[43] has suggested several mechanisms that might explain the findings, and a replication study is currently underway.

The third study has been reported by Fawzy and colleagues.[44,45] This was the first to examine psychological, immune, and disease endpoint data as these related to a psychological intervention. Eighty stage I or II newly treated melanoma patients were randomly assigned to a no-psychological-treatment group or structured short-term (six sessions) group support intervention. The intervention was designed to help patients cope better with the illness and its effects through using drawings that portrayed patients and families. At 6-month follow-up the group receiving the support showed much less mood disturbance and more active coping strategies. The researchers also observed significant differences in immune function of natural killer cell activity in patients in the treatment group as compared with the control group.

These investigators[46] reported 6-year follow-up showed a trend for recurrence for the control group (13/34) and a statistically significant greater death rate (10/34) than for patients in the treatment group (7/34 and 3/34, respectively). Analysis of multiple covariates found only depth of the malignant melanoma lesion and treatment (group intervention) were significant predictors of recurrence and survival. The treatment effect remained after adjusting for depth of the lesion. Higher baseline affective distress and higher baseline active behavioral coping scores were predictive of lower rates of recurrence and survival. Additionally, increases in active-behavioral coping were significantly related to survival; a similar trend was found for recurrence. The authors suggested high baseline affective distress may mobilize coping responses rather than indicating poorer adjustment. The beneficial effects of active-behavioral coping indicated that group interventions need to focus on education, problem solving, and stress management, rather than just on feelings.

In a recent article, Anderson et al.[47] drew on these studies plus extensive investigations by Kiecolt-Glaser and Glaser in psychoneuroimmunology and by Anderson with patients with gynecological cancers to develop a multidimensional biobehavioral model of the effects of cancer stress, compliance, health behaviors, disease parameters, and immunity on disease course. They are currently conducting an intervention study based on this model. They will be examining the relationships between psychological, behavioral, and biologic pathways from cancer stressors to course of disease.

In summary, group intervention studies do support positive results of a group intervention in terms of lessened mood distress and enhanced coping. The study underway by Anderson, Kiecolt-Glaser, and Glaser adds the important measure of quality of life outcomes. This recognizes that not only mood, but all areas of life (functional state, psychological state, social functioning), are affected by cancer and its treatment. The intervention study of Anderson and colleagues will provide further information on the relationship between the immune parameters, psychological stress, and disease outcome. The replication study underway by Spiegel and colleagues will provide insights into which components of an intervention may be most effective for patient adjustment and/or survival.

Proposed model

Figure 1 portrays a model that illustrates the dynamic relationship between cancer, quality of life, and coping. Although cancer is an enormous invasion into the patient's life, the disease is also perceived in the context of other noncancer stressors, such as illness of other family members, developmental tasks, and employment or education issues. These events affect all areas of the patient's quality of life (e.g., physical, emotional, spiritual, social, etc.). Threats or demands affecting one or more areas are appraised and the patient selects coping strategies based on this appraisal. Predictors of both primary and secondary appraisal include individual factors (e.g., age, gender, possibly personality style or self-discrepancy, past coping experiences); disease-related variables (e.g., site and stage of disease, symptoms, type of treatment and side effects, prognosis), and sociocultural variables (e.g., attitudes toward death and dying). The coping strategies selected are either primarily focused on problem solving or on managing emotional reactions, depending on the nature of the appraisal of threat. Implementation leads to an evaluation of outcome in the affected quality of life domain, which leads to a reappraisal of new or different levels of danger/threat. The process then continues. The dotted line represents the possible positive impact of responses such as "a fighting spirit" or support group membership on disease-related variables such as survival.

We suggest that this model facilitates the conceptualization of coping with cancer as a dynamic process that occurs within the broader context of the patient's life experience. It thus allows for research explorations of the impact of other stressors on coping with cancer, as well as further investigation of the relationship between specific coping strategies and quality of life outcomes.

Conclusions

There seems to be agreement that coping with the stress of cancer and its treatment is best conceptualized as a dynamic process involving changing behavioral and cognitive efforts to manage the external and internal stress of cancer. There is some support for the positive effects on psychological adjustment of a "fighting spirit" or "take charge" style in which the patient maintains an attitude of taking charge of the illness in a realistic

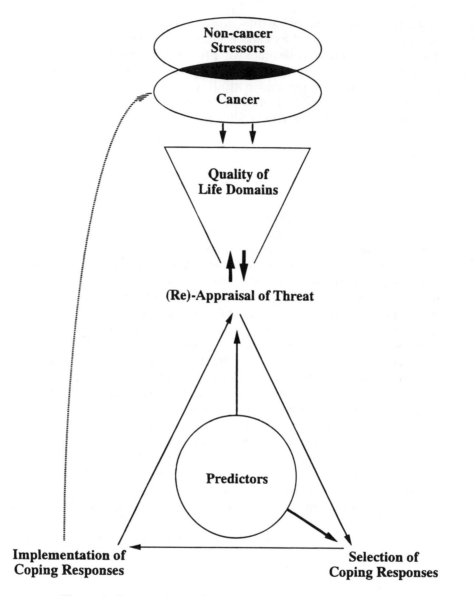

Figure 1 Proposed model of coping with the stress of cancer.

fashion. Longitudinal studies are needed to investigate which coping strategies are most effective as the demands presented change and whether these strategies continue to be context specific or emerge as related to a trait or dispositional style.

Studies of different groups of patients are also needed. Primarily breast cancer patients have been studied, although the work of Fawzy et al.[44-46] in patients with melanoma represents an important exception. Whether males respond differently or whether the relationship between psychological factors, the immune system, and the disease course is the same for all types of cancer is not known.

Studies underway by Spiegel and colleagues as well as Anderson and colleagues should provide new insights into what constitutes effective coping as measured by both its impact on various aspects of quality of life as well as disease course. These will also expand our understanding of components of successful interventions to assist patients to cope more effectively. Finally, coping with cancer occurs often within the context of family or significant others. A number of studies have reported the extent of distress of spouses and suggest the usefulness of examining the entire family to more fully understand the experience of coping with the stress of cancer.[48-51]

Coping with cancer is part of an active and dynamic process, related not only to disease-specific stress, but also to other nondisease events in the patient's life. The overall impact on the patient of cancer stress and coping success may be understood best by assessing outcomes in the many quality of life domains.

References

1. Derogatis, L. R., Morrow, G. R., Fetting, J., Penman, D., Piasetsky S., Schmale, A. M., Henrichs, M., and Carnicke, C. L. M., Jr., The prevalence of psychiatric disorders among cancer patients, *JAMA*, 249, 751, 1983.
2. Freud, S., *New Introductory Lectures on Psychoanalysis*, Norton, New York, 1933.
3. Somerfield, M. and Curbow, B., Methodological issues and research strategies in the study of coping with cancer, *Soc. Sci. Med.*, 34, 1203, 1992.
4. Lazarus, R. and Folkman, S., *Stress, Appraisal, and Coping*, Springer Publishing Co., Inc., New York, 1984.
5. Rowland, J. H., Intrapersonal resources: coping, in *Handbook of Psycho-Oncology*, Holland, J. C. and Rowland, J. H., Eds., Oxford University Press, New York, 1989, 44.
6. Endler, N. S. and Parker, J. D. A., Multidimensional assessment of coping: a critical evaluation, *J. Personality Soc. Psychol.*, 58, 844, 1990.
7. Curbow, B. and Somerfield, M., Use of the Rosenberg Self-Esteem Scale with adult cancer patients, *J. Psychosoc. Oncol.*, 9, 113, 1991.
8. Folkman, S., Lazarus, R. S., Dunkel-Schetter, C., DeLongis, A., and Gruen, R., The dynamics of a stressful encounter: cognitive appraisal, coping, and encounter outcomes, *J. Personality Soc. Psychol.*, 50, 992, 1986.
9. Dunkel-Schetter, C., Feinstein, L. G., Taylor, S. E., and Falke, R. L., Patterns of coping with cancer, *Health Psychol.*, 11, 79, 1992.
10. Jarrett, S. R., Ramirez, A. J., Richards, M. A., and Weinman, J., Measuring coping in breast cancer, *J. Psychom. Res.*, 36, 593, 1992.
11. Cooper, C. L. and Faragher, E. B., Coping strategies and breast disorders/cancer, *Psychol. Med.*, 22, 447, 1992.
12. Cooper, C. L. and Faragher, E. B., Psychosocial stress and breast cancer: the inter-relationship between stress events, coping strategies, and personality, *Psychol. Med.*, 23, 653, 1993.

13. Carver, C. S., Scheier, M. F., and Weintraub, J. K., Assessing coping strategies: a theoretically based approach, *J. Personality Soc. Psychol.*, 56, 267, 1989.

14. Carver, C. S., Pozo, C., Harris, S. D., Noriega, V., Scheier, M. F., Robinson, D. S., Ketcham, A. S., Moffatt, F. L., Jr., and Clark, K. C., How coping mediates the effect of optimism on distress: a study of women with early stage breast cancer, *J. Personality Soc. Psychol.*, 65, 375, 1993.

15. Scheier, M. F. and Carver, C. S., Effects of optimism on psychological and physical well-being: theoretical overview and empirical update, *Cognitive Ther. Res.*, 16, 201, 1992.

16. Mishel, M. H., Padilla, G., Grant, M., and Sorensen, D. S., Uncertainty in illness theory: a replication of the mediating effects of mastery and coping, *Nurs. Res.*, 40, 236, 1991.

17. Pearlin, L. I. and Schooler, C., The structure of coping, *J. Health Soc. Behav.*, 19, 2, 1978.

18. Watson, M., Greer, S., Young, J., Inayat, Q., Burgess C., and Robertson, B., Development of a questionnaire of adjustment to cancer, the MAC Scale, *Psychol. Med.*, 18, 203, 1988.

19. Lazarus, R. S., Coping theory and research: past, present, and future, *Psychosom. Med.*, 55, 234, 1993.

20. Gotay, C., The experience of cancer during early and advanced stages: the view of patients and their mates, *Soc. Sci. Med.*, 18, 605, 1984.

21. Lerman, C., Rimer, B., Blumberg, B., Christinzio, S., Engstrom, P. F., MacElwee, N., O'Connor, K., and Seay, J., Effects of coping style and relaxation on cancer chemotherapy side effects and emotional responses, *Cancer Nurs.*, 13, 308, 1990.

22. Lewis, F. M., The impact of cancer on family: a critical analysis of the research literature, *Patient Educ. Counseling*, 8, 269, 1986.

23. Scheier, M. F. and Carver, C. S., Optimism, coping, and health: assessment and implications of generalized outcome expectancies, *Health Psychol.*, 4, 219, 1985.

24. Friedman, L. C., Nelson, D. V., Baer, P. E., Lane, M., Smith, F. E., and Dworkin, R. J., The relationship of dispositional optimism, daily life stress, and domestic environment to coping methods used by cancer patients, *J. Behav. Med.*, 15, 127, 1992.

25. Billings, A. and Moos, R., The role of coping responses and social resources in attenuating the stress of life events, *J. Behav. Med.*, 4, 139, 1981.

26. Hilton, B. A., The relationship of uncertainty, control, commitment, and threat of recurrence to coping strategies used by women diagnosed with breast cancer, *J. Behav. Med.*, 12, 39, 1989.

27. Mattlin, J. A., Wethington, E., and Kessler, R. C., Situational determinants of coping and coping effectiveness, *J. Health Soc. Behav.*, 31, 103, 1990.

28. Heidrich, S. M., Forsthoff, C. A., and Ward, S. E., Psychological adjustment in adults with cancer: the self as mediator, *Health Psychol.*, 13, 346, 1994.

29. Stanton, A. L. and Snider, P. R., Coping with a breast cancer diagnosis: a prospective study, *Health Psychol.*, 12, 16, 1993.

30. Greer, S., Morris, T., and Pettingale, K. W., Psychological response to breast cancer: effect on outcome, *Lancet*, 2, 785, 1979.

31. Temoshak, L., Personality, coping style, emotion and cancer: towards an integrative model, *Cancer Surv.*, 6, 545, 1987.

32. Cassileth, B., Lusk, E. J., Miller, D. S., Brown, L. L., and Miller, C., Psychosocial correlates of survival in advanced malignant disease?, *N. Engl. J. Med.*, 312, 1551, 1985.
33. Jamison, R. N., Burish, T. G., and Walston, K. A., Psychogenic factors in predicing survival of breast cancer patients, *J. Clin. Oncol.*, 5, 768, 1987.
34. Spiegel, D., *Living Beyond Limits*, Times Books, New York, 1993.
35. Gordon, W. A., Friedenbergs, I., Diller, L., Hibberd, M., Wold, C., Levine, L., Lipkins, R., Ezrachi, O., and Lucido, D., Efficacy of psychosocial intervention with cancer patients, *J. Consult. Clin. Psychol.*, 48, 743, 1980.
36. Cella, D. F., Tulsky, D. S., Gray, G. et al., The functional assessment of cancer therapy scale: development and validation of the general measure, *J. Clin. Oncol.*, 11, 570, 1993.
37. Schay, C. A. C. and Henrich, R. L., Developing a comprehensive tool: the CAancer Rehabilitation Evaluation System, *Oncology*, 4, 135, 1990.
38. Anderson, B., Psychological interventions for cancer patients to enhance the quality of life, *J. Consult. Clin. Psychol.*, 60, 552, 1992.
39. Fawzy, F. I. and Fawzy, N. W., A structured psychoeducational intervention for cancer patients, *Gen. Hosp. Psychiatry*, 16, 149, 1994.
40. Gellert, G. A., Maxwell, R. M., and Siegel, B. S., Survival of breast cancer patients receiving adjunctive psychosocial support therapy: a 10-year follow-up study, *J. Clin. Oncol.*, 11, 66, 1993.
41. Spiegel, D., Bloom, J. R., and Yalom, I. D., Group support for patients with metastatic cancer: a randomized prospective outcome study, *Arch. Gen. Psychiatry*, 38, 527, 1981.
42. Spiegel, D., Bloom, J. R., Kraemer, H. D., and Gottheil, E., Effect of psychosocial treatment on survival of patients with metastatic breast disease, *Lancet*, 2, 888, 1989.
43. Spiegel, D., Psychosocial intervention in cancer, *J. Natl. Cancer Inst.*, 85, 1198, 1993.
44. Fawzy, F. I., Cousins, N., Fawzy, N. W., Kemeny, M. E., Elashoff, R., and Morton, D., A structured psychiatric intervention for cancer patients. I. Changes over time in methods of coping and affective disturbance, *Arch. Gen. Psychiatry*, 47, 720, 1990.
45. Fawzy, F. I., Kemeny, M. E., Fawzy, N. W., Elashoff, R., Morton, D., Cousins, N., and Fahey, J. L., A structured psychiatric intervention for cancer patients. II. Changes over time in immunological measures, *Arch. Gen. Psychiatry*, 47, 729, 1990.
46. Fawzy, F. I., Fawzy, N. W., Hyun, C. S., Elashoff, R., Guthrie, D., Fahey, J. L., and Morton, D. L., Malignant melanoma: effects of early structured psychiatric intervention, coping, and affective state on recurrence and survival 6 years later, *Arch. Gen. Psychiatry*, 50, 681, 1993.
47. Anderson, B. L., Kiecolt-Glaser, J. K., and Glaser, R., A biobehavioral model of cancer stress and disease course, *Am. Psychologist*, 49, 389, 1994.
48. Lewis, F. M., Psychosocial transitions and the family's work in adjusting to cancer, *Semin. Oncol. Nurs.*, 9, 127, 1993.
49. Northouse, L. L. and Peters-Golden, H., Cancer and the family: strategies to assist spouses, *Semin. Oncol. Nurs.*, 9, 74, 1993.

50. Revenson, T. A., Social support and marital coping with chronic illness, *Ann. Behav. Med.*, 16, 122, 1994.
51. Toseland, R. A., Blanchard, C. G., and McCallion, P., A problem solving intervention for caregivers of cancer patients, *Soc. Sci. Med.*, 40, 517, 1995.

Index